Physical Therapy Aide: A Worktext, 2nd Edition

ROBERTA C. WEISS, LVN, ED.D.

Instructional Designer
Allied Healthcare Curriculum Specialist
Vocational Education Teacher Trainer

Delmar Publishers

an International Thomson Publishing company ITP®

Albany • Bonn • Boston • Cincinnati • Detroit • London • Madrid
Melbourne • Mexico City • New York • Pacific Grove • Paris • San Francisco
Singapore • Tokyo • Toronto • Washington

Cover Design: Bill Finnerty

DELMAR STAFF
Publisher: Susan Simpfenderfer
Acquisitions Editor: Marlene McHugh Pratt
Production Manager: Linda Helfrich
Developmental Editor: Debra Flis
Project Editor: William Trudell
Art and Design Coordinator: Richard Killar
Marketing Manager: Darryl L. Caron

Printed in Canada

For more information, contact:

Delmar Publishers
3 Columbia Circle, Box 15015
Albany, New York, 12212-5015

International Thomson Publishing Europe
Berkshire House
168-173 High Holborn
London, WC1 V 7AA
United Kingdom

Thomas Nelson Australia
102 Dodds Street
South Melbourne,
Victoria, 3205 Australia

Nelson Canada
1120 Birchmont Road
Scarborough, Ontario
M1K 5G4, Canada

International Thomson Publishing France
Tour Maine-Montparnasse
33 Avenue du Maine
75755 Paris Cedex 15, France

International Thomson Editores
Sececa 53
Colonia Polanco
11560 Mexico D. F. Mexico

International Thomson Publishing GmbH
Königswinterer Strasfse 418
53227 Bonn
Germany

International Thomson Publishing Asia
60 Albert St.
#15-01 Albert Complex
Singapore 189969

International Thomson Publishing Japan
Hirakawa-cho Kyowa Building, 3F
2-2-1 Hirakawa-cho, Chiyoda-ku,
Tokyo 102, Japan

ITE Spain/Paraninfo
Calle Magallanes, 25
28015-Madrid, Espana

9 10 XXX 04

Library of Congress Cataloging–in–Publication Data
Weiss, Roberta C.
Physical therapy aide : a worktext / Roberta C. Weiss. — 2nd ed.
p. cm.
Rev. ed. of: Your career as a physical therapy aide. c1993.
Includes bibliographical references and index.
ISBN 0-7668-0294-9
1. Physical therapy assistants—Vocational guidance. I. Weiss, Roberta C. Your career as a physical therapy aide. II. Title.
[DNLM: 1. Physical Therapy. 2. Allied Health Personnel. 3. Career Choice. WB 460 W432p 1998]
RM705.W449 1998
615.8'2'023—dc21
DNLM/DLC
for Library of Congress

98–29790
CIP

CONTENTS

PREFACE

This text is written in simple, yet comprehensive, language, and is accompanied by photographs and basic illustrations in order to provide the reader with a well-bounded introduction to the principles and techniques involved with working as a Physical Therapy Aide.

While the author firmly believes that there are many adequate textbooks currently in use that provide information for the advanced learner studying physical therapy, it is the goal of this text to present a manual that meets the very distinct and unique needs of the Physical Therapy Aide or Assistant.

The text consists of sixteen chapters and covers such information as anatomy and physiology of the musculoskeletal, nervous, cardiovascular, and nervous systems, physical therapy modalities, therapeutic and range of motion exercises, and turning, positioning, transferring, and ambulating patients.

To assist readers in their understanding of the subject matter, each chapter is accompanied by behavioral objectives and key words at the beginning and a summary outline and review questions at the end. The four appendixes are included to provide the learner with additional information, such as musculoskeletal terminology, a practice evaluation test, and anatomy and physiology plates of the musculoskeletal system, body directions, and correct postures for standing, sitting, and lifting objects.

Roberta C. Weiss, LVN, Ed.D.
Plantation, Florida

ACKNOWLEDGMENTS

I would like to extend my deepest gratitude and appreciation to all those who have assisted me in the preparation and development of this text book, including:

Ms. Sandy Watson, LPT, Director of the Physical Therapy and Rehabilitation Department at Huntington Memorial Hospital, Pasadena, California, and all the members of her wonderful and caring staff, for the time, energy, and expertise they provided in the preparation of this text.

The individual patients receiving physical therapy treatments at Huntington Memorial Hospital's Physical Therapy and Rehabilitation Department, for all their help and time in providing assistance and a "personal touch," allowing their photographs to be used in this text.

Ms. Marla Keeth, LVN, Coordinator of the Health Careers Academy at Blair High School, Pasadena Unified School District/Los Angeles County Regional Occupational Programs, for her assistance and continued support, in providing time for her health career students to be photographed and work with actual patients, for the preparation of this text.

The many individual Blair High School Health Careers Academy students for their time, expertise and participation in being photographed and kept available for the many hours needed for the photography session involved in the preparation of this text.

Boyd Flinders, II, M.D., orthopedic surgeon and concerned medical practitioner, for his input and knowledge, in the preparation of this text.

Robyn Gilmore, a talented artist, and friend of many years, who worked many hours helping to formulate sketches for future illustrations and photographs for this text.

Bill Ahern, Sales Representative for Delmar Publishers Inc., for all his help and fortitude in finally bringing my work to the "right" people at Delmar Publishers.

Finally, I would like to thank Adrianne Williams (former editor with Delmar) and Debra Flis, Developmental Editor at Delmar, for all of their help and time spent in the preparation of this high quality textbook.

Delmar wishes to acknowledge the following individuals for reviewing the manuscript:

Adrienne Carter
Riverside Community College, Moreno Valle, California

Sandra L. McKenzie
Remington College, Cleveland, Ohio

Donna Shea
Skadron College, San Bernardino, California

Dedication

This book is lovingly and respectfully dedicated to my friend and teacher, Phyllis V. Stilson, RN, whose enduring support and friendship continue to provide me with the vision and skill necessary to develop quality materials for prospective allied health care professionals.

SECTION I

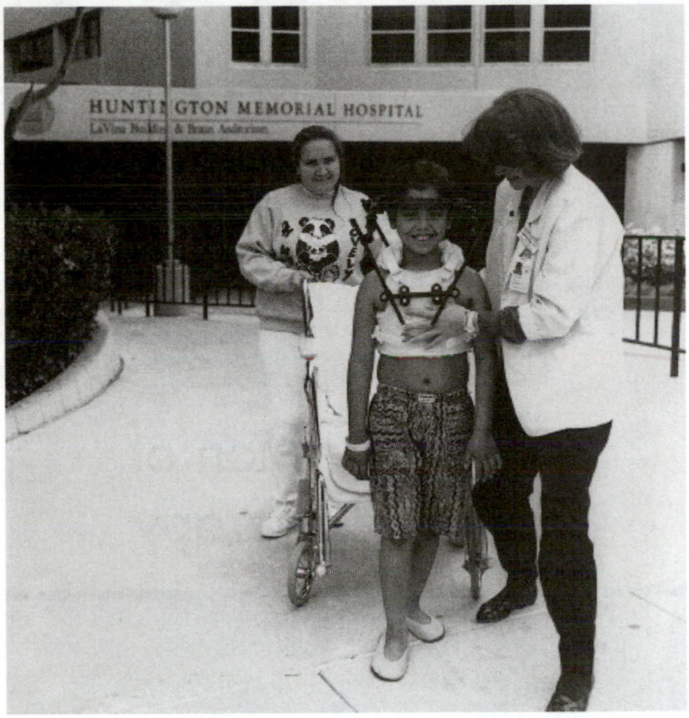

INTRODUCTION TO PHYSICAL THERAPY

1

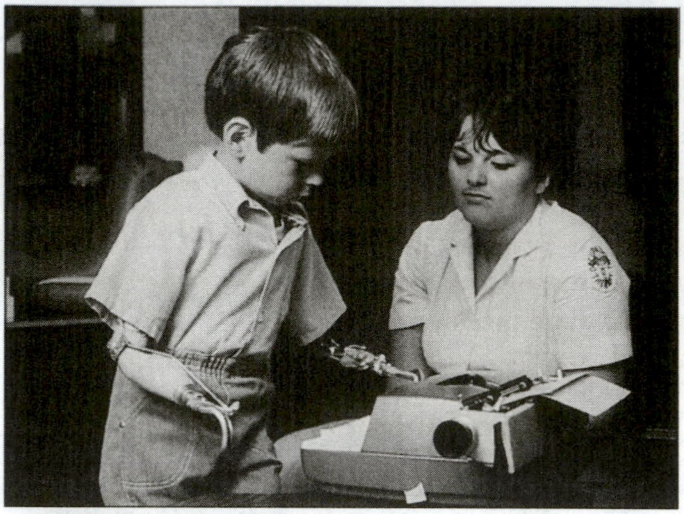

The Profession of Physical Therapy

OBJECTIVES

Upon completion of this chapter, you should be able to:

1. Describe the evolution of physical therapy in the United States from the early 1900s to present day.
2. Discuss how physical therapy became a new occupation.
3. Briefly describe the role Mary McMillan played in the evolution and history of physical therapy.
4. Explain the impact of World War I and World War II on the field of physical therapy.
5. Define the major focus of the rehabilitation team.
6. List the different members of the rehabilitation team and describe the function of each.
7. Discuss the role of the physical therapy aide as it relates to working with patients with physical disabilities.

KEY TERMS

Athletic director
Disability
Exercise physiologist
Occupation
Occupational therapist
Physical medicine
Physical therapist
Physical therapy
Physical therapy aide
Physical therapy assistant
Practitioner
Recreational therapy aide
Recreational therapist
Rehabilitation
Vocational

HISTORY AND EVOLUTION OF PHYSICAL THERAPY

The evolution of physical therapy during the twentieth century can best be grasped by comparing its earliest definition from the 1920s, when the field was first introduced to those definitions and concepts widely used and accepted by modern day practitioners.

During the 1920s, the **physical therapist** was referred to as a trained assistant to the established medical profession. They were only allowed to work in agencies that catered to muscle training, therapeutic massage, hydrotherapy, and mechanical, electro, and, light therapies, and they could only practice under the prescription of a licensed physician. In comparison to the early role of the physical therapist, today's therapist is described as a **practitioner** who, where permitted by law, is responsible for the evaluation, treatment, preventive care, and consultation of patients requiring his experience or expertise in the field of **physical therapy** (Figure 1-1).

Physical Therapy: A New Occupation

In the United States, the use of physical therapy as a specialty area of therapeutic intervention dates as far back as the late nineteenth century, with a sudden increase in its application occurring in the early 1900s. At that time, the use of physical modalities and procedures applied for therapeutic purposes were first used systematically in the United States during the 1890s, in the early treatment programs for infantile paralysis. By 1914, numbers of persons stricken with the disease rose so high, that in an attempt to provide treatment and follow-up care to

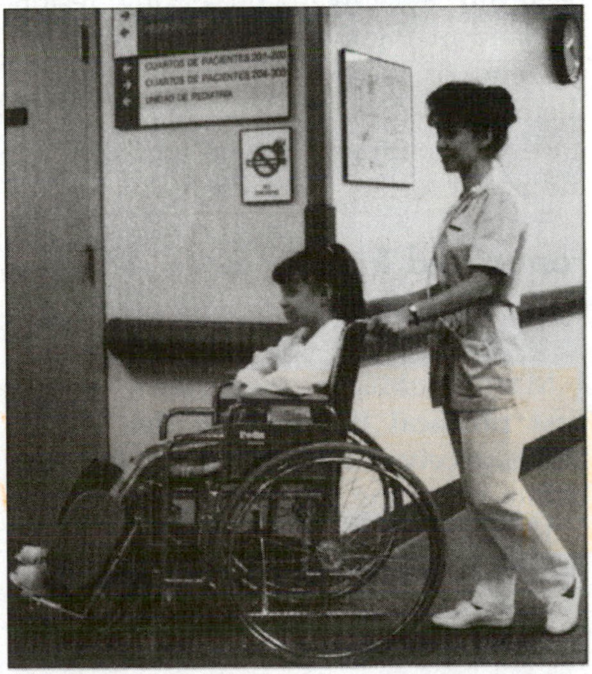

Figure 1-1 Physical therapy aide transporting a patient in a wheelchair.

patients, teams of nonphysician workers were organized under medical direction to provide care to those stricken with the disease. Among the nonphysical personnel on these teams were those who came to be known as physical therapists.

Even though the occupation of physical therapy was not, at that time, a distinct entity, the foundations were being laid for its acceptance as such. By World War I, which forced attention on the use of restoring physical function in injured members of both the military forces and the civilian workforce, the specialty of physical therapy was becoming more widely accepted. Through recognition of the application of physical therapeutics to the needs of military personnel, the specialty branch of medicine known today as physical therapy received a major impetus for becoming a clearly identifiable occupation.

During the earliest years in the evolution of physical therapy, the preservation of human resources was of great importance. During World War I, attention had been directed toward preserving, restoring, and maintaining a fighting force. By the end of the war, however, physical therapy was directed back to preserving and maintaining the workforce, in the industrial society from where it emerged.

Formalized Training for Early Practitioners

Mary McMillan, recognized as the first physical therapist in the United States, received her training in England before returning to the United States in 1915. Because of the high number of personnel needed to provide care to members of the military forces during World War I, other early practitioners in the United States provided the needed services without formal training specific to physical therapy. Preparation for the expanded use of physical therapy fell under the guidance of people whose backgrounds were similar to those practitioners who played a significant role in the early treatment efforts for patients with infantile paralysis. Marguerite Sanderson, a graduate of Wellesley College, and the Boston Normal School of Gymnastics, was one of those practitioners who assisted in the planning and organization of activities that would eventually make physical therapeutics a part of the care provided for military personnel. By 1918, because of Sanderson's work, outlines for a course of study had been developed, and cooperative efforts between the military and personnel in civilian institutions were underway to prepare practitioners who would serve, in a civilian capacity, as Reconstruction Aides in special Reconstruction Hospitals.

A New Title for the Practitioner

As a result of these newly developed training programs, individuals who completed the courses of study were given the title of Reconstruction Aide. In addition, individuals who had prior experience in using physical therapeutics in civilian life were recruited for service with the military as Reconstruction Aides. Practitioners rendering similar service in civilian facilities were referred to as Physiotherapy Aides, Physiotherapy Technicians, and, in some cases, Physician's Assistants. Those individuals who were called "Assistant" were personally trained by a physician to work in his or her private office.

Physical Therapy: 1920 to Present

A national crisis and the usual pressures of an industrial society spawned and supported the development of the occupation of physical therapy during the early twentieth century.

As a result of the great efforts made toward the training of personnel during World War I, greater numbers of physicians and nonphysicians became knowledgeable about the benefits of physical therapeutics. The use of physical modalities as a means to alleviate dysfunction and promote movement spread through the country. By the 1940s, the value of physical therapy would once more be tested through circumstances reminiscent of those that had led to its initial recognition: the polio epidemic and World War II. The challenges were met by once again combining the forces of the military and civilian sectors, and the practice of physical therapy was propelled through a major period of growth.

As a result of treating survivors of World War II, major new concepts in physical therapy began to emerge. Two of these were **rehabilitation** services, both **vocational** and emotional, and the investigation by neuroscientists of the application of neurophysiologic principles in body movement.

During the years immediately following World War II, a new medical specialty, focusing on the use of physical therapeutics, emerged. This new specialization, called "physical medicine," concentrated on caring for the patient through the use of physical properties such as light, heat, cold, water, electricity, massage, manipulation, exercise, and mechanical devices for physical therapy in the diagnosis and treatment of disease.

The rehabilitation concepts that emerged during World War II fostered the growth of the new specialty of physical medicine. The title would eventually become interchangeable with rehabilitation and rehabilitative medicine.

Emergence of the Occupation

Physical therapy as an **occupation** in the United States is clearly an occupation of the twentieth century. It emerged from a need for a specific kind of health service related to the restoration of locomotor function of the human body. Today, physical therapy is listed routinely among the occupations related to health care and is often referred to as an "emerging" profession. The evolution of physical therapy reflect the society in which the occupation has evolved and includes the establishment of standards for education and practice, efforts toward clarifying the scope of practice, and finally, endeavors toward professionalization of the occupation.

At times, progress in the growth of physical therapy has been slow, but it has never halted. At times, its focus may have been diminished, but it has never once been obscured. With each and every renewal of focus on understanding human movements as a basis for alleviating and correcting movement dysfunction, the services of the physical therapy team have been enhanced and the contributions of the individual physical therapy worker has been magnified.

◆ THE REHABILITATION TEAM

How does physical therapy fit into today's health care environment, that is, how is it used in the rehabilitative process? To explain how physical therapy has become the valued profession it is today, we must first begin with the people who work within this rehabilitative process. These individuals are part of what is referred to as the rehabilitation team (Figure 1-2).

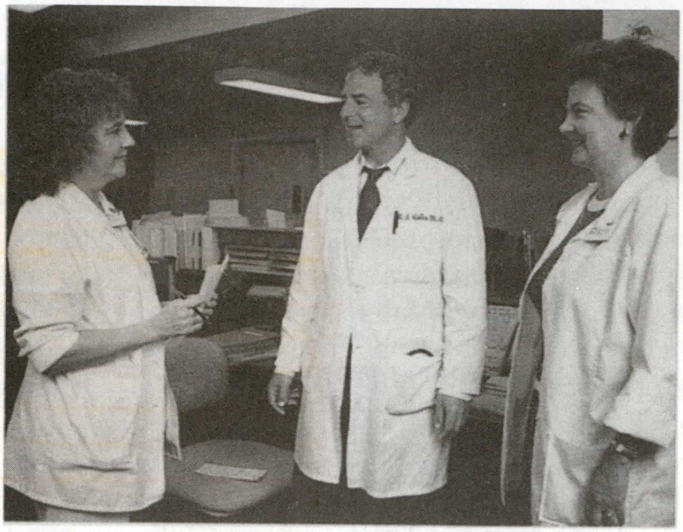

Figure 1-2 Members of the health care delivery team include the physical therapy aide.

The major focus of the rehabilitation team is rendering care to patients after they have begun recovery from an acute or debilitating illness. However, some rehabilitation services, such as special breathing exercises or exercises that help to maintain the patient's range of motion to a specific joint, may be rendered during the acute phase of the illness. After the acute phase of the disease has subsided and the risk to life has passed, many patients face partial or complete loss of function to an extremity or damage to a part of the nervous system that may affect normal body movement and the ability to function in the daily environment. It is important to remember that it is mainly damage to a part of the nervous, vascular, or skeletal system, that is most frequently responsible for causing physical disabilities (Figure 1-3).

Oftentimes, patients are not able to

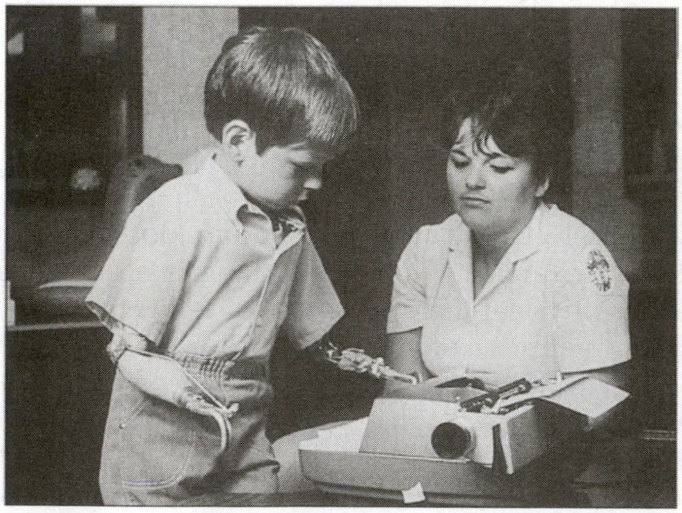

Figure 1-3 The rehabilitation department helps patients return to maximum levels of self care.

return to their homes or places of employment unless they are able to regain some of the functions they have lost. Simple tasks that most of us take for granted, such as being able to walk up and down stairs or dress and undress ourselves, may become monumental stumbling blocks to the patient who has sustained a physical **disability.** Every day we perform innumerable functions with our arms and legs without necessarily concentrating on them. After one loses some function in part or all of an extremity or joint, one becomes acutely aware of how important each part of the body really is. The loss of motion to an ankle or the loss of function in a hand brings about the patient's need for treatment. Such treatment, extensibly, is done by members of the rehabilitation team; the same team that was made up of "reconstruction aides" who only worked as trained assistants to physicians. And not only is the team responsible for caring for the patient's physical needs, but, just as important, it is responsible for helping the patient deal with his or her emotions.

The loss of bodily function sometimes brings with it feelings of inadequacy or despair, and oftentimes, an unwelcome dependence on others. Therefore, a major goal of the rehabilitation team is to assist the patient in minimizing the disability and to help in planning a way of daily living that is optimal for the individual.

Members of the Rehabilitation Team

In addition to the physician-in-charge, there are generally seven key individuals in the rehabilitation team. These include a physical therapist, physical therapy assistant, physical therapy aide, athletic trainer, recreation therapist, recreation therapy aide, and an exercise physiologist. Some teams also include a psychologist or social worker and an occupational therapist.

Physician. The physician in charge is responsible for outlining the rehabilitation program for the patient and for ordering any special physical therapy treatments. This individual has attended medical school and has generally secured a specialty in **physical or rehabilitative medicine**, often with a secondary specialization in psychiatry.

Physical Therapist. The physical therapist has graduated from a four-year-college program with a bachelor's degree, and, in addition to studying physical therapy, has received a postgraduate master's degree in the health sciences. In order to practice, the physical therapist must also be licensed or registered by a state.

The role of the physical therapist is quite extensive and comprehensive. In addition to performing treatments which require special training in therapeutic exercises, hydrotherapy, and electrotherapy, this practitioner is also required to perform procedures dealing with individual muscles and muscular movement.

The physical therapist is also responsible for evaluating the patient and designing an individual therapeutic program. Physical therapists are generally employed in some health agencies, hospitals, nursing homes, fitness centers, and orthopedic offices.

Physical Therapy Assistant. The **physical therapy assistant** is a graduate of a two-year associate or arts or applied sciences community college program. This individual works under the direction of the physical therapist and is responsible for assisting with patient care and per-

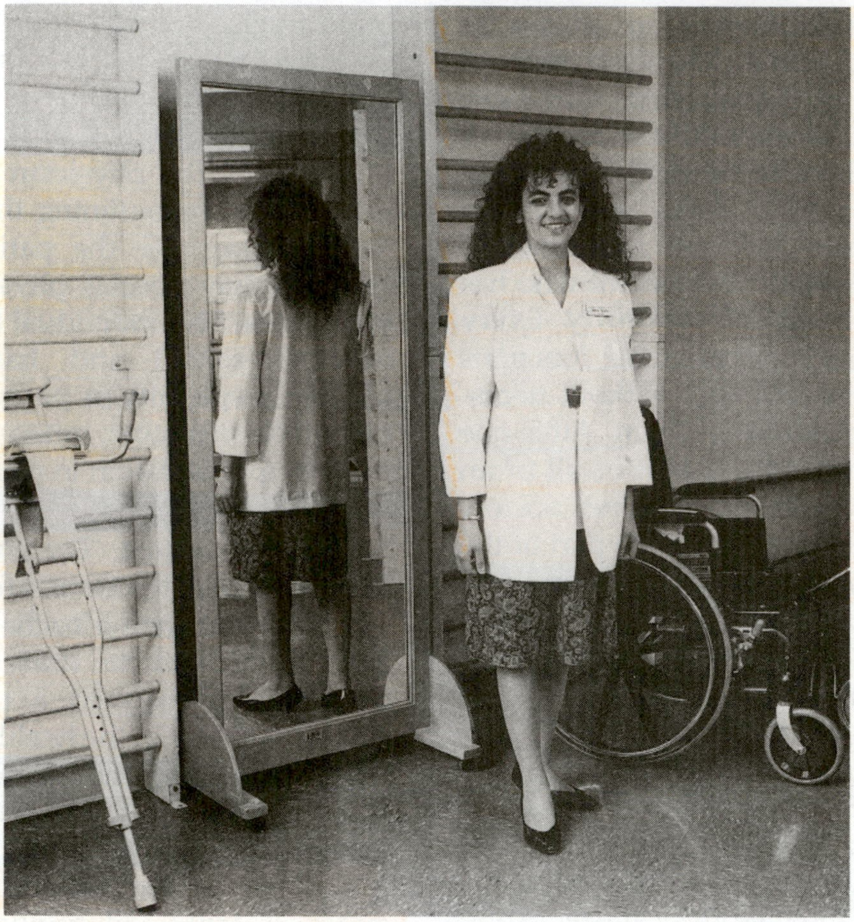

Figure 1-4 The physical therapy aide.

forming selected treatments such as ultrasound. The physical therapy assistant, who is usually employed by home health agencies, nursing homes, hospitals, fitness centers, and orthopedic offices, may also be called upon to assist the physical therapist in evaluating the patient's progress during the treatment.

Physical Therapy Aide. The **physical therapy aide** is generally responsible for carrying out the nontechnical duties of physical therapy, such as preparing treatment areas, ordering devices and supplies, and transporting patients. Working under the direction of the physical therapist, the physical therapy aide may be employed in home health agencies, nursing homes, hospitals, fitness centers, and orthopedic offices (Figure 1-4). Usually, the physical therapy aide receives his or her training in a health occupational education (HOE) program, vocational school, or on-the-job training program.

Athletic Trainer. The **athletic trainer** has graduated from a four-year college program with a bachelor's degree and may or may not be state licensed or nationally certified depending upon the individual state in which he or she is employed. Most athletic trainers are employed by athletic teams in high schools and colleges, sport teams, and fitness centers and are primarily concerned with preventing and treating athletic injuries and providing rehabilitative services to athletes. The athletic trainer may also be responsible for teaching proper nutrition, assessing an athlete's physical condition, giving advice on exercises, and taping or padding players in order to protect body parts from injury.

Recreational Therapist. The **recreational therapist** uses recreation and leisure activities as a means of treating patients' symptoms and thereby improving their physical and mental well-being. This is generally accomplished by the recreational therapist's planning of activities for the patient and then evaluating the patient's progress. Most recreational therapists graduate from either a two-year associate of arts program or a four-year bachelor of science program, and state licensure varies according to type of employment. Recreational therapists may be employed by amusement parks, cruise ships, hospitals, mental health facilities, nursing homes, and rehabilitation centers.

Recreational Therapy Aide. The **recreational therapy aide** is generally trained on the job and works under the direct supervision of the recreational therapist; they are responsible for carrying out activities the recreational therapist has assigned. This individual, who is most often employed by amusement parks, cruise ships, hospitals, nursing homes, and rehabilitation centers, is most often responsible for noting and reporting patients responses and progress to the recreational therapist. Recreational therapy aides also maintain supplies and equipment in good working order and schedule activities for recreation.

Exercise Physiologist. The **exercise physiologist** designs a physical activity program that is tailored to the specific needs of the individual participant. Educational requirements for the exercise physiologist vary with the position, and employment for this member of the rehabilitation team is usually in hospitals, fitness centers, industry, hotels, research, resorts, and freelance consultations.

Occupational Therapist. An **occupational therapist** is a graduate of a school for occupational therapy and has acquired expertise in making special equipment in order to facilitate the performance of a patient's daily activities. This person is responsible for analyzing bodily maneuvers, step-by-step, and for training the patient in such a manner that she is able to compensate for weakness or paralysis of a limb. It is the occupational therapist who is responsible for teaching the patient how to get in and out of a bathtub, or how to set the table for dinner if one arm is damaged, or how to use a weakened arm in order to support the good arm for bimanual activities. The occupational therapist must also design special equipment in order to compensate for the patient's loss of range of motion to a joint.

Social Worker or Psychologist. The social worker or psychologist is also essential for the effective functioning of the rehabilitation team. This person, who has completed either a postgraduate program in medical social work or a doctorate in clinical psychology, has been trained in analyzing patients' emotional needs and reconciling these with the means that their community, or society as a whole, can offer. This individual is also responsible for assisting both patients and the family members of patients in obtaining rehabilitation services or financial support from state or federal agencies, as well as assisting in making arrangements or appropriate referrals for visits by visiting nurses or help from other homebound services.

THE ROLE OF THE PHYSICAL THERAPY AIDE AS A MEMBER OF THE REHABILITATION TEAM

As a physical therapy aide, you are considered an essential member of the health care delivery system. A great part of that responsibility is your actual involvement with the rehabilitation team. Medical rehabilitation is a specialty that concerns itself with the overall improvement of the functional capacity of patients who, for one reason or another, have been left with impaired motion of an arm or leg, or with impaired balance or coordination.

As we have already discussed, the physical therapy aide works under the direction of the physical therapist and may be assigned any number of nontechnical tasks. These may include both clinical and administrative functions, and they are always assigned by the supervising physical therapist. The aide may be asked to teach the patient how to walk with crutches or, after having received proper training, may be directed to apply a heating modality to the patient. The physical therapy aide may also be asked to make appointments, complete insurance billing, or clean the physical therapy equipment.

In order to teach a disabled person how to perform a physical task, the aide must realize that such a task is very challenging for the person. Teaching requires much compassion and patience. Patients may be elderly and the physical impairment may seem insurmountable to them. They may need much encouragement, and they may have to return to their home and friends in order to be successful. As a physical therapy aide, you must never allow yourself to become disappointed when patients do not show any gratitude for all the efforts you have extended to improving their condition. Physical disabilities may arouse bitterness in patients toward their environment. Patients may feel that not enough has been done for them. You may often hear patients say, "I worked all my life and now this happens to me. Why do I have to be a cripple?"

Some of the patients you may encounter may also have some impairment of speech. The decrease in their ability to express themselves may cause patients to feel great frustration and to exhibit feelings of inadequacy. Such a patient may have to write down on paper or use some form of sign language in order to communicate. As a healthcare professional, your patience and understanding may be challenged. It is in this critical situation that you have to call on your human qualities. Show patients that you are concerned and compassionate, but do not become so personally involved that you lose your objectivity and professionalism.

Because patients will look to you for guidance, you must be very careful of what you say in their presence. You should always make sure you are clean and neat, with your uniform or lab coat well kept. You should always be well groomed and appear dignified. It is not only your technical skill but also your personality and appearance that have a beneficial and positive effect on a patient's course of treatment. You should also remember that you may not achieve any improvement in your patient right away, and he or she may become easily discouraged. It will be during this time that the patient will look to you as a professional.

Some patients may ask you questions for which you do not have the answer. In the event that this happens, you should feel free to say no and explain to the patient that you have to confer first with the physical therapist. Never feel compelled to render a therapeutic regimen that you are not familiar with or not accustomed to, or that you are not certain you should do at this particular time. Speak first with your supervisor. If you are asked by a patient to do something that is contrary to the rules of the institution by which you are employed or are in direct conflict with his or her treatment regimen, do not involve yourself. Inform the patient that you are not permitted to do what has been asked. It would not increase the patient's estimation of you if you acted contrary to the rules. If you feel an exception has to be made, you are much better off to first discuss the matter with your immediate supervisor.

As previously stated, a physical disability may change a patient's attitude toward surroundings or toward friends or family members. In some instances, such as patients suffering from Parkinson's Disease, the patient may become very timid. Such a person may need a little extra encouragement. Each activity this patient engages in may take a little longer time and more effort than does the same activity in a patient free of disease, therefore, never try to hurry a patient along. You will find greater rewards for your patience and effort as you see the Parkinsonian patient, or any patient for that matter, liven up under your care and their course of treatment.

Always remember that the aim of assisting patients with physical disabilities is bringing them back to the greatest state of health they can achieve. Such involvement on your part includes aiding the patient to achieve ambulation or completely restore normal strength. Remember, the most important part of your job is to make the patient able to function in his or her home environment without assistance or with minimal assistance from other persons. Your goal, then, is to accomplish the most optimal improvement possible for the specific disability.

Finally, it is important to remember that one of the single most important responsibilities you have is to make patients feel secure and good about themselves. Above all, always try to preserve the patients' dignity and self-esteem. Show patients the same courtesy and dignity you would expect shown to yourself if the roles were reversed.

It is a difficult, yet very rewarding, task to improve the physical disability of another person. One would have to search high and low in order to find a nobler job than that of helping another and easing the burdens of the disabled and physically challenged.

◆ SUMMARY

In this chapter, we discussed the history and evolution of the profession of physical therapy, from the time it first emerged in the early 1990s, through its function in today's highly technological world. We briefly discussed the role Mary McMillan played as physical therapy became a new profession, as well as the impact the two world wars had on the field of physical therapy. We also discussed the role rehabilitation plays in providing patients with physical therapy treatments. Finally, we talked about the role of the physical therapy aide as a member of the rehabilitation team.

◆ ◆ LEARNING ACTIVITY 1-1

Write out the answers to the following questions on a separate sheet of paper.

1. Define rehabilitation.
2. What is the purpose of the team approach to patient care?
3. How many people are generally on the rehabilitation team?
4. Define physical therapy.
5. What is the aim of physical therapy?
6. Where do many physical therapy aides work?
7. What are some of the duties of the physical therapy aide?
8. List at least three character attributes that should be developed by the physical therapy aide.
9. Which health team member is allowed to give patients information about their prognosis?
10. Define ethics.

REVIEW QUESTIONS

1. Who is considered the founder of physical therapy?
2. The use of physical modalities and procedures applied for therapeutic purposes was introduced during 1914 to combat what crippling disease?
3. Who was most responsible for assisting in the planning and organizational activities that eventually made physical therapeutics a part of the care provided for Army personnel?
4. What was the first title given to an individual who completed the newly developed physical therapeutics training classes?
5. What is the specialty of medical rehabilitation concerned with?
6. What is the major focus of the rehabilitation team?

Match the correct answers in Column A with its appropriate response in Column B.

Column A		Column B
1. physician-in-charge	___	teaches patient to work equipment and assist ADL
2. physical therapist	___	responsible for outlining patient's care and treatment
3. occupational therapist	___	acquired advanced training in kinesiology
4. social worker and psychologist	___	analyzes and deals with patient's emotional needs
5. physical therapy aide	___	assists physical therapist in carrying out physical therapy tasks

2

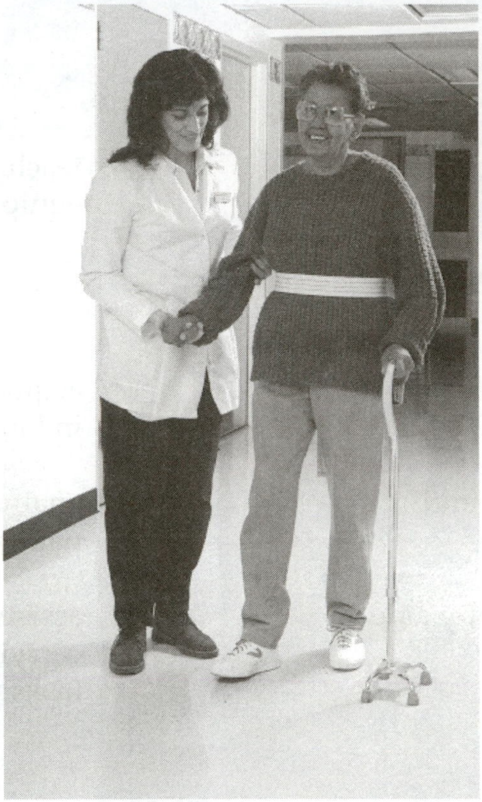

Career Opportunities for the Physical Therapy Aide

OBJECTIVES

Upon completion of this chapter, you should be able to:

1. Discuss career opportunities available to the physical therapy aide.
2. Describe the training required at various levels of health care providers in the fields of physical therapy and physical medicine.
3. Distinguish between divisions within health care facilities.
4. Discuss some of the desirable personal characteristics and technical skills required of a physical therapy aide.
5. Identify several potential duties of the physical therapy aide.
6. List potential employers of the physical therapy aide.

KEY TERMS

Health maintenance organizations (HMOs)
Medical specialist
Vital signs

Throughout our history, periods of time and eras have been given descriptive names in order to indicate what was important during that particular time. For example, when we speak of the Stone Age, we are referring to a time in which little was known except those skills which man needed in order to survive. Now commentators are saying that we live in the Information Age. Computers and electronic technology make a global transfer of data instantaneous. So workers and employees in the health care industry must be versed in information systems for recording, storing, and retrieving data related to the health and wellness of those entrusted to their care. In addition to being skilled in the various clinical skills required of the physical therapy aide (PTA), as a health care provider PTAs will also be expected to use various types of machines, equipment, and computers and information systems, since some are often necessary in order to interpret specific data and information.

HISTORY OF PHYSICAL MEDICINE AND THERAPEUTIC HEALTH CARE SERVICES

Early on in the twentieth century, the clinical or hands-on aspects of a medical practice were quite simple. A doctor performed all the procedures, clinical tests, and treatments on his own, or, in some cases, had only one assistant who helped in all aspects of the practice. More recently, clinical health care providers, particularly those associated with the administration of physical and rehabilitative procedures, have become a necessity in almost all health care facilities and in most private medical practices and clinics. As a result of the great changes made in health care technologies and the ever-increasing role of the physical medicine health care provider, the individual who has been trained in more than one of the physical and therapeutic disciplines and medical services continues to gain more and more authority, along with increased responsibility. There are now exciting possibilities for both variety and specialization in the workplace.

Careers in physical therapy and physical medicine can be found in many areas of the health care industry. Physical therapy, sports medicine and fitness training, chiropractic care, and massage therapy workers can all be found in small and large hospitals, multispecialty clinics and outpatient centers, urgent care centers, private medical offices, private and nonprofit physical therapy centers, fitness centers, clinical trials companies, and health insurance companies. These positions can also be found in skilled nursing facilities, board and care homes, and retirement hotels. An ambitious physical therapy aide may also choose to work for private health care registries, government agencies, and, in some cases, their own business.

No matter where PTAs choose to work, it is important to remember that all members of the physical therapy team are concerned with providing care and treatment to patients who are in need of their services. This includes caring for patients suffering from disorders of the musculoskeletal and nervous systems, as well as others who may be debilitated as a result of diseases affecting other systems of their body. The procedures provided to patients can range from something as basic as taking and recording **vital signs,** which includes blood pressure, temperature, pulse, and respiration, to performing more advanced therapeutic treatments such as assisting someone who is paralyzed how to walk again or providing therapeutic massage on an injured athlete. In addition to the skills necessary for working with weakened bones and muscles, PTAs are also expected to learn and become knowledgeable and skilled in working with other members of the health care team. You will have to learn how to gain access to records about health and treatments and what can and cannot be done with those records.

Training and Education

No matter where you decide to work, the fact that you have selected an occupation in the health care industry says a lot about you and your concern for helping others. Where you ultimately decide to work, however, will depend greatly upon your own unique interests and desires. Only you will be able to make that decision.

To be successful in your position, it is important that you possess the appropriate educational and technical skills, as well as the interpersonal skills necessary to communicate effectively with others. In addition to being a compassionate person, you must also be dependable and punctual. You must be flexible and like being organized. You should be able to work well under pressure and take pride in yourself and the job you are doing. And above all, you must like working with people, and, when doing so, be tactful. You should not have so much pride that you are unable to accept positive criticism, and you must be able to follow rules and detailed instructions.

Most allied health occupations in the field of physical medicine do not require national licensing or certification in order to work in a specific position. However, all assistants and technicians working under the physical medicine umbrella do require a sense of understanding of key therapeutic concepts. Therefore, as a member of this health care discipline, most employers require their workers to have a minimum of a high school diploma or its equivalent. It goes without saying that to be successful in the field of physical medicine you should also have received some advanced technical training in the field you are planning on working in. This generally includes both didactic and theoretical training, as well as many hours of training in the hands-on operations of the medical equipment that you will be working with. It also includes some comprehension and understanding of computer training and basic office machines, medical terminology, and a basic understanding of anatomy and physiology. Most workers receive this training as part of an overall educational program in a vocational or adult school, community college, or as part of a regional occupational program.

PHYSICAL AND THERAPEUTIC ALLIED HEALTH CAREERS

Health care facilities and private medical practices use many different names and titles for their physical and therapeutic workers. Doctors' offices and clinics often hire orthopedic and chiropractic assistants, physical therapy aides, and massage therapists to perform many of the therapeutic procedures required of their patients. Larger health care institutions often have job titles such as physical medicine technicians and rehabilitation technicians. No matter what your job title may be, there are certain tasks that are often common and required to all of these jobs. These include taking and recording vital signs, proper use of medical asepsis and body mechanics, understanding and being able to use the proper medical terminology and medical abbreviations as part of your charting, being able to determine the differences between the anatomical and physiological functions of patients, and having an understanding of such concepts as medical law and ethics, confidentiality, and preserving patient's rights.

During the normal workday, you will come in contact with a wide variety of people. In addition to dealing with the many variations of patients and their individual problems and personalities, you will also interact with members of the nursing staff, doctors and pharmacists, laboratory and radiology technicians, supervisors, housekeepers, hospital volunteers, and many other people who work as members of the hospital staff, as well as visitors seeking understanding and answers about their loved ones. You must always be prepared to communicate with surgeons, who may use very technical terms, as well as patients, some of whom may speak very little English. Such diversity in your work will often create an environment filled with great rewards, while others may seem more challenging and frustrating.

Employment Opportunities

Over the past several decades, employment opportunities for physical medicine workers have expanded far beyond the clinical or medical assistant who was only responsible for assisting the doctor and completing such basic tasks as answering the phone. Where a physician's office once offered the only jobs for someone interested in the field, today the options are much more extensive.

Medical care has never been more expensive or competitive. Insurance companies are not willing to pay for unnecessary procedures. Many different institutions are competing with one another for providing patient services. In today's economy, the health care institution, as well as the private medical practice, must run in a cost-effective manner if it is to survive. Because of the escalating costs of health care and the great demand put on health care providers in today's ever changing, highly technological health care world, there is an increased need to train people in more than one occupation within the same medical discipline.

Ten years ago, it was acceptable to hire one person to complete only one task. In 1987, for example, an employee who was hired to work as a PTA might have only been responsible for transferring a patient in a wheelchair from his hospital room, to the physical therapy department. Today, however, if you were hired into that same position, you might be expected to work in the rehabilitation therapy department, assisting the physical therapist in providing therapeutic massages, or providing a patient with ultrasound therapy.

Today there are many different types of health care facilities and institutions that can be very rewarding places of employment for the physical therapy aide. These include general acute care hospitals, where patients are hospitalized for a short period of time (anywhere from one day to a few weeks), specialized hospitals, which have facilities that provide care for specific problems, such as spinal injury hospitals or facilities for chronic disorders, long-term care facilities, also known as convalescent hospitals, which concentrate on providing care to the elderly, and outpatient clinics, which generally house several doctors with varied specialties combining their practice. Other types of facilities that are available for employment to the PTAs include private physicians' practices, rehabilitation centers, **health maintenance organizations (HMOs),** private fitness clubs, athletic teams, chiropractic offices, and home health care and rehabilitative care agencies.

In addition to working in a health care facility, the physical therapy aide may also seek employment within university medical schools, research centers, pharmaceutical and medical supplies companies, laboratories, insurance companies, and in some cases, even freelance self-employment.

Hospital Organization

As a member of the physical therapy team, if you choose to work in the hospital environment, it is very important for you to understand how today's modern medical facilities function. These facilities must be well organized, with a chain of command that informs each employee as to who his or her immediate supervisor is. Such an organization provides an efficient way for the facility to fulfill its mission and purpose.

An example of a hospital organization chart is shown in Table 2-1. Each service has specialized departments. These departments are determined by the type of service that is provided.

		Board of Directors		
Diagnostic Services	Medical Staff	Administrator	Auxiliary Groups	
Therapeutic Services	Patient Care Services	Nursing Services	Environmental and Equipment Services	General Services
Audiology Cardiology Emergency Rm. Laboratory Neurology Ophthalmology Pulmonary Radiology	Orthopedic Radiology Rehabilitation Renal Dialysis Respiratory Thpy.	Medical Nursing	Engineering Grounds Housekeeping Infection Control Supplies	Adm. & Clerical Dietary Medical Records Pharmacy Personnel Social Work Staff Development

Table 2-1 Organizational Chart of a Health Care Facility

Medical Specialties

If you are working in the hospital or clinic environment, more than likely you will come into contact with many different medical specialties. A **medical specialist** is a physician who devotes himself to a single branch of medical knowledge. You may find yourself working in an area that deals often with one branch of medicine, such as physical therapy. Table 2-2 provides a listing of the definitions of most of the present-day medical specialties and the name of the

SPECIALTY	NAME OF PHYSICIAN	DESCRIPTION OF SPECIALTY
Allergies	Allergist	Deals with diagnosis and treatment of body reactions resulting from sensitivity to foods, pollens, dust, medicine, or other substances
Anesthesiology	Anesthesiologist	Administers various forms of anesthesia in surgery or diagnosis to causing loss of feeling or sensation
Cardiology	Cardiologist	Deals with the diagnosis of treatment of diseases of the heart
Dermatology	Dermatologist	Deals with the diagnosis and treatment of diseases of the skin
Endocrinology	Endocrinologist	Deals with the diagnosis and treatment of diseases of the endocrine system and the hormones produced by the ductless glands
Family Practice	Family Practitioner	Diagnoses and treats diseases by medical and surgical methods for all members of the family
Gastroenterology	Gastroenterologist	Deals with the diagnosis and treatment of diseases of the digestive system
Gynecology	Gynecologist	Deals with the diagnosis and treatment of disorders of the female reproductive system
Internal Medicine	Internist	Diagnoses and treats diseases of adults
Neurology	Neurologist	Diagnoses and treats diseases of the nervous system and brain
Obstetrics	Obstetrician	Cares for women during pregnancy, childbirth, and the interval immediately following
Oncology	Oncologist	Diagnoses and treats cancer
Ophthalmology	Ophthalmologist	Diagnoses and treats disorders of the eye and prescribes glasses
Orthopedics	Orthopedist	Diagnoses and treats disorders of the muscular and skeletal systems
Otolaryngology	Otolaryngologist	Diagnoses and treats disorders of the eyes, ears, nose, and throat
Pathology	Pathologist	Studies and interprets changes in organs, tissues, cells and changes in the body's chemistry to aid in diagnosing disease and determining the type of treatment which may be necessary
Pediatrics	Pediatrician	Deals with the prevention, diagnosis, and treatment of children's diseases
Proctology	Proctologist	Diagnoses and treats diseases of the rectum
Psychiatry	Psychiatrist	Diagnoses and treats mental disorders
Radiology	Radiologist	Uses radiant energy, including x-rays, radium, cobalt, etc., in the diagnosis of diseases
Urology	Urologist	Diagnoses and treats diseases of the kidneys, bladder, ureters, and urethra and of the male reproductive system

Table 2-2 Medical Specialties

physician practicing those specialties.

◆ SUMMARY

In this chapter, we discussed the very involved and rapidly changing field of physical therapy and the various occupations and workers involved in working in this very demanding, yet highly rewarding branch of medicine. We determined that there were many varied career opportunities available to graduates of this field, both in private and public health care agencies and institutions, as well as in other industries, such as fitness centers, athletic teams, and insurance companies and preventative health care maintenance organizations. We also talked about some of the personal characteristics and technical skills that were necessary in order to be successful as a professional member of the physical therapy team, as well as defined the basic level of training for these occupations. Finally, we defined the various types of medical specialties and the name of each of the medical specialists involved in the many branches of medicine, noting that all of these were available to the physical therapy worker as a means to employment.

◆ ◆ LEARNING ACTIVITY 2-1

1. Observe the physical therapy aides in the physical therapy department. Then make a list of all the duties the physical therapy aides have in this department. Make sure you list specific duties under each category and add others.

   Transporting Patients:

   Record Keeping:

   Cleaning:

   Others:

◆ ◆ LEARNING ACTIVITY 2-2

Select one patient seen in the physical therapy department. Then check the patient's treatment chart and medical record to complete the following:

1. List the careers represented on this patient's health care team.
2. Is this patient seen by a physical therapy aide?
3. What are the aide's specific duties regarding this patient?

◆ ◆ LEARNING ACTIVITY 2-3

1. List three careers in the physical therapy department.
2. List at least six duties of the physical therapy aide.
3. In addition to working in an acute care hospital, where else might the physical therapy aide seek employment?
4. In your own words, explain why the physical therapy aide must be in good health and possess a high level of energy.
5. Identify at least two general requirements for the physical therapy aide.
6. Give at least four desirable qualities for the physical therapy aide.

◆ ◆ LEARNING ACTIVITY 2-4

Read the narrative, then write the answers to the numbered questions. You should try to find answers at the health care facility, from classroom information, or from independent research.

Narrative:

Michelle and Thomas are beginning their second week at Greensboro Hospital. In class, Ms. Marlo has assigned investigation of career opportunities for Physical Therapy Aides, and now they are going to do a little investigating on their own about the various career options available to them in the field of physical therapy and physical medicine. Michelle says, "You know Thomas, I am interested in working in a physical therapy department of a large hospital, but I am still confused by the differences in the titles physical therapy aide, physical therapy assistant, and physical therapist.

(1) What are the differences in the training for a physical therapy aide, a physical therapy assistant, and a physical therapists?

Thomas answers, "I'd like to find out more about eventually becoming a physical therapist. But since there are many health occupations included in the category of therapy, I need to know what 'therapy' means."

(2) Define therapy.

Thomas continues. "There are a good many advantages to physical therapy. But in order to earn enough money I'd need a bachelor's or a master's degree, and I'm not sure I want to spend that much time studying." Michelle answers, "But surely you have noted that in general, the longer you train, the more money you will earn." "Well," Thomas replies, "it's a little early for me to make a specific decision, but maybe I'd rather spend the time to go to medical school and become a physician." "That really takes a long time," Michelle answers, "but it certainly would be a challenge."

(3) What training is required to become a physician?

"I need to review the differences in licensure, registration, and certification," says Michelle, "even though I know all of these refer to ensuring competency and skill in a given occupation."

(4) Differentiate among certification, registration, and licensure.

"If I'm going to become a physician, then I need to be thinking about what kind of specialty I might like," says Thomas. "Now there are so many different specialties, I'm going to pay careful attention to the various kinds I hear about while we're in the hospital." "A good idea," Michelle replies, "But so many of them sound alike. I guess the best way to remember them is to concentrate on the prefixes."

(5) Define the following prefixes: a. neuro, b. pedia, c. cardio, d. ophthalmo, d. derma.

REVIEW QUESTIONS

1. What is the name of the services provided for patients within a health care facility that is responsible for treating pathological conditions and diseases?

2. What is the name of the services provided for patients within a health care facility that is responsible for managing the activities of daily living for patients?

3. What is the name of the services provided for patients within a health care facility that is responsible for properly furnishing the facility for safe use by all patients and staff?

4. What is the name of the services provided for patients within a health care facility that is responsible for admitting, feeding, and medicating patients and preserving records which concern both patients and medical personnel?

5. An ______________ is an organization that is comprised of various medical professionals and services to which a patient can subscribe.

6. Give at least three examples of departments that would be found under diagnostic services:

   a. ______________________________

   b. ______________________________

   c. ______________________________

7. Give at least two examples of an auxiliary group working within a health care facility:

   a. ______________________________

   b. ______________________________

8. Under what services would the pharmacy be found within a health care facility?

9. Under what services would staff nurses be found within a health care facility?

10. Under what services would the physical therapy department be found within a health care facility?

3

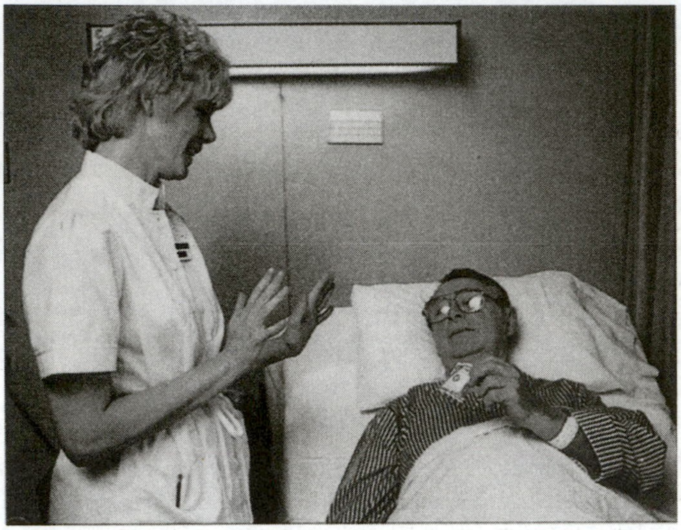

Ethical and Legal Issues Affecting the Physical Therapy Aide

OBJECTIVES

Upon completion of this chapter, you should be able to:

1. Delineate the difference between medical law and medical ethics.
2. Discuss the Patient's Bill of Rights.
3. Discuss the purpose for the need to license medical personnel.
4. Explain the Rule of Personal Liability.
5. Briefly discuss the Good Samaritan Act.
6. Demonstrate an understanding of specific patient consent forms.
7. Discuss the legal implications of a patient's medical record.
8. Discuss ethical and legal issues affecting the field of physical therapy, and briefly explain the Code of Ethics that members of the physical therapy team are morally bound to follow.
9. Identify at least four examples of ethical behavior expected of the physical therapy aides.

KEY TERMS

- Defamation
- Duty of care
- Ethics
- Ethical behavior
- Good Samaritan Law
- Informed consent
- Malpractice
- Medical ethics
- Medical law
- Medical practice acts
- Negligence
- Patient's Bill of Rights
- Reasonable care
- Rule of Personal Liability

The laws and ethical codes of conduct for the medical profession must be understood by all members of the physical medicine team. These laws and **ethics** codes protect all members of the medical profession, as well as the patient and the client.

Medical ethics have been important in the study of medicine as far back as 400 B.C., when Hippocrates wrote the Hippocratic Oath, a document that first developed the standards of medical conduct and ethics. Today, many individual health care professional associations have adopted their own codes of ethics in order to govern their health care workers. Members of the physical therapy team all have ethical codes that provide guidelines for their professional behavior.

The practice of today's medicine exists within a framework of laws. Such laws governing medical practices may vary from state to state, so it is important to know your state's law, as well as federal and local statutes, governing the physical medicine worker.

UNDERSTANDING MEDICAL ETHICS AND MEDICAL LAW

Medical ethics are concerned with whether the physical medicine worker's actions are right or wrong, whereas **medical law** is more concerned with focusing on whether one acted legally or illegally. **Ethical behavior** deals with behavior that is specific and represents the ideal conduct for a certain group. Each group of health care professionals who require a license to function in their position have drafted and adopted a specific code of ethics. These ethics are based upon moral principles and practices. If accused of unethical behavior by a medical worker's professional association, you can be issued a warning, or in some cases, even expelled from the association.

Medical law is concerned with the legal conduct of the members of the medical profession. There are federal, state, and local laws which must be followed, and violation of such laws may subject the offender to civil or criminal prosecution. Professional licenses can be taken away, fines can be levied, and prison sentences can be imposed. Often, the line between what is unethical and what is legal can be unclear. If you, as a member of the health care delivery system, decided, for example, you were going to be rude to a patient, that is unethical behavior. But if you decided to inform the patient's neighbor of his or her disease, that is illegal behavior. In addition, you can also be sued by a patient for **defamation,** which is considered an attack on a person's reputation. This is called *libel* when the defamation is written, and *slander* when spoken.

Another example of the difference between unethical and illegal behavior concerns the viewing of a friend's chart in a part of the hospital where you do not work. If you read it out of curiosity, that is unethical. If you talk about it, that is illegal. If an action is illegal, it is always unethical. However, it can be unethical without being illegal. Remember, ethics represent the highest standards of behavior.

Ethical Behavior

As a member of the physical medicine team, you are responsible for displaying ethical behavior at all times. This means maintaining the highest level of ethical conduct. To accomplish such a task, you should always:

- ❒ respect the rights of all patients to have opinions, lifestyles, and beliefs that are different from your own
- ❒ remember that everything seen, heard, or read about a patient is considered confidential and does not leave the job site
- ❒ be conscientious in doing your work, doing the best you can at all times
- ❒ be ready to be of service to patients and coworkers at any time of the workday
- ❒ let the patient know that it is a privilege for you to assist him or her
- ❒ follow closely the specific rules of ethical conduct prescribed by your employer

◆ THE PATIENT AND THE HEALTH CARE WORKER

The Patient's Bill of Rights

Awareness of the patient's rights is the responsibility of all members of the health care team. Because this is such a vital and important aspect of providing care and treatment to the patient, the American Hospital Association (AHA) felt it was necessary to establish a document which identified what the patient could expect from those individuals who cared for the patient. As a result, the **Patient's Bill of Rights** was adopted by the organization (Figure 3-1). The intent of such a document is to make both members of the health care system and patients aware of what the patient has a right to expect. According to the AHA, the patient has a right to:

- ❒ considerate and respectful care
- ❒ obtain from their physician complete and current information concerning their diagnosis, treatment, and prognosis, in terms that they can be reasonably expected to understand
- ❒ informed consent, which should include knowledge of the proposed procedure, along with its risks and probable duration of incapacitation; in addition, the patient has a right to information regarding medically significant alternatives
- ❒ refuse treatment to the extent permitted by law, and to be informed of the medical consequences of such action
- ❒ have case discussion, consultation, examination, and treatment conducted discretely, and have those not directly involved in the patient's care

American Hospital Association

AHA Policy A Patient's Bill of Rights

This policy document presents the official position of the American Hospital Association as approved by the Board of trustees and House of Delegates.

Management Advisory

Patient and Community Relations

Introduction

Effective health care requires collaboration between patients and physicians and other health care professionals. Open and honest communication, respect for personal and professional values, and sensitivity to differences are integral to optimal patient care. As the setting for the provision of health services, hospitals must provide a foundation for understanding and respecting the rights and responsibilities of patients, their families, physicians, and other caregivers. Hospitals must ensure a health care ethic that respects the role of patients in decision making about treatment choices and other aspects of their care. Hospitals must be sensitive to cultural, racial, linguistic, religious, age, gender, and other differences as well as the needs of persons with disabilities.

The American Hospital Association presents *A Patient's Bill of Rights* with the expectation that it will contribute to more effective patient care and be supported by the hospital on behalf of the institution, its medical staff, employees, and patients. The American Hospital Association encourages health care institutions to tailor this bill of rights to their patient community by translating and/or simplifying the language of this bill of rights as may be necessary to ensure that patients and their families understand their rights and responsibilities.

Bill of Rights*

1. The patient has the right to considerate and respectful care.

2. The patient has the right to and is encouraged to obtain from physicians and other direct caregivers relevant, current, and understandable information concerning diagnosis, treatment, and prognosis.

   Except in emergencies when the patient lacks decision-making capacity and the need for treatment is urgent, the patient is entitled to the oppor-
   tunity to discuss and request information related to the specific procedures and/or treatments, the risks involved, the possible length of recuperation, and the medically reasonable alternatives and their accompanying risks and benefits.

   Patients have the right to know the identity of physicians, nurses, and others involved in their care, as well as when those involved are students, residents, or other trainees. The patient also has the right to know the immediate and long-term financial implications of treatment choices, insofar as they are known.

3. The patient has the right to make decisions about the plan of care prior to and during the course of treatment and to refuse a recommended treatment or plan of care to the extent permitted by law and hospital policy and to be informed of the medical consequences of this action. In case of such refusal, the patient is entitled to other appropriate care and services that the hospital provides or transfer to another hospital. The hospital should notify patients of any policy that might affect patient choice within the institution.

4. The patient has the right to have an advance directive (such as a living will, health care proxy, or durable power of attorney for health care) concerning treatment or designating a surrogate decision maker with the expectation that the hospital will honor the intent of that directive to the extent permitted by law and hospital policy.

   Health care institutions must advise patients of their rights under state law and hospital policy to make informed medical choices, ask if the patient has an advance directive, and include that information in patient records. The patient has the right to timely information about hospital policy that may limit its ability to implement fully a legally valid advance directive.

5. The patient has the right to every consideration of privacy. Case discussion, consultation, examination, and treatment should be conducted so as to protect each patient's privacy.

6. The patient has the right to expect that all communications and records pertaining to his/her care will be treated as confidential by the hospital, except in cases such as suspected abuse and public health hazards when reporting is permitted or required by law. The patient has the right to expect that the hospital will emphasize the confidentiality of this information when it releases it to any other parties entitled to review information in these records.

7. The patient has the right to review the records pertaining to his/her medical care and to have the information explained or interpreted as necessary, except when restricted by law.

8. The patient has the right to expect that within its capacity and policies, a hospital will make reasonable response to the request of a patient for appropriate and medically indicated care and services. The hospital must provide evaluation, service, and/or referral as indicated by the urgency of the case. When medically appropriate and legally permissible, or when a patient has so requested, a patient may be transferred to another facility. The institution to which the patient is to be transferred must first have accepted the patient for transfer. The patient

*These rights can be exercised on the patient's behalf by a designated surrogate or proxy decision maker if the patient lacks decision-making capacity, is legally incompetent, or is a minor.

Figure 3-1 A Patient's Bill of Rights. Reprinted with permission from The American Hospital Association, copyright 1992.

must also have the benefit of complete information and explanation concerning the need for, risks, benefits, and alternatives to such a transfer.

9. The patient has the right to ask and be informed of the existence of business relationships among the hospital, educational institutions, other health care providers, or payers that may influence the patient's treatment and care.

10. The patient has the right to consent or to decline to participate in proposed research studies or human experimentation affecting care and treatment or requiring direct patient involvement, and to have those studies fully explained prior to consent. A patient who declines to participate in research or experimentation is entitled to the most effective care that the hospital can otherwise provide.

11. The patient has the right to expect reasonable continuity of care when appropriate and to be informed by physicians and other caregivers of available and realistic patient care options when hospital care is no longer appropriate.

12. The patient has the right to be informed of hospital policies and practices that relate to patient care, treatment, and responsibilities. The patient has the right to be informed of available resources for resolving disputes, grievances, and conflicts, such as ethics committees, patient representatives, or other mechanisms available in the institution. The patient has the right to be informed of the hospital's charges for services and available payment methods.

The collaborative nature of health care requires that patients, or their families/surrogates, participate in their care. The effectiveness of care and patient satisfaction with the course of treatment depend, in part, on the patient fulfilling certain responsibilities. Patients are responsible for providing information about past illnesses, hospitalizations, medications, and other matters related to health status. To participate effectively in decision making, patients must be encouraged to take responsibility for requesting additional information or clarification about their health status or treatment when they do not fully understand information and instructions. Patients are also responsible for ensuring that the health care institution has a copy of their written advance directive if they have one. Patients are responsible for informing their physicians and other caregivers if they anticipate problems in following prescribed treatment.

Patients should also be aware of the hospital's obligation to be reasonably efficient and equitable in providing care to other patients and the community. The hospital's rules and regulations are designed to help the hospital meet this obligation. Patients and their families are responsible for making reasonable accommodations to the needs of the hospital, other patients, medical staff, and hospital employees. Patients are responsible for providing necessary information for insurance claims and for working with the hospital to make payment arrangements, when necessary.

A person's health depends on much more than health care services. Patients are responsible for recognizing the impact of their lifestyle on their personal health.

Conclusion

Hospitals have many functions to perform, including the enhancement of health status, health promotion, and the prevention and treatment of injury and disease; the immediate and ongoing care and rehabilitation of patients; the education of health professionals, patients, and the community; and research. All these activities must be conducted with an overriding concern for the values and dignity of patients.

A *Patient's Bill of Rights* was first adopted by the American Hospital Association of 1973. The revision was approved by the AHA Board of Trustees on October 21, 1992.

Figure 3-1 A Patient's Bill of Rights (Continued). Reprinted with permission from The American Hospital Association, copyright 1992.

be granted permission by the patient for their presence

- ❒ expect that all communication and records pertaining to his or her care be treated in a confidential manner
- ❒ expect the hospital to make a reasonable response to request for services, and the hospital must provide evaluation, service, and referrals as they may be indicated by the urgency of the case
- ❒ obtain information as to any relationship of the hospital to other health care and educational institutions, insofar as his or her care is concerned, and the relationship among individuals, by name, who are treating the patient
- ❒ be advised if the hospital proposes to engage in or perform human experimentation affecting his or her care or treatment, and the right to refuse to participate in such research projects
- ❒ expect reasonable continuity of care
- ❒ examine and receive an explanation of the bill regardless of the source of payment
- ❒ know what hospital rules and regulations apply to his or her conduct as a patient

LICENSING OF HEALTH CARE WORKERS

The medical profession and many of the individual health care professions are legally regulated throughout the United States by the issuing of licenses and certificates. All fifty states require the licensing of hospitals. The statutes dealing with the individual licensing and certification of the individual health care professionals, are commonly referred to as **medical practice acts.**

Licenses can be revoked or suspended when a medical professional has been found guilty of having violated various statutes involved in the licensing process. Grounds for losing a medical license include serious crimes such as murder, rape, and arson. Crimes of "moral turpitude," such as tax crimes, minor sexual offenses, and false statements while applying for a license, can also be grounds for loss of the license. Other crimes that may cause the worker to have his or her license suspended or revoked include an incapacity due to insanity or excessive use of alcohol or drug addiction.

Protection Under the Law

In the health care environment, both the patient and the health care worker must be assured protection under the law. For the patient, this means being assured of safe care. For the health care professional, it means being protected from irresponsible lawsuits.

The patient is protected by a process known as **duty of care.** This entitles the patient to safe care by making it mandatory that he or she be treated by meeting the common or average standards of practice expected in the community under similar circumstances. The duty of care also provides that the patient be treated with **reasonable care,** that is, protection of the health care professional by law if it can be proven that he or she acted reasonably as compared to fellow workers of the same or similar training in a situation of the same nature. If it is proven that the health care worker failed to meet such a standard and harm comes to the patient as a result, negligence may be proven.

Negligence is the failure to give reasonable care or the giving of unreasonable care. The patient is harmed because the health professional did something wrong or failed to do something that he or she should have done under the circumstances.

The Good Samaritan Law and Medical Malpractice

The **Good Samaritan Law** is a law that addresses the problem of medical malpractice suits for a physician or any trained health care professional who comes upon an accident scene and attempts to render aid to the victim. The law, which has been enacted in some form in all fifty states, encourages members of health care professions to offer treatment without fearing the possibility of a malpractice suit. Laws throughout the country do differ, so it is wise to check the law in your own state in order to determine what professional liability may exist during an emergency situation.

The term **malpractice,** unfortunately, is a term that is familiar to all of us because of the excessive number of lawsuits being filed and settled throughout the country. For the medical worker, it seems that the higher the educational level and requirements of the worker, the greater the likelihood that they may be responsible for their actions.

When used in the medical professions, malpractice refers to any misconduct or lack of skill that results in the patient's injury. A patient who thinks that his or her physician has been negligent in diagnosing and treating an illness or accident may file a medical malpractice claim. Most claims are generally made against physicians, however, any employee working in the health care environment can be named in a malpractice lawsuit. Most insurance companies who issue medical malpractice policies on physicians take into account that the policy will also cover the physician's employees, as well, but medical office or hospital employees may also wish to purchase their own insurance policy, which is usually quite inexpensive.

Physicians are liable for the actions of their employees while the employee is on duty. An example would be a laboratory assistant who accepts a lab specimen from two patients and then mislabels the specimens, consequently causing one patient to be told that his specimen is normal and the other being administered antibiotics. Subsequently, the patient who has been told that everything was alright develops an infection that could have been prevented if the antibiotics had been administered. In this case, the doctor could be sued for the negligence of the employee mislabeling the specimens.

In health care, under the **Rule of Personal Liability,** all individuals are held responsible for their own personal conduct. In a medical malpractice suit, such as the one example previously described, both the physician and the laboratory assistant could be held jointly liable for medical malpractice.

You can also be held jointly responsible if you work for a doctor who is involved in an illegal act, and you are aware of the crime but fail to report it. Physicians must also report crimes that they learn about when practicing medicine, such as a shooting, child or elder abuse, or rape. As a member of the physical medicine team, you can also be held jointly responsible with the physician if you fail to report such crimes. In some cases, protecting patient confidentiality and the patient's right to complete privacy of their records does not apply. Births, deaths, communicable diseases, and crimes are all examples of times when the physician is bound by law to report what has occurred. If you fail to report these types of cases, you may also be held liable.

In some instances, the law is very specific regarding confidentiality and reporting of information. In cases dealing with patients suffering from AIDS, for example, their are laws and regulations which take into account the confidential nature of the patient's illness. However, these regulations seem to be constantly changing, therefore, it is important that you keep current as to the laws and regulations in the state in which you are working regarding confidentiality and patient's records in treating this disease.

Obtaining Patient Consent

When a doctor makes a diagnosis and recommends a specific mode of treatment, the patient has the responsibility whether or not to accept such diagnosis and treatment. The physician has the responsibility of informing the patient in words that he or she can understand as to the risks and alternatives of any suggested procedure. The patient has the responsibility of deciding whether or not to accept all the explained risks. Once it is ascertained that the physician has properly explained the procedure and the patient fully understands it and the risks, a consent form must be signed by the patient, indicating that he or she fully accepts the risk of the procedure. The process is called **informed consent.** As part of your responsibility, you may be asked to prepare the consent form for any type of procedure, whether it is to be performed in the office or in the hospital. Consents are also required before an experimental procedure or prior to any other unusual procedure taking place. Consent forms are also used prior to the administration of any experimental drugs or medication.

In cases where the patient may have difficulty understanding or speaking the English language, the consent form must be translated or prepared in the patient's native language. A patient who has not been properly informed through the informed consent process can sue the physician for malpractice.

Specific guidelines have been established regarding the details and signing of the consent form. These include the following:

- Always make sure that the patient fully understands the consent form and realizes what he or she has signed; patients who are mentally handicapped should be given an explanation that can be understood completely, with as few confusing terms as possible.
- The patient must never be forced to sign the consent form and must not be allowed to sign it under the influence of alcohol or drugs.
- All signatures must be witnessed, dated, and signed in ink, with the full legal names used.
- Any adult over eighteen years of age may sign his or her own consent unless the patient is incompetent and has a guardian, or there is an emergency, in which case, two physicians must sign the consent form.
- Married minors may sign their own consent for treatment.
- Unmarried minors must have a consent signed by one parent or legal guardian, however, consent of both parents is usually suggested; a stepparent may not sign a consent form.
- An emancipated minor, who is under the age of eighteen and who has been declared by a court of law to be legally responsible for his or herself, may sign his or her own consent form.
- Because any break in the skin may be considered an operation, a consent form must be signed in order to avoid liability for battery.
- Telephone consents are valid in an emergency situation, provided that the telephoned consent is witnessed by two people and is immediately followed by a written confirmation.
- A consent is valid for a reasonable time after signing as long as there is no change in the anticipated procedure.

◆ PATIENT MEDICAL RECORDS AND THE LAW

The patient's medical record is considered a legal document and as such is the property of the physician if the patient is an outpatient, and the property of the hospital if the patient has been hospitalized. It is extremely important that these records be as accurate, complete, up-to-date, and as neat as possible in order to protect members of the medical staff from any future litigation, as well as evidence of truth if there is a lawsuit or court case regarding the patient's care or treatment. While all patient's records are considered confidential, any or all parts of it may be summoned and used during a court action. Therefore, most hospitals and private medical practices make it a standard practice to obtain a signed release of information form from the patient when they are first seen or admitted into the hospital.

If you are required to write in the patient's medical records, always remember to use only permanent ink, and never erase an entry. If an error has been made, simply cross the error out using only one line, initial it, and rewrite the correct entry above or next to the original entry. No documentation written in pencil or with erasures are acceptable, and any record with either of these can be automatically rejected as legal evidence.

ETHICAL AND LEGAL ISSUES IN PHYSICAL THERAPY

Practitioners involved in the field of physical therapy have always been concerned about the ethics of their profession. The first code of ethics, which was adopted in 1935 by the American Physiotherapy Association, initially focused almost solely on the duties of the physical therapist, while the sophistication and timeliness of the current American Physical Therapy Association code of ethics stands in stark contrast to earlier guidelines set by its predecessors.

The code of ethics originally adopted by the American Physical Therapy Association in May, 1948 and all its subsequent amendments and principles stand firmly on the premise that such a code is important as a set of broad moral guidelines and as a public document professing the group's moral and ethical commitments to the profession and to the patient. The individual practitioner's commitment to upholding high standards are the best indicators of how the profession as a whole will be judged.

AMERICAN PHYSICAL THERAPY ASSOCIATION CODE OF ETHICS

PREAMBLE

This Code of Ethics sets forth ethical principles for the physical therapy profession. Members of this profession are responsible for maintaining and promoting ethical practice. This Code of Ethics, adopted by the American Physical Therapy Association, shall be binding on physical therapists who are members of the Association.

PRINCIPLE 1 Physical therapists respect the rights and dignity of all individuals.

PRINCIPLE 2 Physical therapists comply with the laws and regulations governing the practice of physical therapy.

PRINCIPLE 3 Physical therapists accept responsibility for the exercise of sound judgment.

PRINCIPLE 4 Physical therapists maintain and promote high standards for physical therapy practice, education, and research.

PRINCIPLE 5 Physical therapists seek remuneration for their services that is deserved and responsible.

PRINCIPLE 6 Physical therapists provide accurate information to the consumer about the profession and about those services they provide.

PRINCIPLE 7 Physical therapists accept the responsibility to protect the public and the profession from unethical, incompetent, or illegal acts.

PRINCIPLE 8 Physical therapists participate in efforts to address the health needs of the public.

AMERICAN PHYSICAL THERAPY ASSOCIATION STANDARDS OF ETHICAL CONDUCT FOR THE PHYSICAL THERAPIST ASSISTANT

PREAMBLE

Physical therapist assistants are responsible for maintaining and promoting high standards of conduct. These Standards of Ethical Conduct for the Physical Therapist Assistant shall be binding on physical therapist assistants who are affiliate members of the Association.

STANDARD 1 Physical therapist assistants provide services under the supervision of a physical therapist.

STANDARD 2 Physical therapist assistants respect the rights and dignity of all individuals.

STANDARD 3 Physical therapist assistants maintain and promote high standards in the provision of services, giving the welfare of patients their highest regard.

STANDARD 4 Physical therapist assistants provide services within the limits of the law.

STANDARD 5 Physical therapist assistants make those judgments that are commensurate with their qualifications as physical therapist assistants.

STANDARD 6 Physical therapist assistants accept the responsibility to protect the public and the profession from unethical, incompetent, or illegal acts.

Morals and Ethics

Morals, or "moral norms," are the attitudes and behaviors that a society agrees upon as both desirable and necessary in order to maximize the realization of things cherished most in that society. At one end of the moral spectrum are minimum rules designed to keep the society from destroying itself. At the other end, are the ideals toward which members can strive in trying to create a perfect society. By adhering to these rules and ideals, we are helped in preserving and fostering the conditions necessary for living together in peace and harmony. While some rules and ideals have changed, others have stood the test of time and have had exceptional staying power.

Morals are generally grouped into several categories, including duties, rights, responsibilities, character traits, and conditions of justice.

Within the framework of health care, some of the basic moral norms are especially important. This is due primarily to the nature of the health care professional and patient relationship. Among them are duties to do no harm, to keep one's promise to patients, and to tell the truth. Rights include the right of patients to their life and the right of health care professionals to be free to make the best possible judgments. Additionally, there are responsibilities of health professionals, patients, and society as a whole, that ought to be taken into account, and character traits, such as compassion, honesty, and conscientiousness, that are valued.

Ethics is related to morals since it is the study of morals and moral judgments. Ethical theories enable a person to reflect on and find resolution to conflicts of duties, rights, or responsibilities.

In health care, we are continuously

bombarded with ethical dilemmas, that question or compromise our own ethical belief system or values. As a physical therapy aide, you can expect, at some point in your career, to encounter one of these "no-win" situations. One such example may be the decision to honor a patient's wishes to have information about his condition, knowing fully well that to provide it would be in direct conflict with the physician's expressed wish that the patient not be told. Another example may be a decision to spend an extra fifteen minutes with a patient who really needs attention, even though it will mean cutting corners with the next patient.

Health care practitioners employed in the field of physical therapy face the wide range of moral problems confronting today's health professions. In their professional role physical therapy aides may not be directly involved in some morally complex situations such as abortion or discontinuing life-support systems; however, they are by no means exempt from many ethical issues affecting the health care industry in general. Most of these issues fall under one of four different areas of concentration: confidentiality, informed consent, interprofessional issues, and issues dealing with justice (see Figure 3-2).

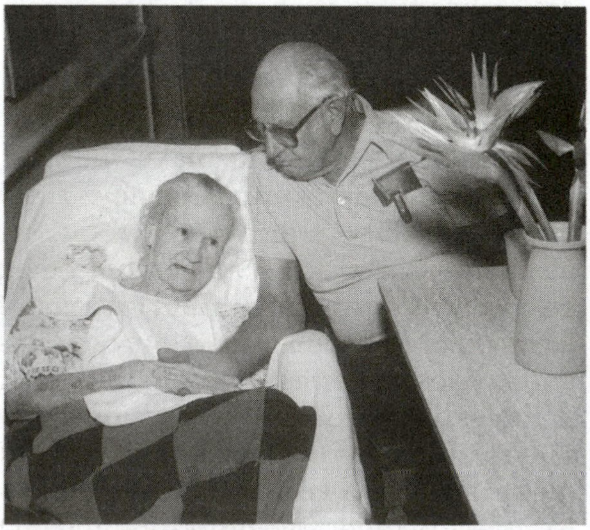

Figure 3-2 Provide privacy for residents and spouses when spouses are visiting.

Confidentiality

In the health care setting, one's commitment to honoring confidences should be considered a momentous challenge, especially when a patient is being seen over a long period of time and by a multitude of professionals, which is usually the case for a patient receiving physical therapy treatments. It is important to keep in mind that most patients expect all health professionals to keep secret the harmful, shameful, or embarrassing information the patient reveals to them. While most health facilities continuously process data and information regarding the patient's state of health from one department to the next, it is always the responsibility of the individual health care worker to be as discrete and protective as possible in order to not defame the patient in any way (Figure 3-3).

Informed Consent

Mechanisms for securing informed consent or obtaining the patient's permission for care and treatment are many, but they, like the concepts surrounding confidentiality, are challenged by long-term treatment and the often complex nature of some health care programs. Seldom does the patient consent initially to becoming a part of a particular program. For example, seldom does the patient consent to the many different kinds of intravenous injections that are tried in the overall goal of rehabilitating him. Today, more than ever, we are seeing physical therapy treatments and evaluation procedures guided more by moral principles and legal constraints,

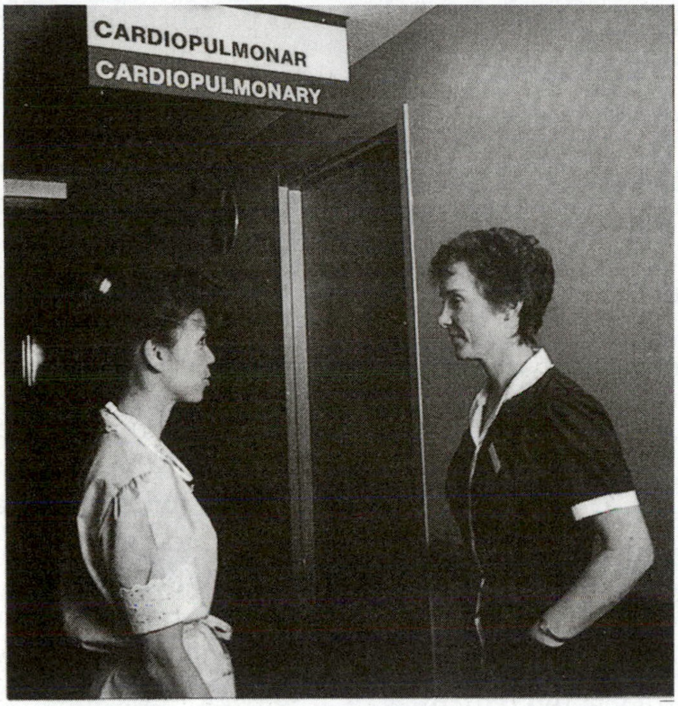

Figure 3-3 Information about patients is confidential and must not be discussed casually with others.

thereby leading to the implementation of the mechanism known as informed consent.

◆ INTERPROFESSIONAL ISSUES

Issues which fall into this category tend to give rise to other types of moral dilemmas befalling the physical therapy worker. For example, many physical therapists and physical therapy aides are justifiably worried that the practice of working in a physician-managed or other privately owned physical therapy clinic may entail built-in conflicts of interest. Other areas, such as the move by many physical therapists toward practice independent of physician referral, have raised consciousness and concern regarding the effect such an arrangement may have on the physician-therapist relationship. At the same time, all members of the physical therapy and rehabilitation team continue to examine ways in which physician-therapist arrangements can be designed to best preserve intraprofessional integrity while better meeting the needs of the patients.

◆ JUSTICE ISSUES

The physical therapy department and the professionals working within its dimensions are not exempt from being involved in agonizing decisions about how to distribute scarce resources according to an acceptable standard of fairness and equity. More and more, the physical therapy worker is being forced to become involved in policy and government in order to help assure that just policies and practices for the field continue to gain support.

MEDICAL ETHICS AND THE PHYSICAL THERAPY AIDE

As a member of the health care delivery team, one of the areas the physical therapy aide is concerned with deals with the subject of medical ethics and how it relates to his or her job as a physical therapy aide. Ethics, as it relates to medicine, is a set of rules that guides or governs the conduct of all individuals who come into contact with patients. These rules, which are moral rather than legal, have been established for the protection of the patient. When you, as a physical therapy aide, assume the responsibility for caring for a patient, you are also agreeing to live up to the ethical code that protects the patient.

Generally speaking, one of the most basic rules of ethics is that life is precious. Therefore, everyone who is involved in the care of patients must put the saving of human life and the promotion of health above all else. For most health care providers, it is not always easy to keep this rule in mind when you are caring for a patient who may be suffering to dying, especially if you know the patient is in pain or has a limited potential for a productive life.

Living in the 1990s, one might say that probably at no other time in history have the questions of medical ethics been under such watchful eyes. Frequently, questions arise that trigger deep-seeded emotional responses—responses that tend to remove the clinician's objective point of view and replace it with a more subjective, emotional reaction. When is life gone from a person on a life support system? How much heroic effort should be given in situations where the patient is dying of a terminal illness? How valid and legally acceptable are living wills which have been written by a terminally ill patient? These and many other medical-legal questions continuously surround us today and will eventually be decided in a court of law.

Still one fact remains very clear, those of us involved in the delivery of health care share a major responsibility, and that responsibility is to preserve life whenever possible, and make comfortable those whose lives may not last much longer.

Now, you may be asking yourself, as a physical therapy aide, what role or responsibility do I play in fulfilling medical ethics? How do the rules or guidelines which govern the medical-legal ramifications of caring for patients affect me on a day-to-day basis? You must always remember that one of the most basic rules that you will be expected to follow will deal with confidentiality; that is, whatever you hear or say within the medical environment must always remain within that environment. While individual circumstances will always arise that will tempt you to "talk shop," you must never break the confidence the health care environment has bestowed upon you. Discussing patients with others not involved with their care is considered gossiping and always is considered ethically wrong.

Talking with Others

Patients, and sometimes others, such as visitors and family members, may question you about the patient's condition, treatment, or prognosis. You must learn to evade such questions and inquiries in a tactful and professional manner. Whenever you are asked such questions, your response should always be the same. You must redirect the inquiry to your supervisor, the nurse, or the physician responsible for the

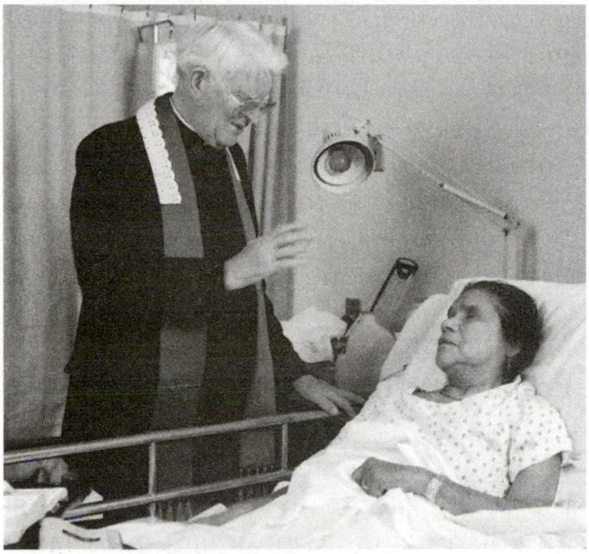

Figure 3-4 A member of the clergy is comforting the patient.

patient's care. Since it is the privilege of each physician to decide how much information should be given to an individual patient, you must never take it upon yourself to answer questions that are not within your realm or scope of responsibility.

Since you may frequently be entering the patient's room, another rule that you are expected to follow is to never discuss a patient's condition while in her hospital room. Even if a patient appears to be unresponsive, she may still be able to hear everything being said (see Figure 3-4).

Tipping

Patients are charged for services they receive while in the hospital; the salary you are paid is included in that charge. Therefore, under no circumstances are you to accept monies or gifts for the services you are expected to perform during your daily work. Tipping within the health care environment is never acceptable. If offered, a firm yet courteous refusal of the money or gift is usually all that is necessary in order to convince the patient of your meaning (Figure 3-5).

◆ MEDICAL ETHICS AND LEGAL ISSUES

While working within the health care environment, there are certain legal issues that you should be familiar with because they will influence your role as a physical therapy aide. These issues deal with negligence, malpractice,

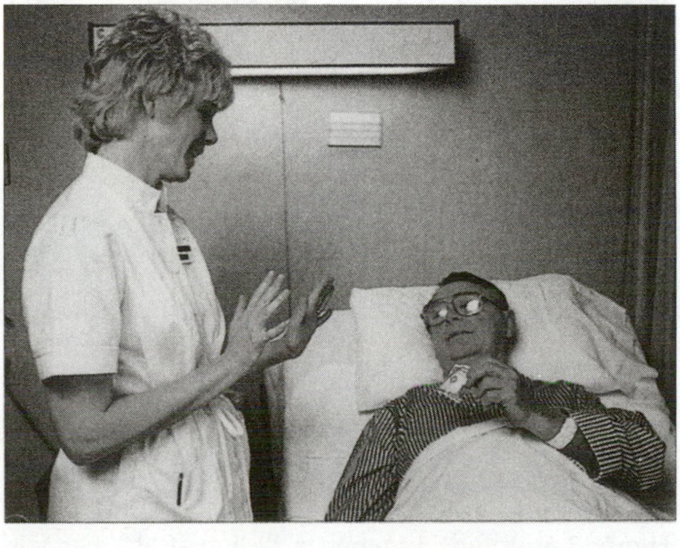

Figure 3-5 Tips must be courteously refused.

reporting illegal and dishonest acts, writing or witnessing a patient's will, and restraining patients—both for their own safety and against their will.

Negligence

When a health care provider fails to give care that is required by the job he has been hired and trained to perform, that provider is guilty of negligence. For example, if the hospital in which you are employed has a policy that states the physical therapy aide cannot ambulate the patient without a waist belt, and you do so anyway, you would in fact be guilty of negligence since you did not follow proper hospital policy in carrying out your task. Remember, whether you perform a procedure in the wrong manner or for the wrong reason, you are always accountable for your own actions (Figure 3-6).

Malpractice

Malpractice occurs when a health care provider improperly delivers care or provides the care without having had proper training or formal instruction. Applying hot packs to a patient without a doctor's order or applying them without proper instruction on how they are to be applied, would be considered malpractice.

Writing or Witnessing a Patient's Will

Sometimes patients ask members of the health care team to write or witness a will. You should note that all matters of this nature should be promptly reported to your supervisor since writing or signing a patient's will is a legal matter for which you are not trained. As a physical therapy aide, you will not have problems if you simply follow the hospital's or medical facility's policies regarding these procedures. Remember, perform only those services that you have been taught and know the proper lines of authority whenever a case arises in which you are asked to do some-

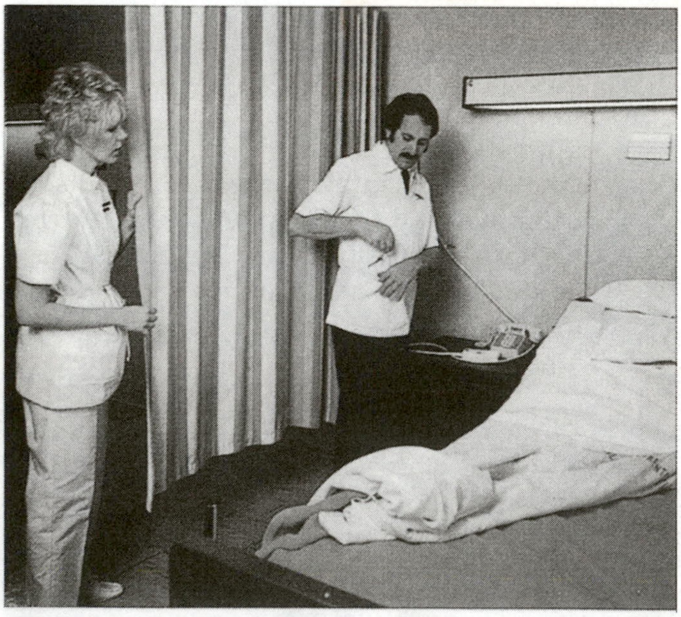

Figure 3-6 Failing to report a dishonest act that you observe makes you guilty of aiding and abetting.

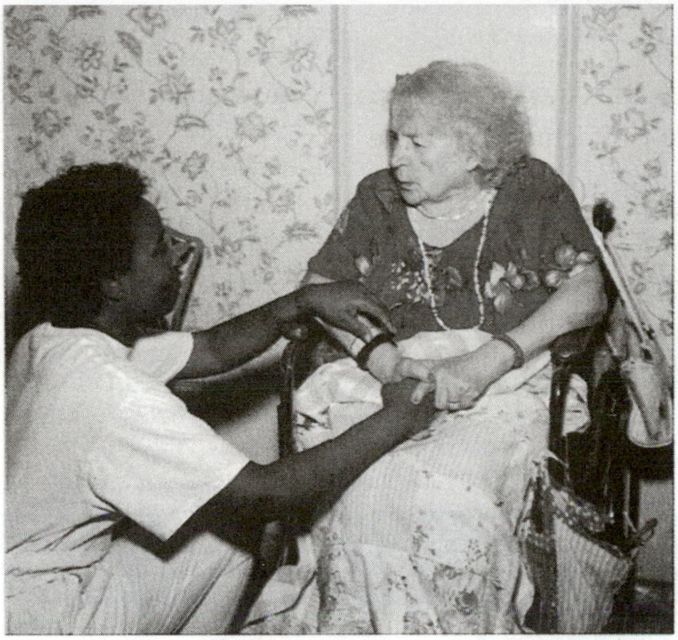

Figure 3-7 Perform those services within your scope of practice.

thing which is not within your scope of practice (Figure 3-7).

Restraints

In some instances it may be necessary to restrain the movements of patients. Whenever restraints are employed, always remember that they must be applied in accordance with a specific doctor's order. Such an order indicates the extent of the restraint and the rationale for its application.

As a physical therapy aide, you should not be called upon to apply restraints since they are generally applied by nursing personnel for the sole purpose of protecting the patient or to protect others from the patient. Application of these restraints without the proper authorization or justification can constitute false imprisonment. Whenever you are required to work with a patient who does have restraints applied, always remember to follow good common sense and safety when moving the patient about. If the restraints must be untied or removed during a procedure, always remember to make sure they have been properly reapplied when you have completed your task.

All persons providing care to the patient must voluntarily agree to live up to the medical ethical code. This code protects the patient by prohibiting the discussion of personal matters and by assuring the preservation of life and the promotion of health. Patients receive care based on their need, not their ability to pay: therefore, the acceptance of tips or gifts is never permitted. Remember, as a member of the health care team, you have legal responsibilities—responsibilities that include no toleration of negligence, malpractice, or dishonest acts. There will never be concern about legal complications as long as prudent judgment is exercised and policies are followed.

◆ SUMMARY

In this chapter, we discussed the ethical and legal issues affecting both the health care field in general and the specialty area of physical therapy. First we discussed the differences between medical law and medical ethics. We also talked about the patient's bill of rights, and the role each member of the health care team plays in protecting those rights. We briefly discussed the rule of personal liability and the Good Samaritan Law. We described the legal implications of a patient's medical record and specific patient consent forms. Finally, we discussed the ethical and legal issues affecting the physical therapy aide, including the Code of Ethics, which members of the physical therapy team are morally bound to follow.

◆ ◆ LEARNING ACTIVITY 3-1

Objective:

To research literature for information regarding ethical problems and to analyze, synthesize, and evaluate the information in a written report.

Directions:

Review the list of current ethical concerns and discuss the list in class. Choose one topic for a research project. Use a minimum of three references and write a three-page report. Justify your position on the issue chosen, and be prepared to present your views in class.

- ❒ Moral obligation to work at a task dependably, cheerfully, and punctually.
- ❒ Acceptance of each patient as a person of value who happens to have a medical problem, regardless of race, gender, economic circumstances, or sexual preference.
- ❒ Quality care for incurable and incompetent patients.
- ❒ Influence of the legal and insurance and managed care professions on cost and quality of patient care.
- ❒ Patient's bill of rights: suggest modification, or discuss whether or not there is a need for such a document.
- ❒ The problem of total honesty in dealing with terminally ill patients.
- ❒ Living wills and transplants.
- ❒ Responsibility concerning drugs in the clinical facility.
- ❒ Care of infectious patients with incurable diseases.
- ❒ Care of the indigent patient: How much and at what cost?

◆ ◆ LEARNING ACTIVITY 3-2

Objective:

To encourage students to apply information from the classroom to out-of-class situations.

Directions:

Read the narrative, then write answers to the numbered questions. You should try to find answers at the health care facility, from classroom information, or from independent research.

Narrative:

Jean and Betsy are just leaving Jackson Hospital to return to class when they meet a fellow student, Harry Johnson, who is observing in the physical therapy department. He is very excited and stops for a minute to tell them, "I just saw a patient who is a famous celebrity, being helped to walk because he has had a stroke. He's that patient in Room 301. It really is a pretty good example of helping a patient to ambulate, and after all, he is a famous person." Jean looks at Betsy and says, "What should we do? I know that Harry is so excited about seeing someone famous in the hospital, that he completely forgot about confidentiality." Betsy says, "I don't know exactly."

(1) What should the students do?

On their way back to school, Betsy says, "Remembering the ethical thing to do isn't always easy, is it? Ms. Smith told me about the time she was censured because she helped a patient out of a bed too soon before the doctor had written an order to get her up."

(2) What might have happened if the patient had fallen out of bed while getting up and then decided to pursue the matter?

Jean says, "I guess it is hard to know sometimes. Did you hear about the time Dr. Jones stopped to help at an accident involving ten cars and then was sued for malpractice? Even though he followed a standard procedure to treat one of the injured, the victim felt he might have recovered more quickly if Dr. Jones had followed a slightly different first aide procedure. The judge refused to hear the case because it fell under the Good Samaritan Law, but still, Dr. Jones was pretty unhappy."

(3) How does the Good Samaritan Law protect providers to emergency care?

Then Betsy turns to Jean and asks, "Well, what should a health professional do if he or she sees a life-threatening accident, just drive on by and avoid becoming involved, even though the patient may die?"

(4) What should he or she do?

REVIEW QUESTIONS

1. In what year was the first code of ethics adopted by the American Physiotherapy Association?
2. Briefly define what a moral is.
3. List the five categories morals are grouped into.
4. What is the difference between a moral and a moral norm?
5. Briefly define ethics.
6. What are the four main areas of concentration ethics are concerned with in health care?
7. Medical ethics involves rules that are ________, rather than __________.
8. __________ deals with a health care provider failing to give the care expected or required.
9. Not reporting illegal or dishonest acts may be considered __________ __________ __________ the crime.
10. What is always required when restraints are applied to a patient for his or her safety?
11. A medical code of ethics __________ the patient by prohibiting discussion of personal matters related to him or her.
12. A patient's __________ is a document which states what a patient has the right to expect during his or her medical treatment.
13. Briefly define the Good Samaritan Law.
14. __________ pertains to any attack on a person's reputation.

    a. ethics
    b. negligence
    c. defamation

15. __________ pertains to any member of the health care delivery system failing to perform or to do something for a patient that another person of the same training and position would do under the same or ordinary circumstances.
    a. negligence
    b. defamation
    c. malpractice

16. __________ pertains to any care provided to a patient which is below an expected standard and which can result in injury.
    a. negligence
    b. defamation
    c. malpractice
17. Briefly define what is meant by duty of care.
18. When the written word is used to defame someone, it is called __________; when the spoken word is used to defame someone, it is called __________.
19. Give at least two examples of ethical behavior:

    a. ____

    b. ____

4

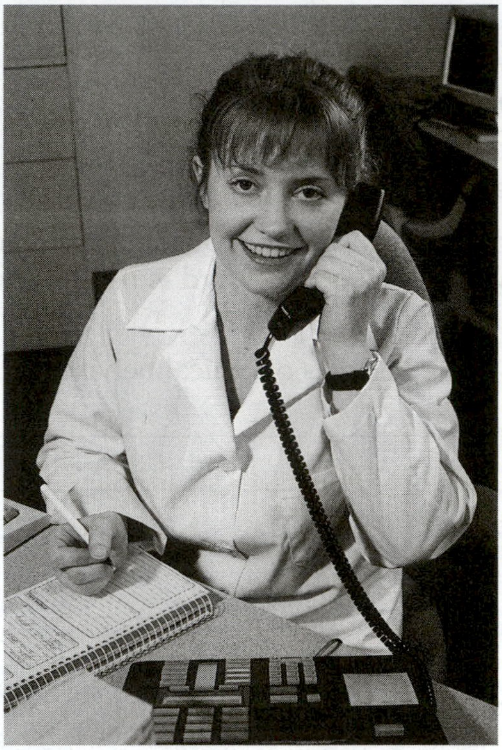

Communicating Effectively

OBJECTIVES

Upon completion of this chapter, you should be able to:

1. Describe how effective communication occurs.
2. Identify the various forms communication takes in the health care environment.
3. List the three components of effective communication.
4. Explain the concept of empathy.
5. Explain the concept of tact.
6. Explain the concept of patience.
7. Differentiate between verbal and nonverbal communication and explain the components of each.
8. Discuss the role communication plays in the physical therapy setting.
9. Discuss the proper use of the telephone.
10. Explain how to properly screen telephone calls.
11. Discuss the importance of proper telephone etiquette.
12. Explain how to use the "hold" button of a telephone.
13. Discuss the importance of proper appointment scheduling and describe the procedures for completing it in the physical therapy setting.

KEY TERMS

Appointment book
Appointment log
Atmosphere
Communication
Diplomacy
Empathy
Environment
Etiquette
Nonverbal communication
Oral communication
Patience
Screening
Tact
Understanding
Verbal communication

Depending upon the facility in which you work, occasionally you may be called upon to complete tasks involving the administrative or clerical duties necessary in caring for patients receiving physical therapy treatments. While the majority of skills you undertake generally take place in the clinical setting, you may also be asked to perform basic administrative tasks such as greeting patients, screening and answering the telephone, and appointment scheduling. Whether you are asked to perform a clinical task or one that requires an administrative skill, you must always remember that at the base of all patient or office-oriented duties is the most basic skill of all—effective communication.

Before we discuss the actual mechanics of effective communication, however, we must first take a look at how communication occurs.

Do you remember the very first time you walked into a room of strangers, yet, for some reason, you felt as though the people gathered there seemed to care about you? Did the warmth and feelings of friendliness from the others radiate to you? As a member of the health care team, the **atmosphere** just described is as much a responsibility of the physical therapy aide as it is all the other members of the team. In order to create an **environment** in which the patient feels at ease and comfortable, in which she feels a genuine sense of interest and understanding, the key ingredient, effective communication, must be achieved.

In health care, communication is based upon interpersonal skills, or interaction among people. It is a way in which we relate to one another, in which we are able to empathize, reassure, and offer comfort in stressful situations. It is also a way in which we are better able to help one another feel good about themselves.

Communication in the health care environment usually takes many forms and it generally involves projecting concern for others through one's tone of voice, words, and actions. Because patients sometimes experience a high degree of stress when they see a doctor or therapist for treatment, words of friendliness, encouragement, and courtesy help put them at ease. Because emotional sensitivity is often higher when a person is sick or incapacitated, it is important that you project a positive attitude, using good manners and respect for others whenever you are called upon to communicate. Always remember to choose your words carefully, use a soothing tone of voice, and above all, display a professional manner. In the following case scenarios, consider how the words and actions demonstrate that the physical therapy aide cares for the patient.

Case Scenario #1:

Good morning, Ms. Smith. May I take your coat? I'll put it in this corner so you won't forget it when you leave."

Important Points:

a) The physical therapy aide makes Ms. Smith feel that her coat is important.
b) The physical therapy aide assumes partial responsibility for remembering the coat, which establishes a "we are in this together" attitude that will carry over to other aspects of the patient's care.

Case Scenario #2:

"Good afternoon Mr. Greene. How are you feeling today? I hope the pain in your knee has disappeared. Oh, it's worse today, swollen and inflamed? I'm sorry to hear that, but the physical therapist will check it carefully."

Important Points:

a) The physical therapy aide through words and tone of voice, tells the patient, "I care about you."
b) The physical therapy aide remembers the patient's problem, which makes the person feel important.
c) The physical therapy aide reassures the patient about the care he will receive.

PARTS OF EFFECTIVE COMMUNICATION

For effective communication to occur, the communicator must consider three important concepts. These include the use of empathy, tact, and patience.

Empathy involves the ability to understand another's feelings and the sensitivity to be able to respond to those feelings. Put more simply, it means being able to put yourself in another's place. An empathetic physical therapy aide is able to understand and offer comfort when dealing with relatives or friends of patients because they are worried. Consider the physical therapy aide's behavior in the following case scenarios. Then ask yourself if you believe the physical therapy aide communicates empathy.

Case Scenario #3:

"Mrs. Gomez, I understand how concerned you are because you think Linda has not responded to the treatment. Sometimes it takes several days for improvement to show."

Important Points:

a) The physical therapy aide tries to reassure the parent.
b) The physical therapy aide does not make any promises about the condition improving quickly.

Case Scenario #4:

"Don't worry, Joanne. If you can't do the exercises today, we'll try again tomorrow."

Important Points:

a) The physical therapy aide sets the patient at ease and does not embarrass her because she can not do the exercises today.

b) The physical therapy aide gives the patient an alternative by indicating that she may do the exercises the next day.

Tact refers to saying or doing the proper thing at the proper time. When a person is tactless, we say that the individual has "put his foot in his mouth." A tactful person is always diplomatic and uses good judgment when working with other people. Most of us would never think of saying to a friend, "Your hair does not look good today," or "That outfit makes you look fat." In a physical therapy office, the situations requiring tact may be less personal but are no less important. The patient who owes money must be tactfully reminded to pay; the patient who disturbs the reception area by talking loudly needs to be asked to speak more quietly.

Most people know the difference between tact and tactlessness and therefore strive to be tactful. Unfortunately, however, physical therapy aides who do not understand the effect of tactless comments and actions may jeopardize their jobs. Consider the following case scenarios. Then ask yourself if you thought the physical therapy aide handled the situation tactfully.

Case Scenario #5:

"Mrs. White, could you ask your son, Ben, to play a little more quietly? I'm concerned that his noise may be bothering some of our other patients. If you like, I will get him some books to read.

The parent makes a defensive comment: "Yes, I know the adults are talking, too, but their conversations aren't very loud. If necessary, I'll ask them to speak more quietly."

Important Points:

a) The physical therapy aide tactfully explains why the child's noise is a problem.

b) The physical therapy aide remains in control while tactfully explaining that other patients will be asked to lower their conversations if necessary.

Case Scenario #6:

"I'll leave the room while you undress, Mr. James. Please remove your slacks and cover yourself from the waist down with this sheet. The physical therapist will be in to check your knee. You may wear your shirt."

Important Points:

a) The physical therapy aide, who is aware of the patient's modesty, leaves the room while he undresses.

b) The physical therapy aide provides the patient with explicit instructions about which clothes should be removed.

c) The physical therapy aide tells the patient the type of examination to expect.

Perhaps no other human relations skill is as important to a physical therapy aide as the third component of effective communication, known as **patience.** Being patient means that you do not become angry or visibly annoyed when a patient blames you for a long wait before an appointment. It also means not being curt when a person asks several times, "How much longer before my treatment?"

Patience often involves waiting—waiting for people to undress or dress, to give you information, or to pay their bill. You may want to hurry them, interrupt their sentences, or speed things up so you can move on to the next task. When you feel yourself becoming impatient, you must maintain your self-control, breathe deeply, smile, and look for realistic ways in which you can remedy the problem. Consider the following case scenario.

Case Scenario #7:

The reception area of the office is crowded because an emergency patient required 20 minutes of the physical therapist's time. Although waiting patients were understanding and gracious about the emergency when it occurred, they are now complaining to one another about the delay, and several have become irritable. One patient asks if he can be placed ahead of others because he has planned to go to a baseball game after his treatment.

"Mr. Adams, I'm sorry you have been delayed, but I know you understand how important it is for the therapist to see emergency patients at once. Only two people remain ahead of you, and they, too, want to leave. Your wait will not be much longer, at most 30 minutes. You may reschedule the appointment if you like."

Important Points:

a) The physical therapy aide recognizes that the patient's point is valid and that the wait has been long.
b) The physical therapy aide tries to give the patient a time frame for any additional wait and offers an alternative to waiting.
c) The physical therapy aide does not place this patient ahead of others.

◆ TYPES OF COMMUNICATION

There are two basic types of communication. They include the use of words that we form into sentences, known as **oral** or **verbal communication,** as messages that do not use spoken words, called **nonverbal communication.** Expressions such as "a look that would kill," "red-faced in anger," or "love written all over her face," are examples of messages delivered without words. It is important to remember that when you work with patients, you must be careful that your verbal and nonverbal communication sends the same message; otherwise, you may confuse, hurt, or offend someone. Consider the following case scenario. Do you think the physical therapy aide's verbal and nonverbal messages agree?

Case Scenario #8:

A physical therapy aide who is engaged in a telephone conversation ignores a patient who stands at the reception desk and waits several minutes. After finishing the call, the physical therapy aide looks at the patient, picks up a medical record, and reviews it while talking to the patient. The physical therapy aide then leaves the room while talking over her shoulder to the patient who remains standing.

"Good morning, Mr. Brown. How are you this morning. As you feeling better? I'll be right back."

Oral Communication

Oral communication, as we already stated, refers to oral messages and includes face-to-face encounters, announcements, questions, off-hand remarks, telephone conversations, gossip, and other forms of communication. Successful communication depends on correct word choices and on the listener's understanding of what is being said.

There are many factors that influence the communication process and affect understanding between communicators. These include one's level of education, economic status, prior experiences, and cultural heritage. Since there is no absolute universal meaning for words existing in the minds of people, each defines words based upon his or her own influencing factors. The greater the difference in one's background, the more difficulty he or she may encounter in understanding another person.

An area in which many health care professionals get into trouble involves using medical or technical terms beyond the scope of the patient's understanding or background. Some people use technical words to impress the listener or to prove their superior knowledge. New employees or recent graduates often feel important by using big words to show how smart they are. If you are confident in your education, you will recognize that use of medical words does not necessarily demonstrate knowledge, and you should not display a wide vocabulary at the expense of another's understanding or comfort. Consider the following case scenario.

Case Scenario #9:

"Mrs. White, here is a pamphlet on living with low back pain that the physical therapist asked me to give to you. It will help you to understand your illness. You will notice from the pamphlet that weakness of the leg muscles is an early symptom."

This physical therapy aide knows that the patient will not understand medical language and use laymen's language to discuss the medical condition. A less informed physical therapy aide might have communicated in the following manner:

"Mrs. White, here is a pamphlet on rheumatoid arthritis of the lumbosacral region that the physical therapist asked me to give to you. The etiology of this disease is unknown, however, the pamphlet will help you to understand your illness. You will notice from the pamphlet that the atrophy of the leg muscles is an early symptom."

Nonverbal Communication

Nonverbal communication, as we have already discussed, refers to messages sent without words or in addition to words. It includes facial expressions, touch, tone of voice, listening, eye contact, gestures, appearance, manner, time, body language, silence, and other nonverbal behavior. Every individual person sends and receives hundreds of nonverbal messages daily. They enhance the communication process and should be used by both the sender and the receiver in order to confirm verbal messages.

Nonverbal communication is important to any relationship, and this is especially true with people who are sick, uncomfortable, or anxious. When we hear the statement, "What is not said may be more important than what is said," we should understand that this makes reference to the significance to nonverbal behavior. As a physical therapy aide, your competence in using and interpreting nonverbal behavior will oftentimes determine the degree of success you enjoy in your relationship with others.

◆ COMMUNICATION IN THE PHYSICAL THERAPY SETTING

Now that we have spent some time discussing the components of communication and how the process of effective communication occurs, let's talk about how and when communication occurs in the physical therapy setting.

Using the Telephone

In any clinical or administrative setting, the telephone is generally considered the most important line of public relations. Because you create an impression each and every time you talk on the telephone, it is extremely important that the techniques you use are correct.

Proper use of the telephone usually depends upon many different skills, since the impression you create on it, for the most part, tends to influence a patient or any other caller, it is most important that you always remember to be tactful, diplomatic, courteous, professional, and firm, but flexible. You should also be capable of making decisions, as well as willing to accept responsibility for making those decisions.

In addition to developing such essential skills as using a correct tone of voice, being pleasant, clear and distinct, and using correct grammar, there are very specific abilities you must acquire that are necessary for proper telephone techniques.

To begin with, you should always answer the telephone promptly. In addition, try to answer with a smile. This helps the caller to feel secure in your response, as well as helping you to create a pleasant voice. Even though the caller may not be able to see this gesture, he or she will be able to detect it in your voice.

Another important skill necessary in correct telephone usage is identifying both yourself and the office or department in which you are working. And never use slang when you answer the telephone. A "Good morning, this is Ms. Jones," or "Dr. Smith's office, can I help you," generally goes a lot farther than being rude or short with the caller (Figure 4-1).

Whenever you are talking on the telephone, it is also important to keep the receiver firmly against your ear and put the mouthpiece approximately one inch away from the center of your lips. This usually helps the caller receive the best transmission of your voice.

Screening Telephone Calls

In some hospitals or physical therapy agencies, you may be responsible for **screening** telephone calls. This has to do with determining which calls should be transferred to the physical therapist or the appropriate person and which can be handled by you or another worker in the department. You will find that most departments or agencies have their own or policy regarding the screening of telephone calls. Refer to Procedures 1 and 2.

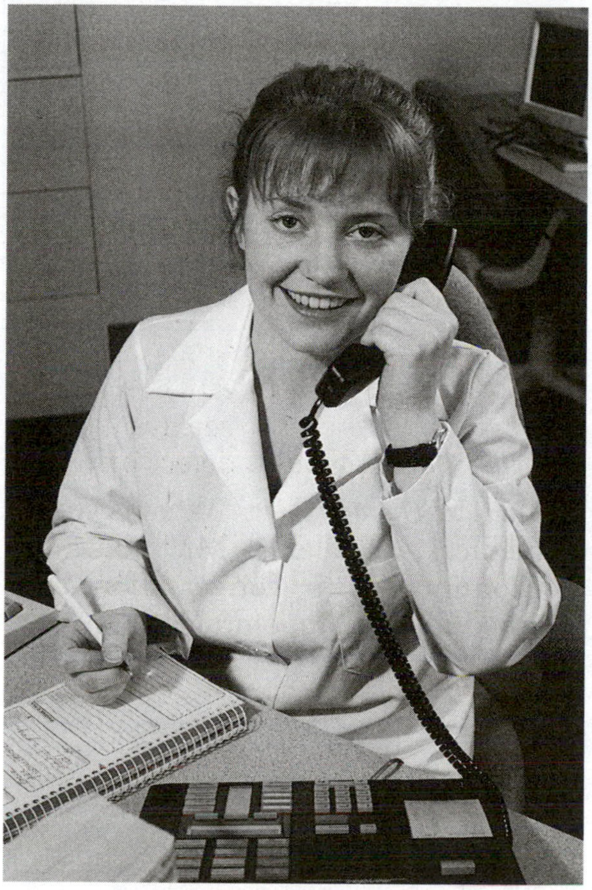

Figure 4-1 A smile conveys a positive attitude.

In order to properly screen calls, it is important for you to determine the purpose of the call. Many patients simply ask to talk with a particular person. By asking the caller, "May I help you?" or "May I tell Ms. Smith why you are calling?" generally helps in determining the nature of the call.

Screening telephone calls may also involve evaluating emergency situations and then dealing with them appropriately. In some cases, for example, a patient may be upset even though there is no real emergency. By asking pertinent questions and remaining calm, you may be able to determine what is a real emergency and what is not. Most emergencies are referred to the appropriate person if she is available. If that individual is not available, you should obtain important information regarding the nature of the call, so that you can help the caller obtain help from the correct source. In most cases, hospitals and medical facilities usually have a procedure to follow for emergency situations that might occur when an appropriate person is not available.

PROCEDURE #1: Using the Telephone

1. Assemble your equipment. This includes a telephone message pad, a pen or pencil, and a telephone setup.
2. Answer the telephone promptly and with a "smile."
3. Identify yourself and the facility to the caller.
4. Ask the caller his or her name and the purpose of the call.
5. Watch your tone of voice, manners, grammar, and responses.
6. Deal with the call or refer it to the appropriate person.
7. Close the conversation with saying "Thank you for calling."
8. Gently replace the receiver in its cradle.
9. Immediately record the message, noting the time and date of the call, the caller's name, a brief message and your initials.

PROCEDURE #2: Screening Calls

When required to screen telephone calls, consider the following procedure:

1. Ask the person's name and the reason for the call.
2. Ask questions that clarify the reason for the call.
3. Handle the call personally if you can.
4. Transfer the call to another staff member when appropriate.
5. Get details for a callback message if the physical therapist should return the call.

Typical Telephone Screening Situations

When screening incoming telephone calls, consider the following scenarios. At the completion of each scenario, ask yourself, as the person answering the call, would you have responded in the same or similar manner.

Case Scenario #10: Incoming Call to Make an Appointment

Physical Therapy Aide: "Valley Physical Therapy Center. May I help you?

Caller: "I'd like to talk to the head physical therapist."

Physical Therapy Aide: "I'm sorry, the head therapist, Ms. Smith, is with a patient at the moment. May I ask who is calling?"

Caller: "This is John Jones."

Physical Therapy Aide: "Are you a patient of Ms. Smith's?"

Caller: "Yes."

Physical Therapy Aide: "Would you like to make an appointment with Ms. Smith?"

Caller: "Yes, I would.

Physical Therapy Aide: "What is your medical problem, Mr. Jones?" (Continue with conversation by scheduling an appointment.)

Case Scenario #11: Incoming Call for Billing and Insurance

Physical Therapy Aide: "Ms. Jones office. May I help you?"

Caller: "This is Jose Garcia with AAA Insurance Company. I would like information about the charges for your patient, Robert Brown."

Physical Therapy Aide: "Mr. Garcia, I will transfer your call to Ms. Short, who is in charge of insurance payments for our office."

Case Scenario #12: Incoming Call for "Personal" Business

Physical Therapy Aide: "Good morning, physical therapy department.

May I help you?"

Caller: "Mr. Black, please."

Physical Therapy Aide: "I'm sorry, Mr. Black is with a patient. May I ask who is calling?"

Caller: "This is a personal call. I'm a friend of his."

Physical Therapy Aide: "Mr. Black usually returns his calls just before lunch. If you leave your name and number, I will ask him to return your call."

Caller: "It's Jane Good at (818) 555-1234."

Telephone Etiquette

It is always important to use discretion and **etiquette** whenever you are required to use the telephone. You would never say "The physical therapist is out to breakfast," or "The therapist isn't in yet and I don't know when she'll be in." Statements such as "The therapist is not available at present," or "I expect Ms. Smith to return at 4:30 p.m., may I take a message?" are more appropriate.

Whenever you are about to end a telephone conversation, it is always appropriate to close with "Thank you for calling," and then say good-bye. This should be followed by your gently replacing the receiver in the telephone cradle and, if possible, allowing the caller to hang up first.

If your facility requires that messages be taken for persons not available, you should always make sure that the message is taken accurately and that the time and date of the call is recorded appropriately. Telephone messages should always contain the name of the caller; his or her telephone number, with the area code; a brief summary of the reason for the call; the action taken, if any; and the initials of the person taking the call. Remember too, that it is important to always keep a memo pad and a pen or pencil close to the telephone in order to record messages. If a copy of the telephone call is necessary for the patient's record, you may also use carbon paper and a ballpoint pen in order to record the information. Refer to Procedure 3.

Dealing with Problem Calls

Problem calls may occur in any health agency. Some people may refuse to give their name or discuss the purpose of their call. At times, they may even try to intimidate you or make threats toward you or your coworkers. Always try to remain calm and control your temper and attitude, and never hesitate to tell the caller that the person he or she is asking for is unable to answer the telephone. While it may be difficult, try to remain polite yet firm in dealing with this type of situation. If a patient does give his or her name but refuses to state the purpose of the call, remember that this type of situation also requires tact. If ever in doubt, you can always put the patient on "hold" and check with the individual the caller wants. It is then up to that person whether or not to take the call.

Putting the Caller on Hold

The term holding refers to the telephone's capability of keeping a call waiting on one line while a second call is on another line. The two callers do not hear one another's conversations. When a call is placed on hold, the telephone line is blocked, making the line unavailable to incoming and outgoing calls. Asking a person to hold is necessary at times, however, the hold function can be

PROCEDURE #3: Taking Callback Messages

Since physical therapists do not routinely answer telephone calls, you will generally be required to take callback messages. To take such a message, consider the following procedure:

1. Write the date and time of the call.
2. Write the name of the person called.
3. Ask the caller's name and telephone number.
4. Ask whether the caller will telephone again.
5. Write down the complete message.

Always remember to ask for specifics if the message is unclear. Complete the task by adding your initials as the person who took the call (Figure 4-2).

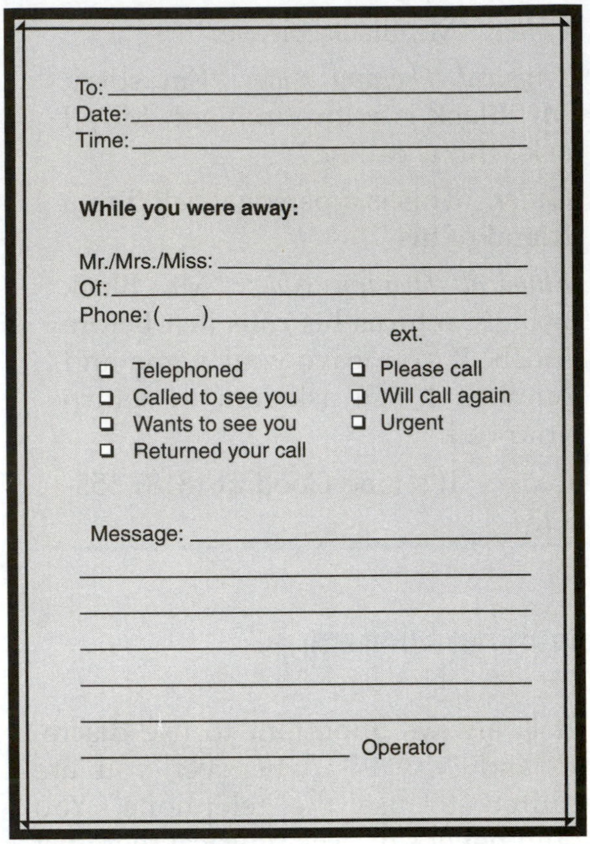
To: ______
Date: ______
Time: ______

While you were away:

Mr./Mrs./Miss: ______
Of: ______
Phone: (__) ______ ext.

- ❑ Telephoned
- ❑ Called to see you
- ❑ Wants to see you
- ❑ Returned your call
- ❑ Please call
- ❑ Will call again
- ❑ Urgent

Message: ______

______ Operator

Figure 4-2 An example of a telephone message pad.

abused if it is used too frequently or if callers are kept waiting too long. You should use the "hold" function when the person being called cannot come to the telephone immediately or when the person answering the telephone is busy with another call.

If you find that you have to put the caller on hold or if you know there will be a slight delay before the appropriate person answers the call, always make sure you inform the caller of this fact. Never leave a caller on hold for long periods of time, and if there is a delay, offer to take the caller's number and have the individual return the call.

◆ APPOINTMENT SCHEDULING

Another important administrative task that you might be responsible for completing and that generally goes along with using the telephone has to do with scheduling appointments for patients who are to receive physical therapy treatments. Such appointments may either be for treatments that the patient will receive at the bedside, if he is confined to the hospital, or may be for outpatient visits, either in the physical therapy department of the facility or in a private physical therapy office or center.

The most important point to remember

when scheduling appointments is that efficient operation of the department or office depends on the correct scheduling of appointments, an activity that requires clear thinking and good judgment. Whether appointments are scheduled by hand in a daybook or with the help of a computer using scheduling software, the entire staff depends on a smooth flow of patient traffic in order to maintain a workable schedule. Appointments must be made so that they allow sufficient time for each patient's treatment, yet without wasteful time gaps. Refer to Procedure 4.

Generally speaking, one of the most frequent complaints heard from patients who are required to come into the department or the office has to do with them having to spend a great deal of time sitting in a waiting room before they are scheduled for their treatment. In order to avoid this as much as possible, a carefully planned **appointment book** can be used.

Appointment books vary from facility to facility (Figure 4-3). However, most of them contain one-half page for each day. Time is usually blocked off in quarter hour periods in order to ensure that all time can be used wisely. Try to become familiar with the type of book or **appointment log** your facility uses, and get to know what block of time each line represents.

Since you will always want to make sure that appointments are not scheduled with individuals who are not available, try to take an organized approach to appointment scheduling. Before scheduling any appointments, make sure you block out periods of time when the individual is not available. Such time may include lunch, meetings, or even afternoons in which the person may be off or out of the office. The easiest way to block out the period of time is to place a big "X" through those times so that no errors of scheduling can occur.

Another important point to using the appointment book is to always make the appointments in pencil. In this way, if an appointment must be canceled, names can be erased and the time can be rescheduled for another patient. Since

PROCEDURE #4: Scheduling an Appointment

If required to schedule appointments, the following procedure should be considered:

1. Assemble your equipment. This includes the appointment book and a pen or pencil.
2. Check the appointment book or log and note how much time each line represents.
3. Place the day of the week and date on the top of each of the daily columns.
4. Block off those periods of time when the person for whom the appointments are being scheduled will not be in. Cross through the block with a large "X."
5. Schedule the appointment in the correct time slot. Include the patient's correct name, his or her physician's name, and the telephone number. Include the reason for the appointment.
6. Double-check your entry.

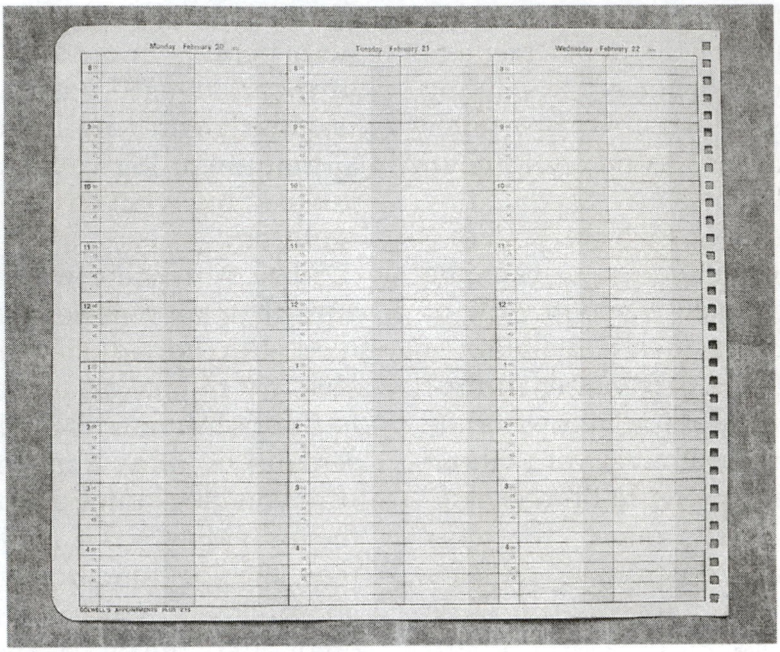

Figure 4-3 A sample appointment book.

not all facilities may follow this policy, you should always follow your individual facility's procedure for this particular practice.

When you are required to schedule appointments for patients, you should also have a pretty good understanding of how long specific therapies might take. If, for example, you know a patient is coming in for an ultrasound of the lower back, followed by hot packs to the area, you should check with the therapist or the posted schedule, if one exists, about how long such a procedure takes prior to making the appointment. If you discover that this procedure takes approximately forty-five minutes to an hour, you would not want to schedule another patient during that time.

Even though most facilities or physical therapy departments generally have a posted schedule that indicates which patients are coming in for specific therapies, always try to get the patient to tell you why he is coming in. By doing this, you can double-check your schedule and if necessary, make any corrections to the appointment book prior to the patient's coming in. In order to do this, however, you should also make sure that when the patient calls you get her telephone number, which is then written in pencil next to her name under the scheduled appointment time.

Since appointment scheduling on the telephone with the patient is more often done in a private physical therapy facility than in a hospital physical therapy department, when the patient does call for an appointment, you should make sure that you have the necessary information before closing your conversation. This includes obtaining the patient's full name, as well as the name of the physician ordering the treatment; the reasoning for coming into the office, that is, what type of treatment is to be given; and the patient's telephone number. As we have already discussed, by securing the patient's telephone number and putting it directly into the appointment book, it may save time, later, if the patient's appointment has to be canceled or rescheduled.

After you have obtained all the required information from the patient, make sure you repeat the date, day of the week, and the exact time of the appointment. By repeating both the date and day of the week, you provide the patient with a double check and thereby prevent needless errors in the long run. Once you have completed your conversation with the patient, make sure that you mark the full amount of time in the appointment book.

If a patient calls to cancel an appointment, always try to be polite and understanding. Ask the patient if he or she would like to reschedule the appointment. Since the original appointment was written in pencil, you may then erase it and record al the new information in the correct day and block of time.

Chronic problems of rescheduling generally occur in all health care agencies. If a specific patient becomes a chronic offender, there are several methods of dealing with the problem. One method involves scheduling this patient at the end of the day. If he does not appear, this will not affect other patients or schedules as much. Some offices send bills for time scheduled. In these facilities, patients must be told in advance that if they cannot keep the appointment, they must notify the office within a specified period of time, usually twenty-four hours prior to their appointment, or they will be charged for the missed appointment. Some departments or private offices, also note broken appointments as "no shows" on the patient's chart. Usually, the final decision as to how to deal with these situations rests upon the individual in charge.

The proper scheduling of appointments takes time and practice. If you find that your position requires that you schedule appointments, always make sure that you review your facility's individual policy regarding their system, and once reviewed, make sure you follow the facility's method appropriately.

◆ SUMMARY

In this chapter, we discussed how to communicate effectively. We talked about the parts of effective communication, as well as the roles empathy, tactfulness, and patience play in our everyday communication with others. We talked about the two types of communication; verbal and nonverbal. Finally, we discussed the importance of effective communication in the physical therapy setting, including proper use of the telephone and appointment scheduling techniques.

◆ ◆ LEARNING ACTIVITY 4-1

Read the narrative, then write answers to the numbered questions. You should try to find answers at the health care facility, from classroom information, or from independent research.

Narrative

Mrs. White is talking with Jeff and Liz as they take a break. "Now Jeff, I know you've learned how to complete a job application and a resume, and how to write a letter of resignation, but there is another important area to discuss, and that's how to get along on the job after you're hired." Jeff says, "I hadn't thought of that, but I guess you're right. I know that I must get along well with my supervisor and with my coworkers.

(1) Who else should I be concerned about in a health care facility?

Jeff thinks for a minute and says,

(2) "How can I get along with a patient who is ill, worried, perhaps in pain, and expect him to be concerned about getting along with me?"

Liz says, "I think I can get along with patients and families, but what worries me is how to get along with coworkers. They've been so nice to me here, but in another hospital I suspect they'll be less helpful."

(3) What are some ways to help get along with your coworkers?

Then Jeff says,

(4) "What are some other ways in which I can ensure that I will not lose my new job?"

A new job does sound pretty scary, but being aware of ways to get along on the job and with other employees will make it easier.

◆ ◆ LEARNING ACTIVITY 4-2

Read the narrative, then write answers to the numbered questions. You should try to find answers at the health care facility, from classroom information, or from independent research.

Narrative
Rob and Robyn are now observing in the outpatient clinic at Riverside Hospital. Here patients from the community come for treatment and return home. But some are admitted to the hospital if they need more care. Rob says to Robyn, "Many of these patients are indigent."
(1) What does "indigent" mean?

Robyn replies, "Indigent means very poor, but notice that even though most of these patients cannot pay the entire cost of their medical care, the personnel treat them with the same respect and courtesy as the paying patients in the hospital. Do you remember that Ms. Marlo reminded us that in patient care, all patients should be treated the same. Economic status, race, or social status should make no difference."

As they are standing in the clinic, an elderly woman comes up to Robyn and asks, "Do you remember when I was here last Thursday? The doctor gave me some red medicine and it did make me feel a lot better, but I can't remember what it was. Will you look on my chart and tell the doctor what it was so I can get some more?" Robyn is surprised, then she remembers—of course, she has on a uniform and the patient assumes that she must know all about everything in the clinic. She tells the patient, "Wait here just a minute and I'll find someone to help you."
(2) Why didn't Robyn try to help the patient herself?

Rob then says, "If some of these patients are unable to pay for medical services, where does the money come from to maintain the clinic?" Robyn has just asked Ms. Marlo the same question, so she is ready with an answer. "There are city, county, state, and federal programs paid for with tax dollars that help pay for those who cannot afford it. Also, there are many civic organizations and foundations that pay for specific kinds of care." Mrs. Kelly, the charge nurse for the clinic, comes over just in time to hear the conversation and says, "And we couldn't get along without our volunteers who work here. These dedicated people spend many hours without pay, doing tasks that are time-consuming but that do not require actual medical expertise."

Then Mrs. Kelly says, "Let's go to the treatment room where they are caring for a patient who is receiving an ultrasound treatment for his low back pain. Rob follows her, but before he gets there he can hear the patient talking a little wildly and incoherently. He is a white male, about forty-five years old, dressed in dirty clothes, and obviously without a bath or a haircut for a long, long time. Dr. Osgood sees Rob and says, "Here's a person who mixed his drugs and may never be the same again. I don't share his values, but I sure hope we can help him to get rid of his back pain."

(3) What is meant by "values?"

Next, Mrs. Kelly takes Rob and Robyn to another part of the clinic. On the way they overhear two aides talking about the orderly. "I just can't stand him, he thinks he's so smart!" The other replies, "But he does his work well, and you can certainly depend on him to be where he's needed. Maybe we could find a way to let him know we would get along with him better if he wouldn't be so condescending to us."

(4) How could these aides approach this problem?

◆ ◆ LEARNING ACTIVITY 4-3

Read the narrative, then write the answers to the numbered questions. You should try to find answers at the health care facility, from classroom information, or from independent research.

Narrative:

Keesha and James have been observing in the Business Office of the physical therapy department for the past two days, and among other things, Ms. Collins, the business manager, is showing them the various kinds of communication equipment used in the hospital. She reminds them that communication has become complicated because there are so many sophisticated methods of sending and receiving messages. She says, "Let's tour the hospital and see how many types of communicating devices we can find. Then we'll come back here and talk about the patient's chart as a means of communicating."

James and Keesha are happy to move around. For the past two days, they've been learning about charts and how they are used. First they go to 12A, a postoperative unit. Most of the patients here are recovering satisfactorily. They each have a pillow speaker.

(1) How is a pillow speaker used for communication?

They find Janet Greene, a quadriplegic, in the next unit. She is able to move only her head, but her pillow speaker is modified so that she can activate it just by deep breathing. In the next room, where Jon Smith is in a cast from the shoulders down, the pillow speaker is modified so that it is activated when Jon rolls his head against it. All of these modifications give patients a feeling of some independence and control.

As they walk down the hall, Keesha and James hear an intercom system calling Dr. Jonas.

(2) What is an intercom system?

(3) Give an example of a situation in which everyone in the hospital should be contacted.

James and Keesha had no idea there were so many different ways to contact persons in the hospital. But Mrs. Collins says, "And we haven't even been to ICU and CCU yet. But while we're here, notice that in the bathroom there is a call button placed where the patient can easily reach it."

(4) Why is it necessary to have a call button in each bathroom?

James says, "Surely patients feel more confident knowing that someone is tending them all the time, but what are all these computer screens and printers used for?" Mrs. Collins answers, "We just couldn't get along without our data processing system."

(5) Name any information that is transmitted by data processing.

Keesha continues, "Now I see why data processing is used so extensively in the business office." "You're right," says Mrs. Collins. "Whenever a patient comes into the PT department for a treatment, their chart comes right along with them. When the patient is discharged, the chart then goes to the hospital record room, where it is kept for a period of five years. Those charts you have seen at the charge desk are sent to our record library where they are eventually stored on microfiche. But the information on the charts can easily be called up on the computer for study and discussion. Charts are one of our most valuable forms of communication." James asks,

(6) "How can a record be considered a form of communication?"

Then James says, "Is it a form of communication when people wear their individual beepers?" "Of course," replies Mrs. Collins. "They are just one more way to send and receive messages. The little individual beepers you are talking about are commonly used when a person who moves about a lot and in an unpredictable pattern needs to be able to communicate with some other particular place. For example, if a doctor needs to keep in touch with his or her office, or the engineer with the engine room, a beeper is very efficient. They can "answer" the beeper by telephoning the switchboard. The operator will know whom they should contact for their messages."

James asks, "What about the callboard down by the switchboard? Who uses that?"

(7) What is a callboard?

"So we've mentioned several means of communication used in most health care facilities," says Mrs. Collins.

(8) "Can you think of any other besides yelling to each other?"

REVIEW QUESTIONS

1. Define oral and nonverbal communication and explain why each is valuable.
2. Why do you think a physical therapy aide should choose his words carefully when interacting with patients?
3. Define empathy and explain how it differs from sympathy.
4. Define tactfulness.
5. Define patience.
6. Explain the circumstances in which putting a caller on hold would be acceptable.
7. Briefly explain the procedures for screening telephone calls.
8. List at lease five pieces of information needed for a callback message:
   a. ______________________________
   b. ______________________________
   c. ______________________________
   d. ______________________________
   e. ______________________________
9. Explain how you handle the following calls:
   a. A patient asks to speak to the bookkeeper who is on another line.
   b. Another physical therapy aide, who is busy, receives a personal call.
   c. A patient asks to talk with the physical therapist.
10. What would you do if the following situations occurred during regular office hours?
    a. A patient who has an 11:00 A.M. appointment does not appear.
    b. The physical therapist is behind schedule by forty-five minutes.

5

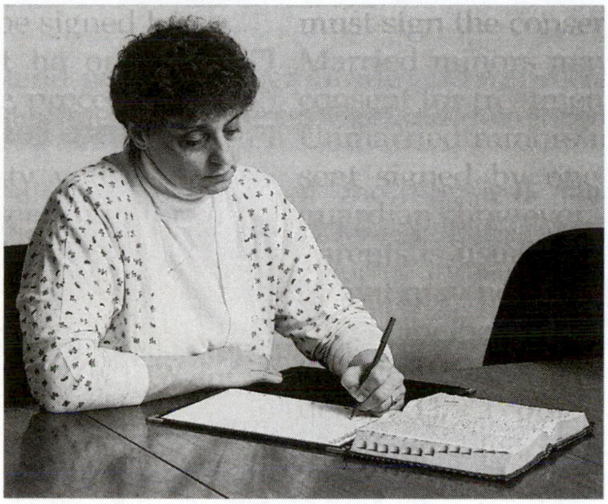

Medical Terminology and the Medical Record

OBJECTIVES

Upon completion of this chapter, you should be able to:

1. Identify specific prefixes, suffixes, and root words related to medical terms.
2. List common medical abbreviations used in the health care environment.
3. Identify body structure terms related to positions, directions, anatomical planes, posture, and types of movement.
4. Explain the importance and uses of the medical record.
5. Distinguish between subjective, objective, assessment, and plan information on a patient's medical record.

KEY TERMS

Prefix
Root word
SOAP notes
Suffix

PREFIXES, SUFFIXES, AND ROOT WORDS

The discussion of medical terminology will help you to understand the many terms commonly used in medicine and in your individual department. The prefixes and suffixes of many medical terms give definite information about the meaning of the term. If you know these prefixes and suffixes, it will be a lot easier to understand many medical words. A **prefix** is a word fragment placed in front of the basic or root word (Table 5-1). A **suffix** is a word fragment added at the end of the basic or root word (Table 5-2). The **root word** is the main body of the word, that is, the part that usually gives the meaning to the word (Table 5-3).

There are no specific rules governing the pronunciation of medical terms. A medical dictionary will give you some suggestions as to the pronunciation of words, however, in many hospitals and medical facilities, these pronunciations will vary among professionals and individual departments.

PREFIX	MEANING	WORD EXAMPLE	MEANING OF EXAMPLE
a-, an-	without	apnea	without breath
ab-	away from	abnormal	away from the rule
		abduct	away from the midline of the body
ad-	toward	adduct	toward the midline of the body
albus-	white	albinuria	white or colorless urine
ambi-	both	ambidextrous	uses both hands with equal ease
anti-	against	antisepsis	preventing growth of bacteria
bi-	two; both	bilateral	pertaining to two sides of the body
circum-	around	circumrenal	around the kidneys
cyano-	blue	cyanosis	bluish skin color due to lack of oxygen
endo-	in; within	endocardium	inside layer of the heart
epi-	upon; over	epidermis	outside layer of the skin
erythro-	red	erythrocyte	red blood cell
ex-, exo-	out; away	extension	movement widening angle between two adjoining parts
glyco-	sweet; sugar	glycosuria	sugar in the urine
hyper-	above; excessive	hypertension	abnormally high blood pressure
hypo-	below	hypotension	abnormally low blood pressure
inter-	between	intervertebral disc	cartilage found between most vertebral bones
leuko-	white	leukocyte	white blood cell
lith-	stone	lithotomy	removal of a stone
nephro-	kidney	nephrology	study of the kidney

Table 5-1 Common Prefixes and Their Meanings

SUFFIX	MEANING	WORD EXAMPLE	MEANING OF EXAMPLE
-algia	pain	neuralgia	pain along course of a nerve
-ectomy	cutting out	thyroidectomy	surgical removal of the thyroid
-iasis	condition of	lithiasis	formation of a stone
-itis	inflammation	endocarditis	inflammation of the endocardium
-logy	study of	cardiology	study of the heart
-pathy	disease	osteopathy	disease of the bone
-phobia	fear	hydrophobia	fear of water
-plasty	repair	rhinoplasty	surgical correction of the nose

Table 5-2 Common Suffixes and Their Meanings

◆ USING MEDICAL ABBREVIATIONS

Many abbreviations for words and phrases are used in the treatment of patients to save time and space. As a member of the physical medicine team, you must learn these abbreviations so that you can follow directions and communicate with other health care workers (Table 5-4). Since the physical medicine profession has adopted many abbreviations that are commonly used by health care professionals in writing their notes in the patient's medical record, it is very important that you study and learn these common abbreviations so that you will be able to easily recognize their meanings.

◆ BODY STRUCTURE AND MEDICAL TERMINOLOGY

The human body may be compared to a smooth-running machine. It has many parts that must work together in order to promote good health, growth, and life itself. The body is a combination of organs and systems, which are supported and protected by a framework of bones known as the skeleton. The muscles working upon the skeleton provide for the movements as we work and play each day. All of this is then protected by an external covering known as the skin, which is considered the largest of all our body organs. You will need to know the various parts of the body and how to describe them in medical terms.

ROOT	MEANING	WORD EXAMPLE	MEANING OF EXAMPLE
cardia	heart	carditis	inflammation of the heart
costa	rib	costalgia	pain in a rib
gastro	stomach	gastroenteritis	inflammation of the stomach
neuro	nerve	neuralgia	pain along a nerve
oto	ear	otitis	inflammation of the ear
pedi	foot	pedicure	care of the feet
phlebo	vein	phlebitis	inflammation of a vein
pneumo	lung	pneumonectomy	surgical removal of a lung

Table 5-3 Common Root Words and Their Meanings

COMMONLY USED ABBREVIATIONS	MEANING
aa	of each
ad lib	as desired
AIDS	acquired immune deficiency syndrome
amt.	amount
ASHD	arteriosclerotic heart disease
ax	axillary
BM	bowel movement
BP	blood pressure
BRP	bathroom privilege
c	with
C	Celsius (Centigrade)
Cal	calorie
cc	cubic centimeter
CHF	congestive heart failure
cm	centimeter
CO	coronary occlusion
CNS	central nervous system
CPR	cardiopulmonary resuscitation
CVA	cerebrovascular accident (stroke)
DC	discontinue; discharge
DOA	dead on arrival
Dx	diagnosis
EKG	electrocardiogram
elix	elixir
F	Fahrenheit
Fx	Fracture
gm (GM)	gram
gtt	drops
hema	blood
hemi	half
H&P	history and physical
Ht.	height
Kg	kilogram
L	liter
m	minim
MI	myocardial infarction (heart attack)
ml	milliliter
NG	nasogastric
NPO	nothing by mouth (nil per os)
O.D.	right eye
O.S.	left eye
O.U.	both eyes
O2	oxygen
OOB	out of bed
oz	ounce
P	pulse
PID	pelvic inflammatory disease
PM	afternoon
Post-op	after surgery
Pre-op	before surgery
Pt.	patient
PO	by mouth (per os)
P.R.N.	whenever necessary, or as needed
QNS	quantity not sufficient
QS	quantity sufficient
R	respiration
Rx	prescription (recipe)
Semi	half
Sig	write (let it be labeled)
SOB	shortness of breath
S.O.S.	if necessary
SSE	soapsuds enema
ss	half
STD	sexually transmitted disease
Stat	immediately
T	temperature
T.O.	telephone order
TPR	temperature, pulse, respiration
tr	tincture
ung.	ointment
URI	upper respiratory infection
V.O.	verbal order
wt.	weight
>	greater than
<	less than
♀	female; woman
♂	male; man
S	without

ABBREVIATIONS RELATED TO TIME	MEANING
a.c.	before meals
A.M.	morning
b.i.d.	twice a day
h	hour
h.n.	tonight
h.s.	bedtime; hour of sleep
noct.	night
p.c.	after meals
q.d.	every day
q.h.	every hour
q.2h	every 2 hours
q.i.d.	four times a day
q.o.d.	every other day
t.i.d.	three times a day
t.i.n.	three times a night

Table 5-4 Common Medical Abbreviations and Their Meanings

DEPARTMENT ABBREVIATIONS	MEANING
CCU	Coronary Care Unit
CS; CSR	Central Supply; Central Supply Room
EENT	Eye, Ear, Nose, and Throat
ER	Emergency Room
GI	Gastrointestinal Department
GYN	Gynecology Department
ICU	Intensive Care Unit
LAB	Laboratory
MICU	Medical Intensive Care Unit
NICU	Neonatal Intensive Care Unit
OB	Obstetrics
OR	Operating Room
PEDI	Pediatrics
P.T.	Physical Therapy
R.T.	Respiratory Therapy
X-Ray	Radiology

Table 5-4 Common Medical Abbreviations and Their Meanings (Continued)

The human body is divided into five specific *cavities* or compartments: thoracic, abdominal, pelvic, cranial, and spinal (Figure 5-1). Within the thoracic cavity are the lungs, heart aorta, and the thymus gland. The brain lies within the cranial cavity, while the spine is located within the spinal cavity. The abdominal cavity contains the stomach, liver, gallbladder, small intestine, colon—or large intestine—spleen, and the pancreas. The reproductive organs and the urinary bladder are all located within the pelvic cavity. Various structural units make up the body. Cells, tissues, and organs are organized into individual systems. These systems include the skeletal, muscular, nervous, circulatory, digestive, respiratory, urinary, reproductive, and endocrine.

◆ ANATOMICAL POSITION

Many terms are used t describe the body and to identify the position, direction, and location of the parts of the body. In addition, these terms are also used to describe various medical characteristics of the body, such as the location of incisions or injuries on the body. In order for the health care professional to be able to read the patient's medical record and thus have a mental picture of the patient's condition, all descriptive terms are based on an accepted standard position. This standard is known as the *anatomical position* (Figure 5-2). In this position, the person is standing erect, facing forward, with the head and trunk aligned, the arms straight by the sides with palms facing

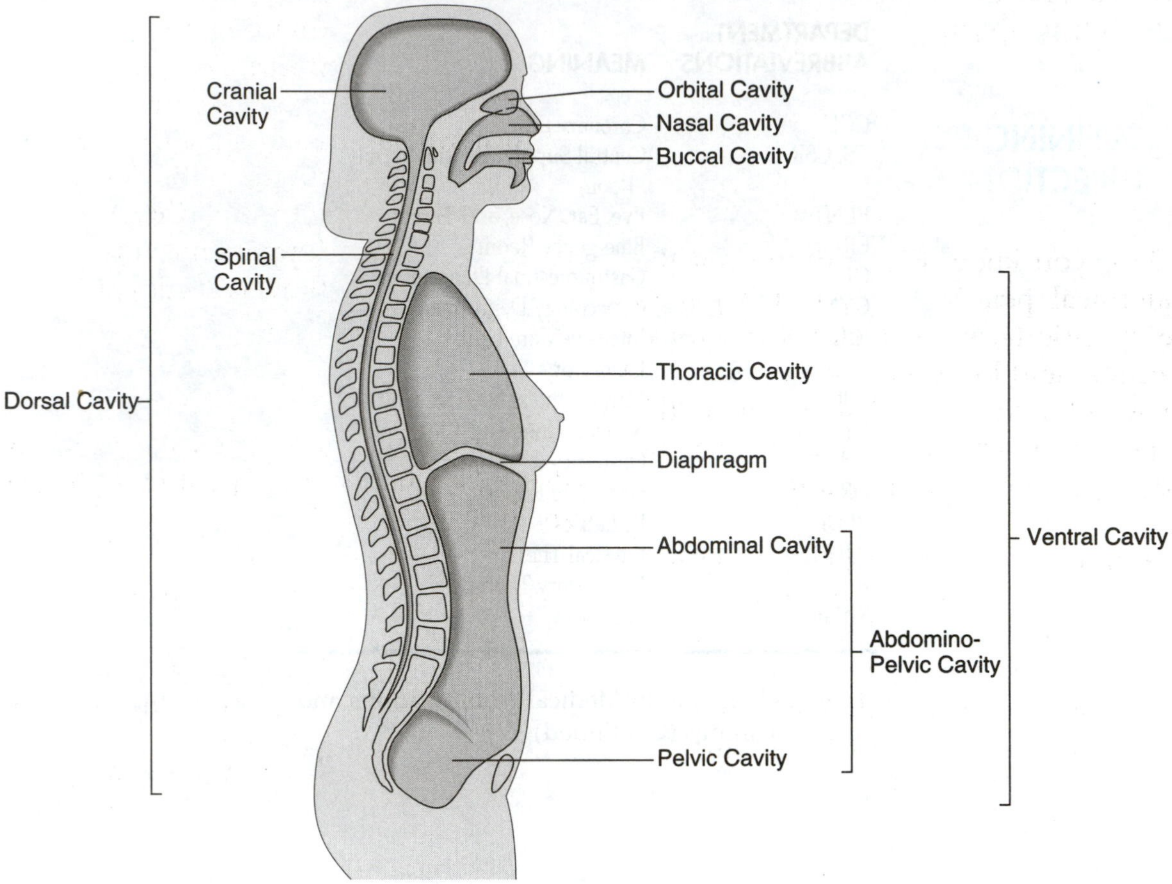

Figure 5-1 Lateral view of body cavities.

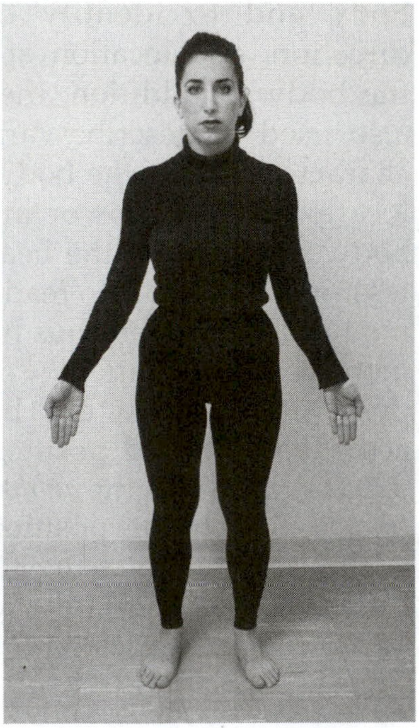

Figure 5-2 In the anatomic position, the person is standing, facing forward, with palms forward.

forward, and the legs straight with the feet slightly apart.

◆ DEFINING POSITION AND DIRECTION

Once you know the definition of the anatomical position, you can begin to use specific terms to describe position, direction, and location.

The following is a list of all of the terms which are used to describe the body's position and direction:

- ❒ anterior — toward the front or in front of; ventral
- ❒ posterior — toward the back or in back of; dorsal
- ❒ medial — nearest the midline
- ❒ lateral — away from the midline or toward the side
- ❒ internal — inward or inside
- ❒ external — outward or outside
- ❒ proximal — nearest the point of reference
- ❒ distal — farthest away from the point of reference
- ❒ superior — above
- ❒ inferior — below
- ❒ cranial — toward the head
- ❒ caudal — toward the tail

Defining Anatomical Planes

There are specific terms used to describe and identify structures, areas of the body, and certain types of movement of the extremities. These include:

- ❒ sagittal — an imaginary plane that runs parallel to the long axis of the body dividing it into right and left sections
- ❒ frontal — an imaginary plane that runs through the side of the body dividing it into anterior (front) and posterior (back) sections
- ❒ transverse— an imaginary plane dividing the body into superior (upper) and inferior (lower) sections

Defining Anatomical Postures

There are specific terms used to describe anatomical postures. These include:

- ❒ erect — standing position
- ❒ supine — lying down
- ❒ prone — lying flat on the stomach, with the face down
- ❒ side-lying— lying with the body positioned on either the left or right side

Defining Types of Movement

There are specific terms used to describe various types of body movement. These include:

- ❒ flexion — bending at a joint
- ❒ extension — straightening at a joint; unbending
- ❒ abduction — moving away from the center of the body
- ❒ adduction — moving toward the center of the body
- ❒ rotation — rolling a part on its own axis, such as the turning of the head
- ❒ pronation — moving the palm from the anatomical position into a position with the palm facing

posteriorly or backward

- supination — moving the palm into the anatomical position facing anteriorly or forward
- eversion — turning the foot outward
- inversion — turning the foot inward

It is very important to remember that not all joints can perform all motions. The immovable joints are, of course, incapable of performing any of them. Of the freely moving joints, only the ball-and-socket joints, such as the hip and the shoulder, can perform all motions. The hinge joints, such as those found at the knee and the elbow, are only able to flex and extend.

◆ UNDERSTANDING THE PATIENT'S MEDICAL RECORD

Memory, at its very best, is often times fleeting and inaccurate. Medical records fill the need by containing accurate and detailed facts. These facts serve as a basis for the study, evaluation, and review of the patient's medical care.

Patient's medical records have been found among the earliest writings of Egyptians and Hindu literature. Until modern times, however, no effort was ever made to keep patients' histories in any type of systemic order. These records are of the greatest importance to the physician while the patient is under his or her care. They are also extremely valuable if the patient returns for treatment after several years. For the patient, the record has a historical value, as it is the document that forms his or her case history.

A patient's history also has great statistical value. For instance, it may be of use to the physician in evaluating a specific type of treatment, or to find out the incidence of a particular disease. The record may also be used as the basis for a lecture, an article, or a textbook. Further, patients' histories have legal importance. They may be summoned as a legal document and used in a court of law either to uphold the rights of the doctor if he or she is involved in litigation, or they may be used to confirm the claim of the patient if the doctor is called as a witness.

The medical record is used by health care practitioners to exchange information or as a means of communication. The physician, nurses, and other personnel contribute information to the record. A doctor may change a patient's care if the nurse has observed a change in the patient's condition. Likewise, after reading the notes written by the physical therapy aide, a nurse may plan specific nursing care that will allow the patient the greatest degree of comfort toward the prevention of any future musculoskeletal symptoms.

There are many different types of printed forms available for keeping medical records. Some hospitals print their own forms. Preprinted forms are useful because they save time. They also assist the recorder in remembering questions he or she wants to ask. They are a way to accurately record the details of the patient's care and treatment.

The physician is always the person who initiates the treatment by checking the appropriate referral blanks or writing directions or orders for treatment in a narrative form. The request for a lab test or an electrocardiogram, for example, is then sent to the cardiovascular department or the laboratory, as soon as possible, so that the procedure or lab test can be scheduled and carried out. Usually, the hospitalized patient and the chart are brought to the department from the nursing unit. Information relating to how the testing or procedural goals are being accomplished, and the patient's response to the procedure, is then recorded in the medical record after the test or procedure has been completed.

Charting Notes in the Medical Record

Most large health care facilities and individual medical practices document the patient's care and treatment in the medical record by utilizing a four-point system known as **SOAP notes**. The SOAP abbreviation refers to the four methods in which the patient's care is identified, assessed, and ultimately, carried out. The S stands for subjective symptoms that the patient may be presenting, and includes any information the patient says, family remarks made regarding the patient, and any other information stated by other health care providers. The O refers to any objective information, tests, or treatments that may have been provided for the patient, as well as any observations or measurements made by a member of the health care team. The assessment, or how well the patient is responding to a given treatment, is abbreviated by the A. It includes any documentation or notes made by the patients' provider. And the P, which pertains to the plan, is what needs to be done or what will be done for the patient based on the objective and subjective findings and the assessment.

Not all hospitals or individual departments will use the SOAP note format. Your department may choose to set up its own method of keeping records. Some departments use 5-by-8-inch file cards and record only the visits of the patients. Others may use an 8-by-11-inch file folder that encloses individual progress notes. In any case, the SOAP format is a good way of organizing your written data, no matter what type of forms the department uses.

Writing in the Medical Record

Since the patient's medical record is considered a legal document, it should always be written in ink. The information should be factual and have meaning. Notes must be accurate, without any spelling or grammatical errors. And any errors must be properly corrected by drawing one line through the error, with the person making it writing his or her initials to verify that an error has been made. You must never scratch out mistakes or use correction fluids. Remember, too, that all information within the medical record is confidential. This means that the record should not be used for any other reason but as a means of exchanging information between members of the professional medical staff.

◆ SUMMARY

In this chapter, you were introduced to medical terminology and the medical record. In doing so, we determined that a basic knowledge of medical terms will make you more knowledgeable about your patient's condition and thus allow you to read medical reports and records with greater understanding. As you continue to gain experience in the field of physical medicine, you will recognize the importance of using proper terms and abbreviations to save time and space when documenting patients' responses to medical treatments.

◆ ◆ LEARNING ACTIVITY 5-1

Using Medical Terminology

Using the abbreviations in your textbook, rewrite each of the following paragraphs.

1. This patient is a twenty-two-year-old female. She has come to the hospital complaining of back pain. The doctor has done all tests available and has diagnosed the disorder as muscle spasm due to overexertion this past weekend. The physician has ordered physical therapy as follows:

   "Hot packs and ultrasound three times each week. Include exercise and a home program. See the patient for at least two weeks, and then report to the doctor on the patient's condition."

2. This patient is a fifty-nine-year-old male with bilateral above-the-knee amputations. He has a history of diabetes and myocardial infarction. He was in the coronary care unit during his stay in the hospital after his myocardial infarction. His last admission to the hospital was in 1990 when he was admitted to the medical intensive care unit for observation after complaining of blackouts, usually after meals. No central nervous system problems were identified.

   "Physical therapy will be seeing the patient for ambulation and exercise. He should wear the above-knee prostheses and must use a walker for all activities of daily living. Full-weight-bearing is allowed on the lower left extremity, but only partial-weight-bearing should be attempted on the right lower extremity. Please be sure to monitor his blood pressure and any complaints of shortness of breath."

◆ ◆ LEARNING ACTIVITY 5-2

Medical Abbreviations

Using your textbook, write the correct meaning for each of the following abbreviations.

1. TO
2. Wt
3. Gm
4. Gtt
5. L
6. Stat
7. OOB
8. QNS
9. Rx
10. NPO
11. QS
12. Oz
13. <
14. >
15. EENT
16. Ad lib
17. TPR
18. cc
19. kg
20. ml
21. PO
22. R
23. BP
24. OR
25. PT
26. CCU
27. ICU
28. PEDS
29. Aa
30. BRP

◆ ◆ LEARNING ACTIVITY 5-3

Medical Terms You Should Know

Match the following terms with their correct definitions.

I. General Terms

a. Ambulation
b. Rehabilitation
c. Plinth
d. Supine
e. Prone
f. Therapy
g. Erect
h. Laterally recumbent
i. Modality
j. Physical

_________ 1. The body is lying horizontally flat on the back.
_________ 2. Ability to walk; not confined to bed.
_________ 3. Exercise and treatment table.
_________ 4. To cure or heal.
_________ 5. To restore patients to their most effective condition.
_________ 6. The application of a physical agent to help the patient's healing process.
_________ 7. Pertaining to such agents as heat, light, water, exercises, sound, and electrical energy.
_________ 8. The body is in a standing position.
_________ 9. The body is lying horizontally with the face and trunk down.
_________ 10. The body is lying horizontally on either side.

II. Types of Body Motion

a. Abudction
b. Adduction
c. Extension
d. Eversion
e. Flexion
f. Inversion
g. Pronation
h. Rotation
i. Supination

_________ 1. Turn upward.
_________ 2. Away from the body midline.
_________ 3. Turn around, turn the head.
_________ 4. Straightening the joint.
_________ 5. Bending a joint.
_________ 6. Turn outward.
_________ 7. Turn down.
_________ 8. Turn inward.
_________ 9. Toward the center of the body.

III. Direction

a. Distal
b. Inferior
c. Proximal
d. Superior

_________ 1. Above the transverse plane.
_________ 2. Below the transverse plane.
_________ 3. Nearest the point of attachment.
_________ 4. Farthest from the center, farthest from the trunk.

◆ ◆ LEARNING ACTIVITY 5-4

Identifying Root Words Pertaining to Systems

Find and circle the 43 root words in the word find puzzle. The words may be vertical, horizontal, diagonal, or backwards. List the root words in the numbered spaces. Write a sentence using each word on a separate piece of paper.

Example: **arthro** — I do hope this pain in my wrist is not **arthritis.**

1. arthro
2. carpal
3. chondro
4. costa
5. cranio
6. dactyl
7. my (myo)
8. osteo
9. pedi
10. spondyl
11. chol
12. entero
13. gastro
14. hepato
15. procto
16. pyloro
17. stoma
18. angio
19. arterio
20. cardi (io)
21. hema (hemo, hemato)
22. phlebo
23. thromb
24. vena
25. cerebro
26. encephalo
27. meningo
28. neuro
29. ophthalmo
30. oto
31. cysto
32. nephr (o)
33. ren (o)
34. pleur (o)
35. pneum (o)
36. pulmon
37. cervi
38. hyster
39. mamma
40. mast
41. oophoro
42. orchido
43. salpingo

Word Find Puzzle: Root Words

A	R	T	H	R	O	S	T	E	O	R	E	T	B	E
N	C	C	O	S	T	A	A	N	N	E	P	H	R	O
G	A	S	T	R	O	L	B	C	O	N	C	R	T	I
I	R	D	C	E	F	P	L	E	U	R	O	O	P	D
O	P	K	O	H	C	I	J	P	H	T	G	M	A	R
L	A	O	R	U	E	N	N	H	S	M	E	B	N	A
T	L	O	P	Z	W	G	O	A	V	H	Q	P	O	C
A	B	Z	E	C	R	O	M	L	O	R	O	L	Y	P
O	F	C	E	C	E	E	L	O	O	P	H	O	R	O
G	D	R	O	E	T	F	U	H	E	P	A	T	O	P
N	V	A	M	R	S	L	P	S	C	Y	S	T	O	H
I	E	N	U	L	Y	T	C	A	D	N	L	H	G	T
N	N	I	E	D	H	C	H	O	N	D	R	O	S	H
E	A	O	N	T	O	I	R	E	T	R	A	P	S	A
M	Y	O	P	R	T	O	B	E	L	H	P	A	O	L
A	P	E	D	I	C	O	R	B	E	R	E	C	P	M
S	T	O	M	A	M	M	A	O	D	I	H	C	R	O

◆ ◆ LEARNING ACTIVITY 5-5

Identification of Word Parts

Using your textbook and medical dictionary, write the definition of the italicized word in each sentence.

1. We're afraid that Jane has an *osteoma* of the left tibia.
2. Mr. Sanchez can't stand straight because of his *spondylitis*.
3. I'm worried about the asthmatic's *brachypnea*.
4. I think I'll specialize in *neurology*.
5. That tackle will need *chondroplasty* on his left hand.
6. I hope this new drug will help Pam's *myalgia*.
7. That little person has *dysarthrosis*.
8. Mrs. Green is an eighty-year-old woman with *osteoporosis*.
9. The athlete will undergo an *arthroscopy* of his right knee.
10. Ms. Smith will need a *prosthesis* after surgery.
11. I think I'd like to work for an *orthopedic* surgeon.
12. The PTA is part of the *rehabilitation* team.
13. Please assist Mr. Jones with his *range of motion* exercises.
14. Jimmy is a six-year-old boy who has *muscular dystrophy*.
15. Mr. Thomas will require a below-the-knee *amputation*.

REVIEW QUESTIONS

1. Briefly explain the purpose of a medical record.

2. The medical record serves as a _________ tool among members of the health care team.

3. List five reasons for keeping an accurate medical record:
   a. ____________________ d. ____________________
   b. ____________________ e. ____________________
   c. ____________________

4. Briefly explain the difference between a medical record and a hospital chart.

5. A patient's medical record or chart is considered a _________ document.

6. Identify the two basic types of charting used by most medical facilities.
   a. ____________________
   b. ____________________

7. What does the abbreviation SOAP refer to?
8. What do the "ABCs" of charting refer to?
   a. ____________________
   b. ____________________
   c. ____________________

9. Briefly explain how to correct a charting error.

10. What is the main purpose for using medical terms?

11. The ____________________ is located at the beginning of a word, and the ____________________ is located at the end of the word.

12. Match the following terms with their meaning:

cardio	gallbladder
gastro	white
leuko	stomach
arthro	heart
cholecysto	joint

13. Match the following suffixes with their meaning:

emia	tumor
itis	to cut into
oma	blood
ectomy	to remove a part
otomy	inflammation

14. Match the following abbreviations with their meaning:

amb	nothing by mouth
ADL	whenever necessary
NPO	four times a day
PRN	ambulate
QID	activities of daily living

15. Match the following abbreviations with their meaning:

cc	milligram
gtt	centimeter
kg	drop
mg	cubic centimeter
cm	kilogram

16. Match the following regular times with twenty-four-hour clock time:

11 P.M.	2400
8 A.M.	1900
2 P.M.	2300
12 midnight	0800
7 P.M.	1300

SECTION II

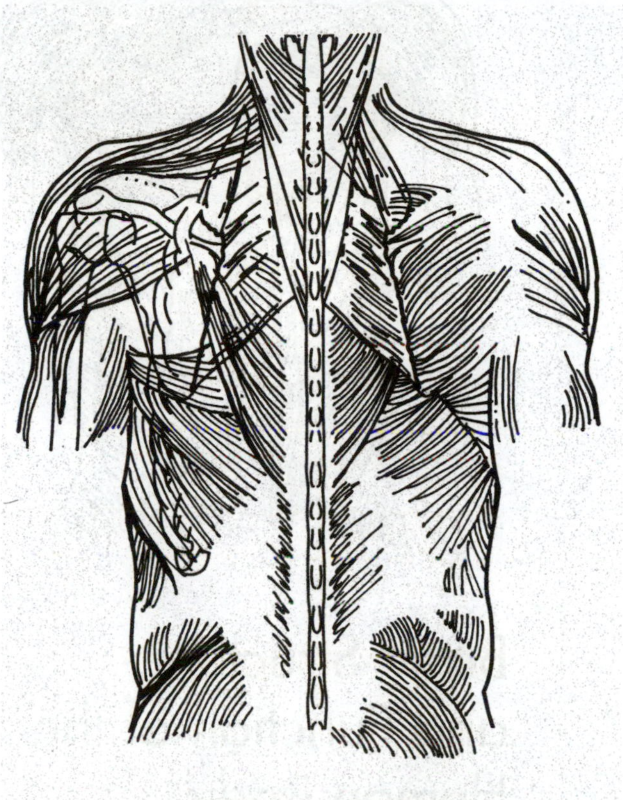

SCIENTIFIC PRINCIPLES

6

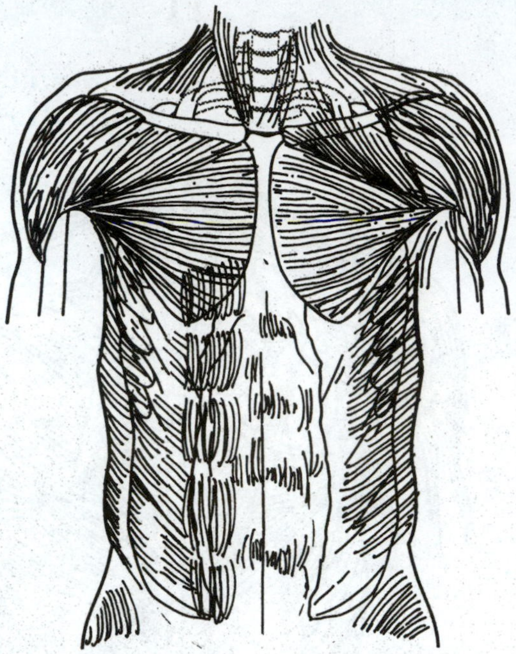

Basic Structure and Function of the Human Body

OBJECTIVES

Upon completion of this chapter, you should be able to:

1. Identify the various systems of the human body, and briefly explain the individual structures, components, and functions of each.
2. Identify common disorders of each of the systems of the body.

KEY TERMS

Acromegaly
Appendicitis
Arthritis
Cerebrovascular accident
Constipation
Diabetes mellitus
Diarrhea
Dislocation
Dysmenorrhea
Erythrocytes
Fertilization
Fracture
Leukocytes
Ligaments
Nephritis
Orchitis
Paralysis
Urinary calculi

UNDERSTANDING THE HUMAN BODY

The human body is a miraculous piece of work which consists of many individual structures, organs, and systems, all of which work both independently and as part of a team whose overall goal is the ongoing preservation of life. While you may not be involved in the actual hands-on care and treatment of patients, other than those suffering from a disorder or injury of the musculoskeletal system, as a member of the physical medicine health care team, it is still important for you to have a basic understanding of the rest of the individual systems that make up the human body so that you can better comprehend why patients seek medical care in the first place. Grasping a basic knowledge of these very important concepts, will almost guarantee you the ability to perform your job in a much more efficient and effective manner.

SYSTEMS OF THE BODY

The human body is comprised of nine body systems. These include the musculoskeletal system, the digestive system, the circulatory system, the respiratory system, the nervous system, the integumentary system, the urinary system, and the reproductive system.

The Musculoskeletal System

The musculoskeletal system, which is made up of all the bones and muscles of our body, provides us with the ability to stand erect, while at the same time, protects us from falling and injuring ourselves (Figure 6-1). The three types of muscles found in this system include *skeletal*, or voluntary muscles, which are connected to bone and which make it possible for voluntary movement, such as walking or picking up an object off the floor; *smooth*, or involuntary muscles, which cannot be controlled by our will, but rather, by the autonomic nervous system, and which include such muscles as those found in the digestive and respiratory systems; and *cardiac* muscle, which makes up the heart wall.

When all the bones of the body come together, they make up the skeleton (Figure 6-2). When this occurs, the skeleton has three general functions: movement, because skeletal muscles are

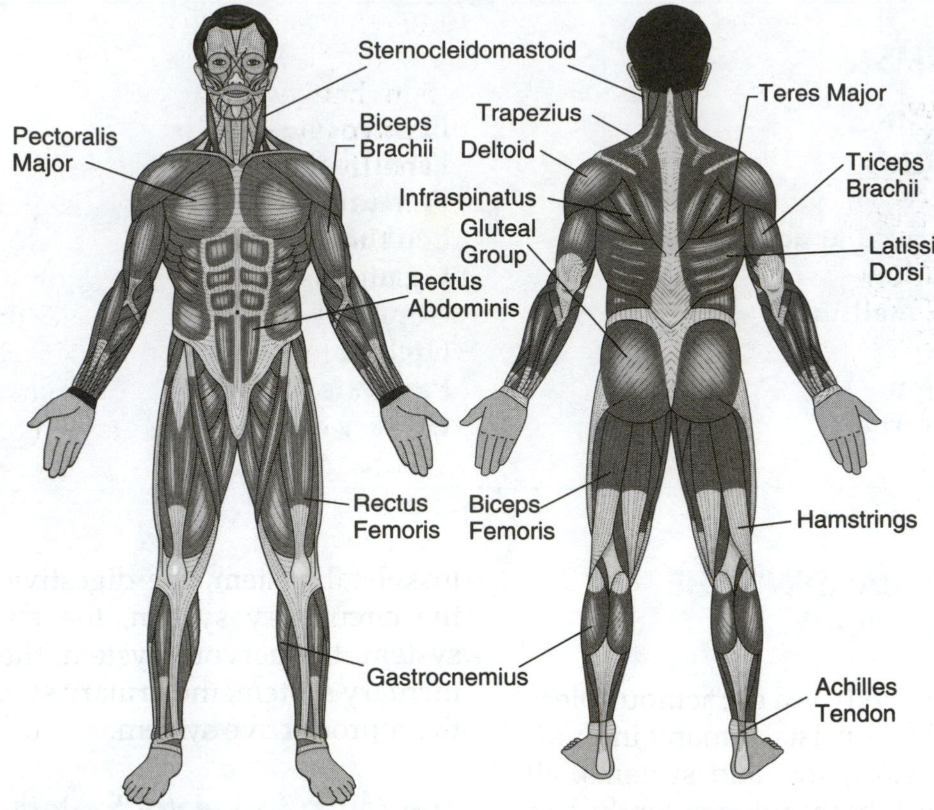

Figure 6-1 The muscular system.

attached to bones; support of the body, and protection of our vital organs, such as the heart or our liver.

The point at which two bones come together is called a *joint*. There are many different kinds of joints, each with a different function, some joints allow us to bend our elbow, fingers, or knees. These are called hinge joints. Another type of joint is called an immovable joint, such as the junction of the bones of the adult skull. This joint helps protect our brain.

Tendons and ligaments are actually parts of the musculoskeletal system. Tendons attach muscles to bones, while **ligaments** hold the bones together at the joints.

The most common injury or disorder of the musculoskeletal system is a **fracture**, which is any break in a bone. While there are several different types of fractures, the most commonly seen include *simple fractures*, which occur without resulting in a break in the skin, *compound fractures*, which involve breakage of soft tissues and result in the broken bone protruding through the skin, and *greenstick fractures*, which are incomplete breaks in the bone fibers and occur most often in children.

In addition to fractures, the most common disorders and injuries to the musculoskeletal system include dislocations, sprains, and strains. A **dislocation**, which is almost always accompanied by torn or stretched ligaments, is a bone injury in which a bone is moved from its normal position in a joint. A *sprain* is an injury that occurs when a joint moves too far, thus resulting in overstretching or tearing of the ligaments. Back sprains or sprained ankles are common types of injuries. Muscle *strains* result from simply overworking the muscles. They are usually accompanied by a great deal of

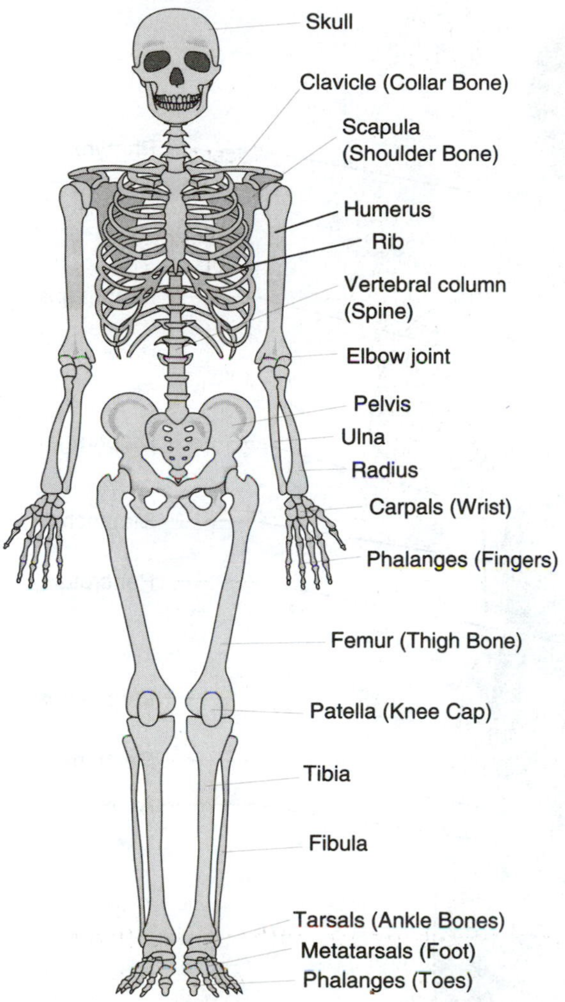

Figure 6-2 The skeletal system, also called the skeleton.

soreness and pain.

A disease considered quite common to the musculoskeletal system is **arthritis.** It is a disorder involving an inflammation of the bones at the joints, which is often accompanied by pain and swelling of the joints. Arthritis is most often seen in older patients.

The Digestive System

The digestive system includes the mouth, throat, esophagus, stomach, small and large intestines, and closely associated glands and organs (Figure 6-3). Its function is to digest food, or to change it from an insoluble to a soluble form. This is accomplished through a process of action between the chemicals and the digestive juices.

The first part of the digestive tract is the mouth. Here the food is ground up and then torn apart by the teeth. Digestion begins in the mouth as saliva mixes with and then acts on the food. The food then passes through the throat or pharynx as it is swallowed and eventually goes through the esophagus to the stomach. Food remains in the stomach from four to six hours. During this time, it is churned by the action of smooth muscles in the stomach and is then mixed with digestive juices secreted by glands in the stomach.

Food passes from the stomach into the small intestine, which is about twenty feet in length and is arranged in coils and loops held in place by a thin sheet of tissue, called the *mesentery.* The small intestine is divided into three parts. The first part is called the *duodenum,* which is eight to ten inches long. The second part is called the *jejunum,* which is six to nine feet long. The final part of the small intestine is called the *ileum.* Most digestion occurs in the duodenum. Bile from the liver and pancreatic juice from the pancreas empty into the duodenum. These juices, along with the secretion of glands in the small intestine, carry on most of the digestion of the food. The digested food is then absorbed from the lining of the small intestine and enters the bloodstream.

After food has been carried through the small intestine, the undigested food residue eventually moves into the large intestine. The large intestine consists of the *cecum,* the *appendix,* the *ascending, transverse,* and *descending colons,* the *rectum,* and the *anus.* The last part is the external opening of the digestive system. Food is not digested in the large intes-

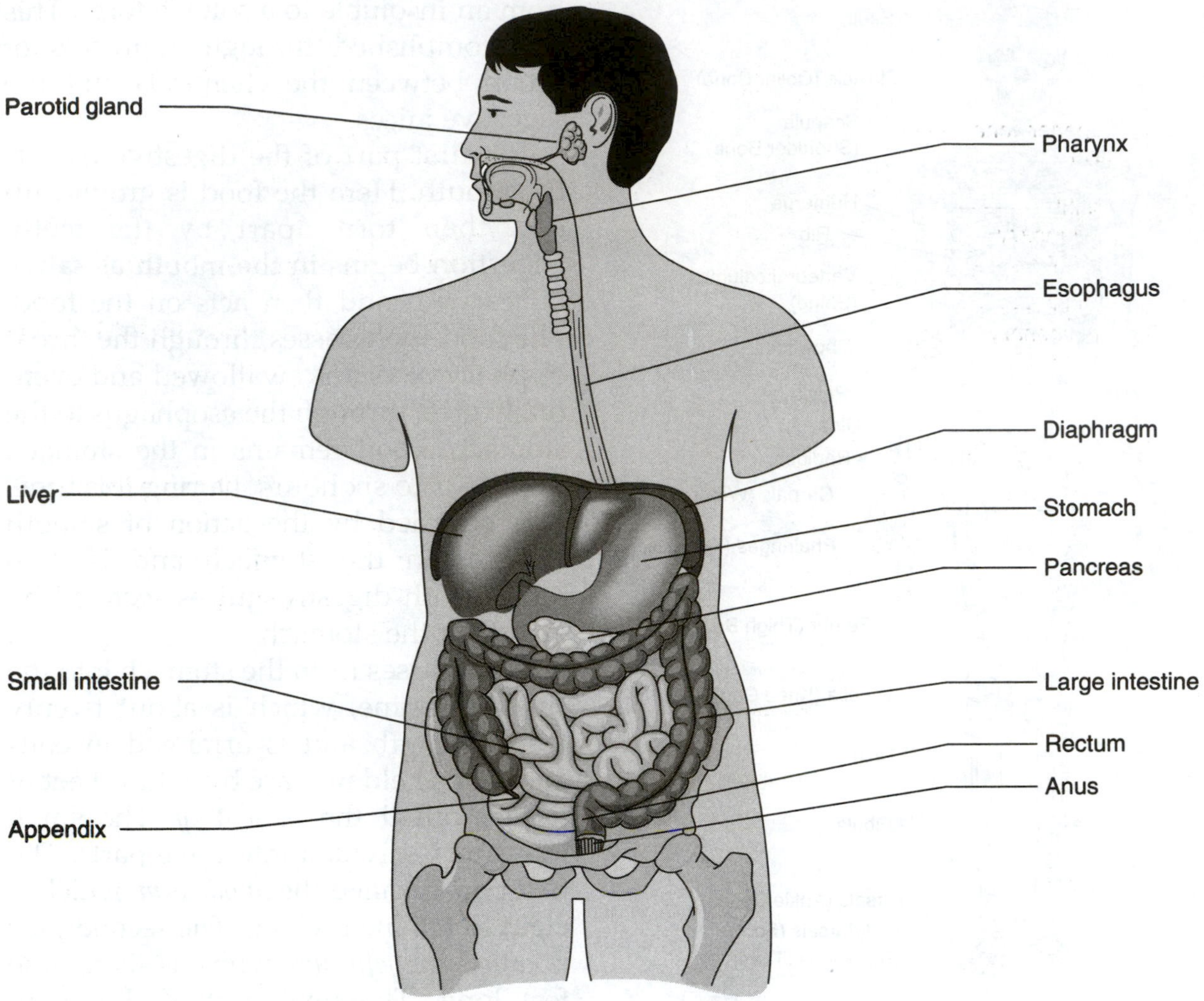

Figure 6-3 Major structures of the digestive system.

tine, but water and minerals are absorbed here. The food is moved through the entire digestive tract by wavelike contractions of the intestines, called *peristalsis*.

Disorders and diseases of the digestive system are very common. Many of these include inflammatory conditions. Those most often seen include **appendicitis,** which is an inflammation of the appendix, cirrhosis, which is a chronic disease of the liver often caused by excessive intake of alcohol, **constipation** and **diarrhea,** gastritis, an inflammatory condition of the lining of the stomach, and heartburn, which is a burning sensation experienced in the stomach. Other conditions seen frequently include hepatitis, which is an inflammation of the liver, nausea, and ulcers, which occur in an area of the stomach or small intestine where the tissues are gradually disintegrating.

The Circulatory System

The circulatory system is made up of the heart, blood vessels, and blood (Figure 6-4). Its main function is to send the blood throughout all parts of our body, carrying with it digested food and oxygen, and then return blood to

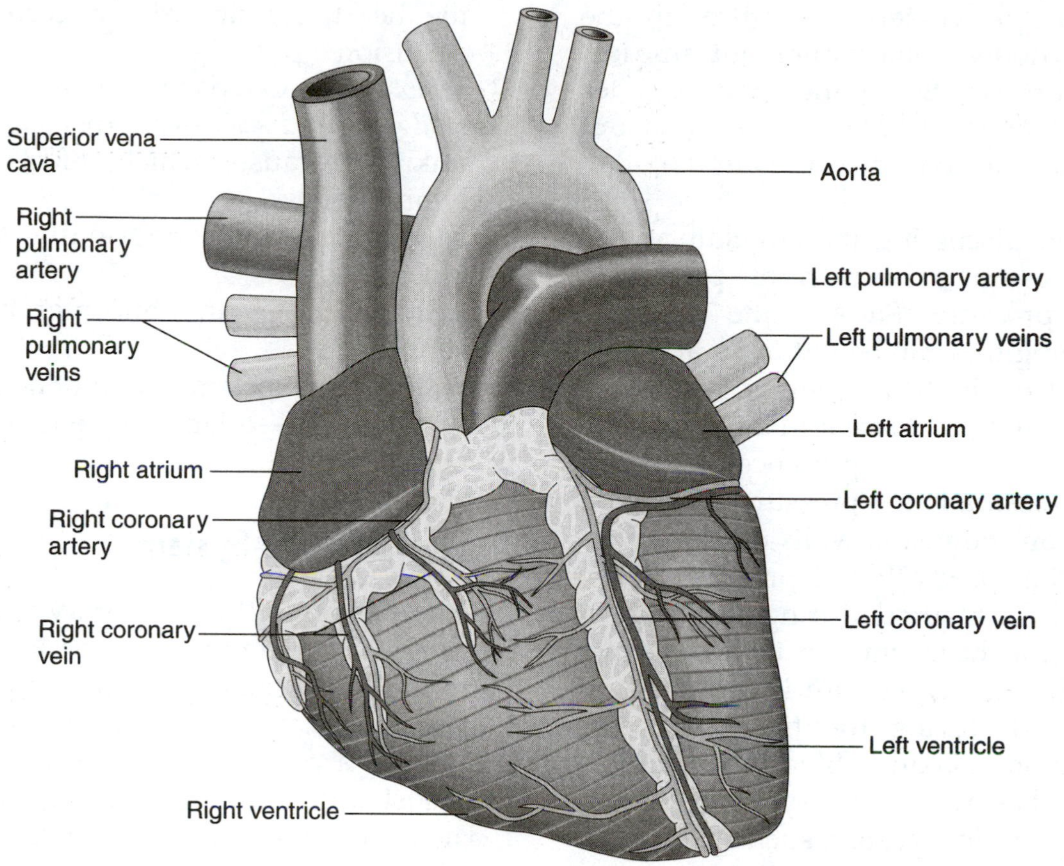

Figure 6-4 External view of the heart.

the heart carrying waste products of metabolism.

The heart is a hollow, cone-shaped organ that is about the size of your fist when it is closed. It has four separate chambers and is located in the center of the chest cavity with the tip pointing slightly to the left. It is well protected by the ribs and sternum. The function of the heart is to pump blood to every part of the body.

Blood vessels of the circulatory system include the *arteries,* which carry blood away from the heart; *veins,* which return the blood to the heart; and *capillaries,* which are small vessels that connect arteries to veins. The blood vessels you are most likely to find discussed at your facility are the *aorta,* which is the largest artery of the body and is located along the spinal column, and the *coronary arteries* and veins that supply the heart.

The blood that is carried throughout the body is a very complex fluid. It is made up of red blood cells, called **erythrocytes,** white blood cells, called **leukocytes,** and platelets. The red blood cells carry oxygen to every cell in the body. The white blood cells destroy pathogenic bacteria and thereby help the body to combat diseases caused by bacterial infection. Platelets are involved in the clotting mechanism of blood.

The lymphatic system is also part of the circulatory system. Lymph is a clear, colorless fluid that is formed in tissue spaces throughout the body. It collects in tiny lymph capillaries and is eventually carried to even larger lymph vessels until finally it empties into the blood.

The lymph vessels pass through the lymph nodes, which filter out any foreign particles. Sometimes lymph nodes become infected because they filter out bacteria that may then invade the node itself.

When discussing the circulatory system, we must also mention pulse and blood pressure. *Pulse* is the rhythmic throbbing that can be felt in an artery as a result of the heart beating. The pulse rate, rhythm, and strength are all indicators of health or the presence of disease. *Blood pressure* is the pressure that blood exerts on the inside walls of blood vessels. The *systolic* blood pressure is the pressure measured during the time in which the heart muscle is contracting. *Diastolic* blood pressure is the pressure measured during the time the heart muscle is relaxing. Blood pressure is reported as two figures, systolic pressure over diastolic pressure, such as 120/80.

Many patients coming into the medical office or being admitted into the health care facility will have diseases and disorders of the circulatory system. The most common of these include the following:

- ❒ *anemia*—a condition in which the blood is deficient in the number of red blood cells or in hemoglobin
- ❒ *arteriosclerosis*—a condition in which there is a thickening, hardening, and loss of elasticity of the blood vessels
- ❒ *congestive heart failure*—a condition which occurs when there is a failure of the heart to maintain an adequate output of blood in order to meet the demands of the body
- ❒ *coronary occlusion*—an obstruction of a coronary artery
- ❒ *myocardial infarction*—also referred to as a heart attack, in which damage to the heart muscle has occurred as a result of diminished blood supply to the heart muscle from a coronary occlusion
- ❒ *hemorrhage*—extensive loss of blood
- ❒ *Hodgkin's disease*—a disease of unknown cause, which affects the lymph nodes
- ❒ *hypertension*—an abnormally high blood pressure
- ❒ *heart murmur*—an abnormal heart sound
- ❒ *phlebitis*—an inflammation of a vein
- ❒ *varicose veins*—dilation of veins, often occurring in the legs

The Respiratory System

The function of the respiratory system is to bring air containing oxygen into the body and, at the same time, eliminate carbon dioxide and water. Each body cell must have a constant supply of oxygen and must also get rid of carbon dioxide.

The structures of the respiratory system include the *nasal cavities,* the *sinuses,* the *pharynx,* which is the throat, the *larynx,* or voice box, which contains the vocal chords and make speech possible, the *trachea,* which is the short tube extending from the larynx to the bronchi, the *bronchi,* which lead to the *lungs,* which are a pair of lobed organs found in the thorax or chest cavity, and the *diaphragm,* which is a sheet of muscle that separates the abdominal and chest cavities (Figure 6-5). The contraction of the diaphragm forces air into the lungs. The pleura is the membrane that covers the lungs and lines the chest cavity.

Air is brought into the lungs as the diaphragm contracts. It then passes through the nasal cavity, the pharynx, larynx, trachea, bronchi, and finally into the lungs. The actual exchange of oxygen with carbon dioxide takes place through the thin cell walls of the alveoli by the process of diffusion. Oxygen from the alveoli actually enters the blood and

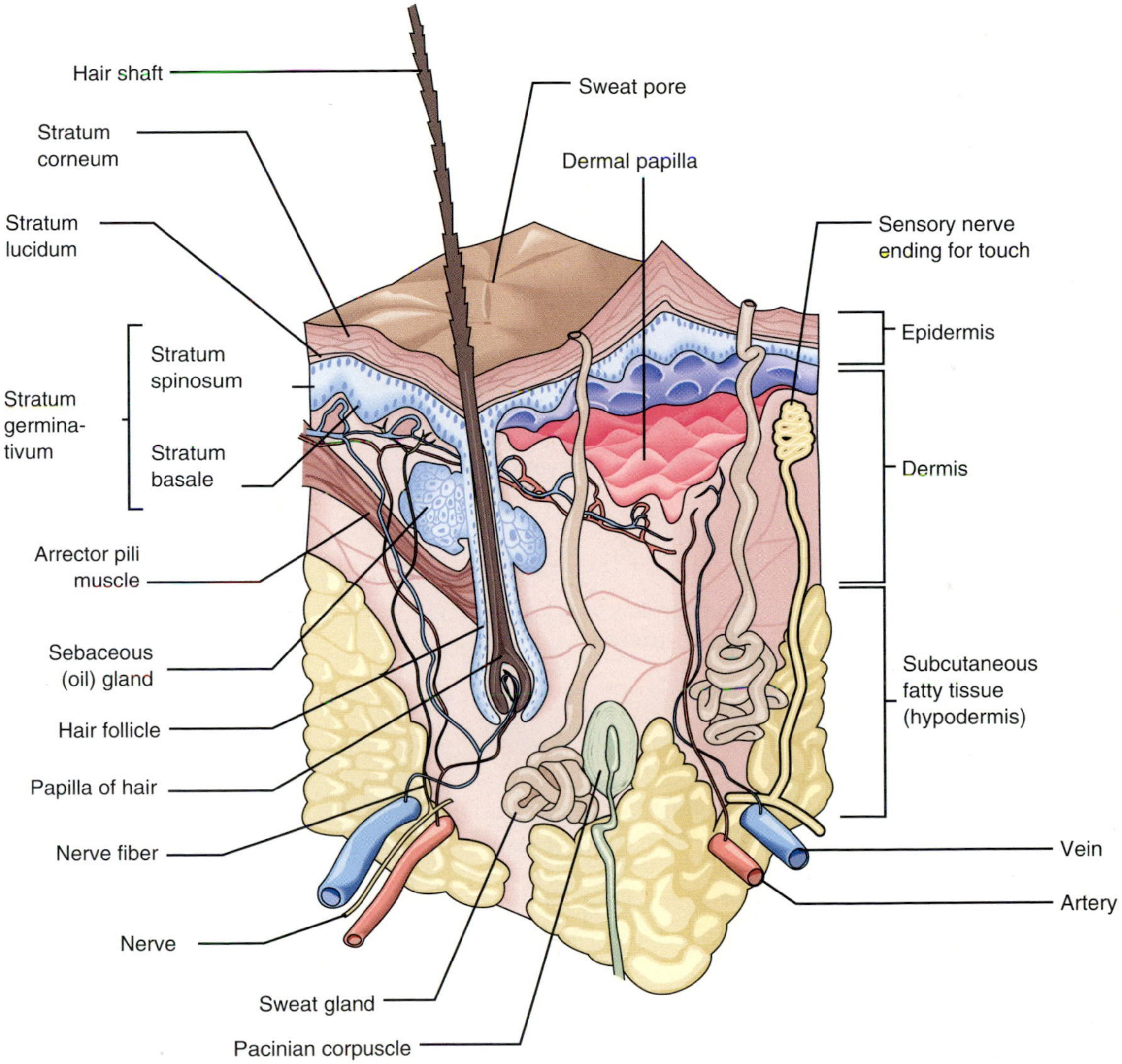
Hair shaft
Sweat pore
Stratum corneum
Dermal papilla
Stratum lucidum
Sensory nerve ending for touch
Stratum spinosum
Epidermis
Stratum germinativum
Stratum basale
Dermis
Arrector pili muscle
Sebaceous (oil) gland
Subcutaneous fatty tissue (hypodermis)
Hair follicle
Papilla of hair
Nerve fiber
Vein
Artery
Nerve
Sweat gland
Pacinian corpuscle

Plate 1 Cross Section of Skin

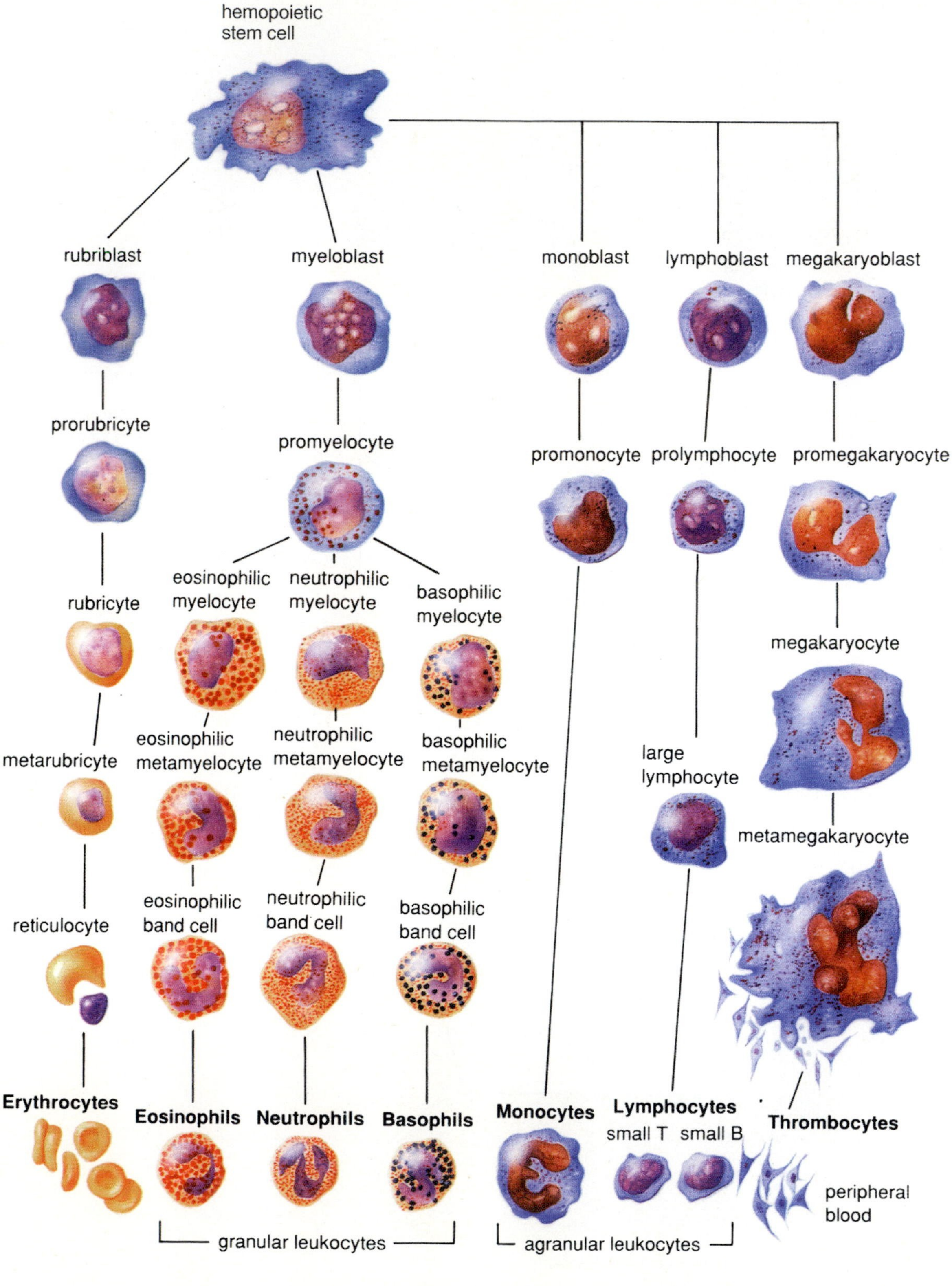

Plate 2 Blood Cells and Platelets

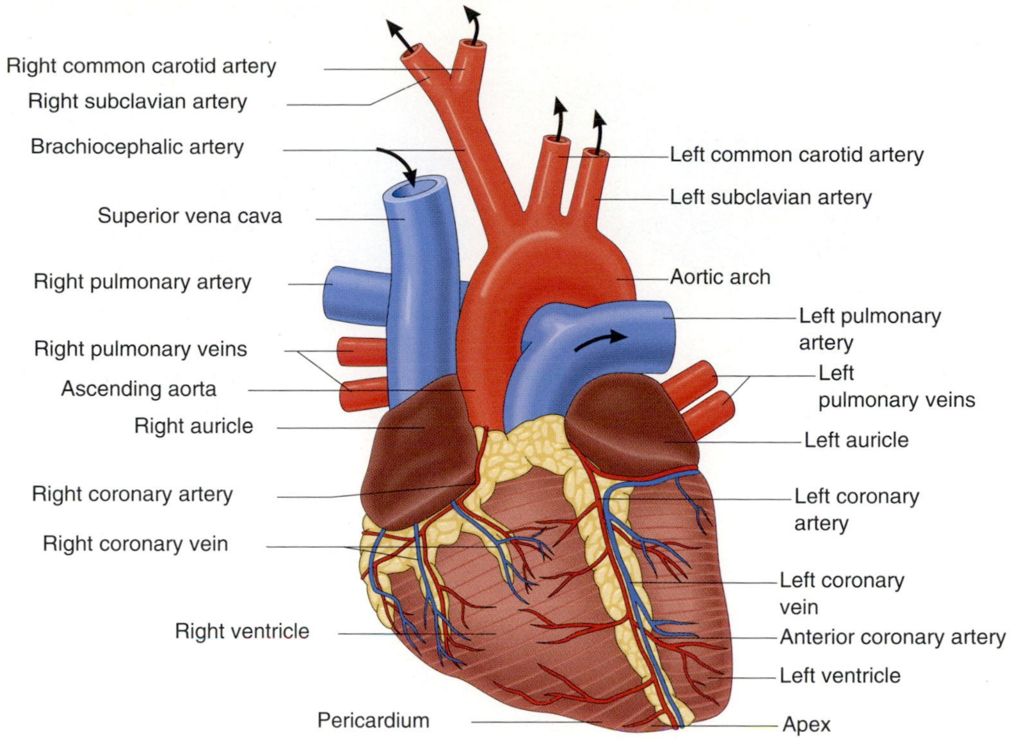
Right common carotid artery
Right subclavian artery
Brachiocephalic artery
Superior vena cava
Right pulmonary artery
Right pulmonary veins
Ascending aorta
Right auricle
Right coronary artery
Right coronary vein
Right ventricle
Pericardium
Left common carotid artery
Left subclavian artery
Aortic arch
Left pulmonary artery
Left pulmonary veins
Left auricle
Left coronary artery
Left coronary vein
Anterior coronary artery
Left ventricle
Apex

Plate 3 Front View of Heart

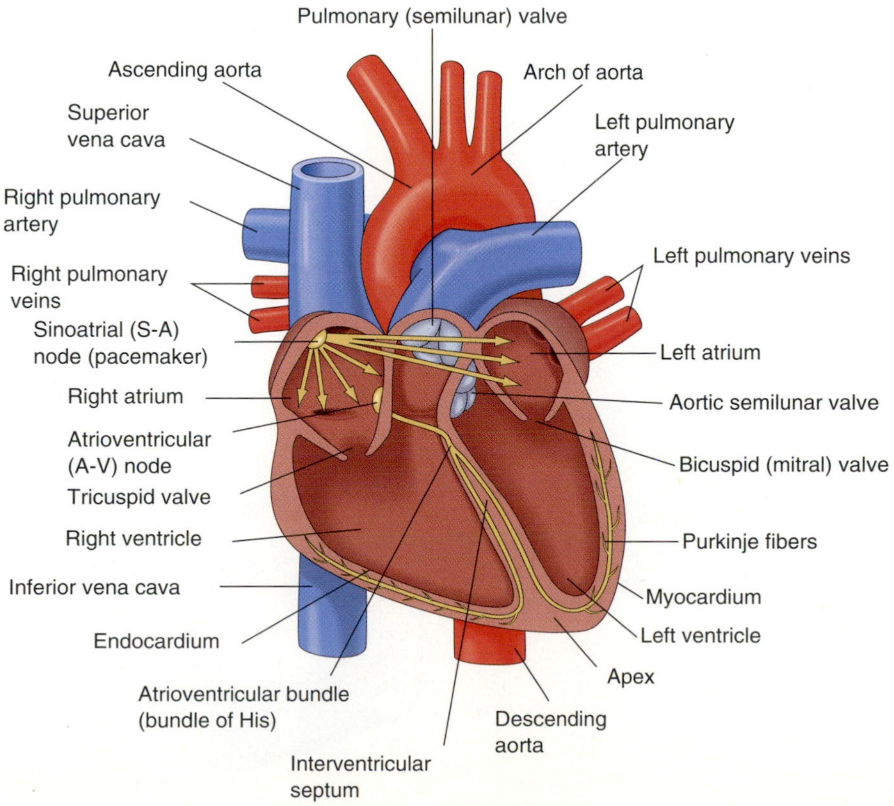
Pulmonary (semilunar) valve
Ascending aorta
Arch of aorta
Superior vena cava
Left pulmonary artery
Right pulmonary artery
Left pulmonary veins
Right pulmonary veins
Sinoatrial (S-A) node (pacemaker)
Left atrium
Right atrium
Aortic semilunar valve
Atrioventricular (A-V) node
Bicuspid (mitral) valve
Tricuspid valve
Purkinje fibers
Right ventricle
Myocardium
Inferior vena cava
Left ventricle
Endocardium
Apex
Atrioventricular bundle (bundle of His)
Descending aorta
Interventricular septum

Plate 4 Conductive Pathways

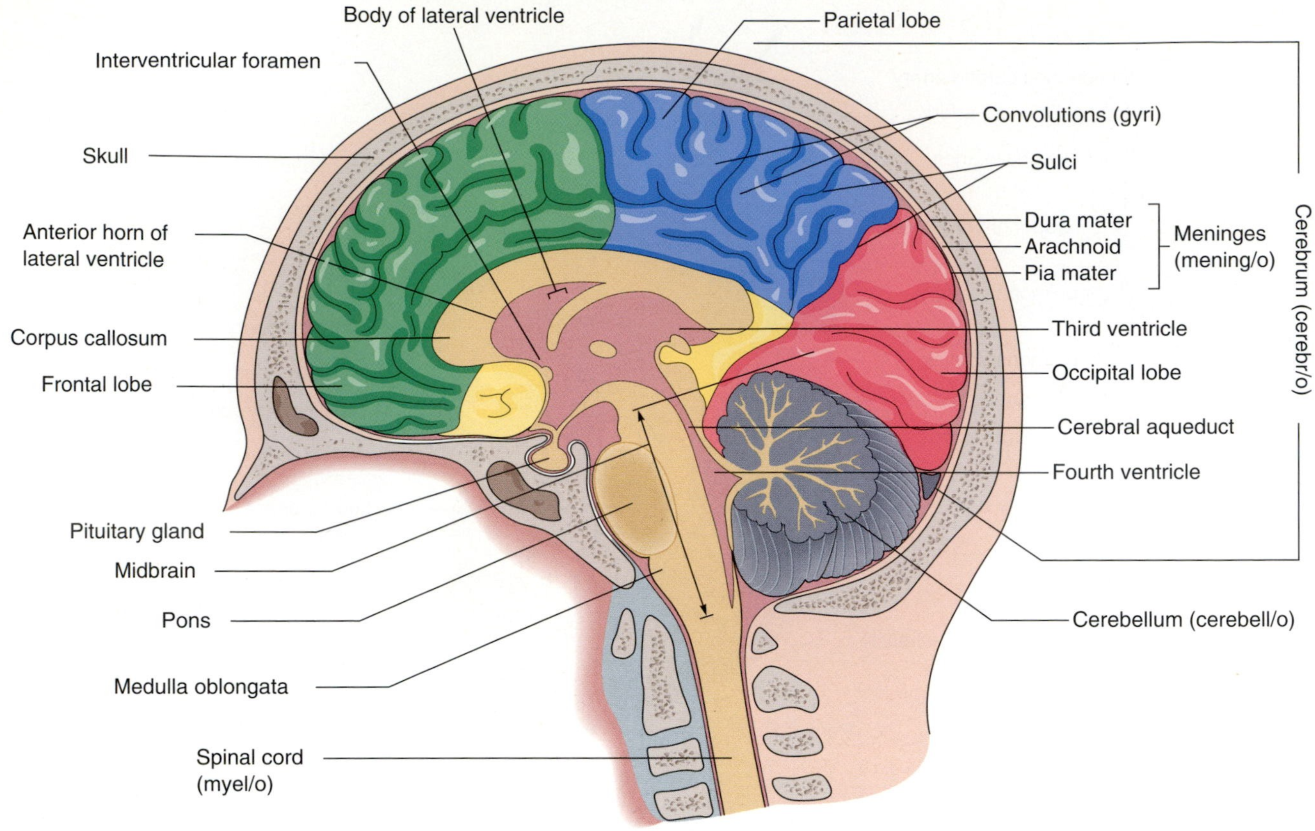
Body of lateral ventricle
Parietal lobe
Interventricular foramen
Convolutions (gyri)
Skull
Sulci
Anterior horn of lateral ventricle
Dura mater
Arachnoid
Pia mater
Meninges (mening/o)
Cerebrum (cerebr/o)
Corpus callosum
Third ventricle
Frontal lobe
Occipital lobe
Cerebral aqueduct
Fourth ventricle
Pituitary gland
Midbrain
Pons
Cerebellum (cerebell/o)
Medulla oblongata
Spinal cord (myel/o)

Plate 5A Section of Brain

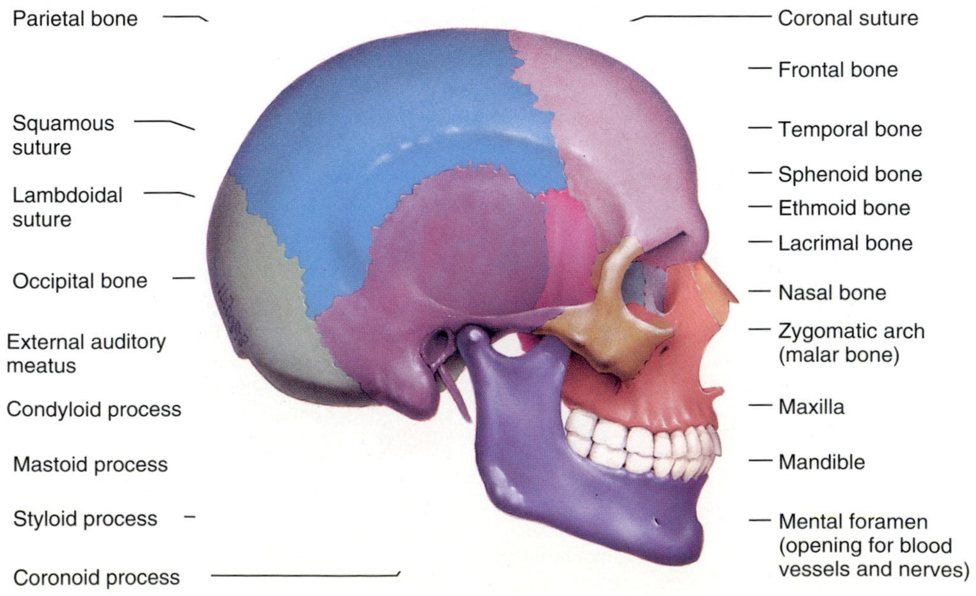
Parietal bone
Coronal suture
Frontal bone
Squamous suture
Temporal bone
Sphenoid bone
Lambdoidal suture
Ethmoid bone
Lacrimal bone
Occipital bone
Nasal bone
External auditory meatus
Zygomatic arch (malar bone)
Condyloid process
Maxilla
Mastoid process
Mandible
Styloid process
Mental foramen (opening for blood vessels and nerves)
Coronoid process

Plate 5B Lateral View of Cranium

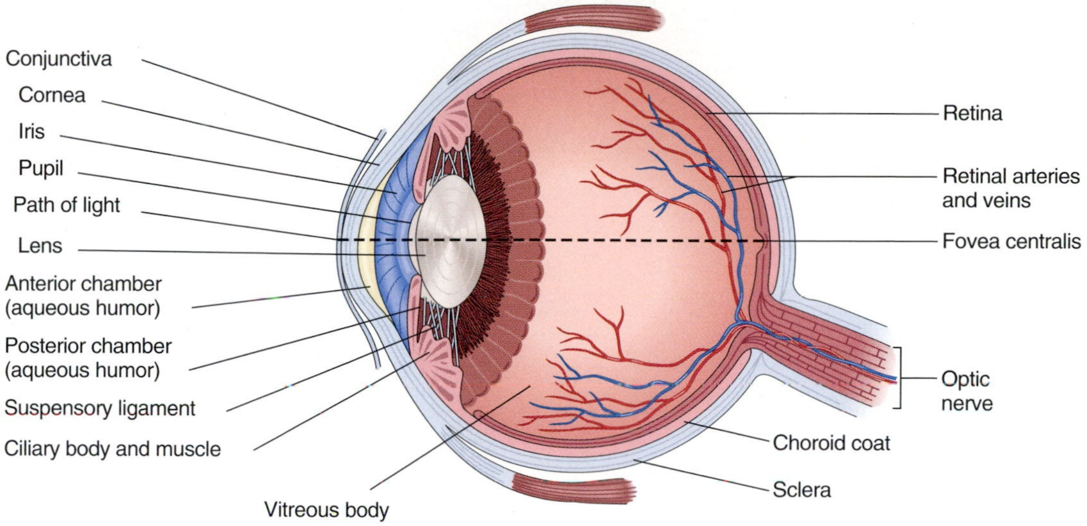
Conjunctiva
Cornea
Iris
Pupil
Path of light
Lens
Anterior chamber
(aqueous humor)
Posterior chamber
(aqueous humor)
Suspensory ligament
Ciliary body and muscle
Vitreous body
Retina
Retinal arteries
and veins
Fovea centralis
Optic
nerve
Choroid coat
Sclera

Plate 6A Eye Structure

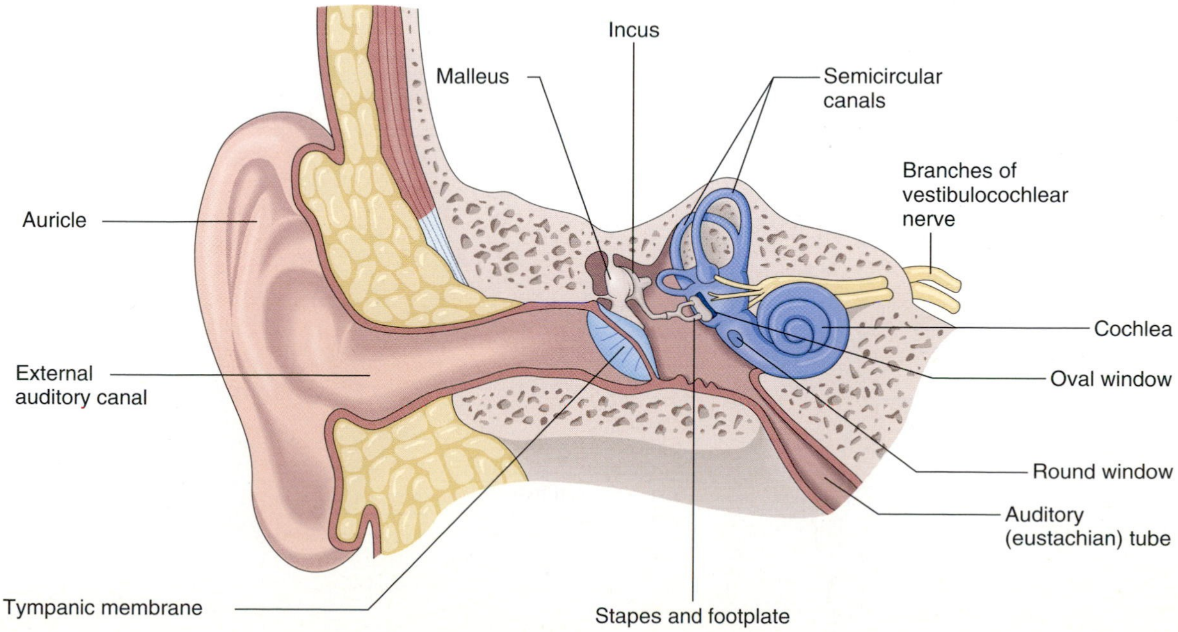
Incus
Malleus
Semicircular
canals
Branches of
vestibulocochlear
nerve
Auricle
Cochlea
Oval window
External
auditory canal
Round window
Auditory
(eustachian) tube
Tympanic membrane
Stapes and footplate

Plate 6B Ear Structure

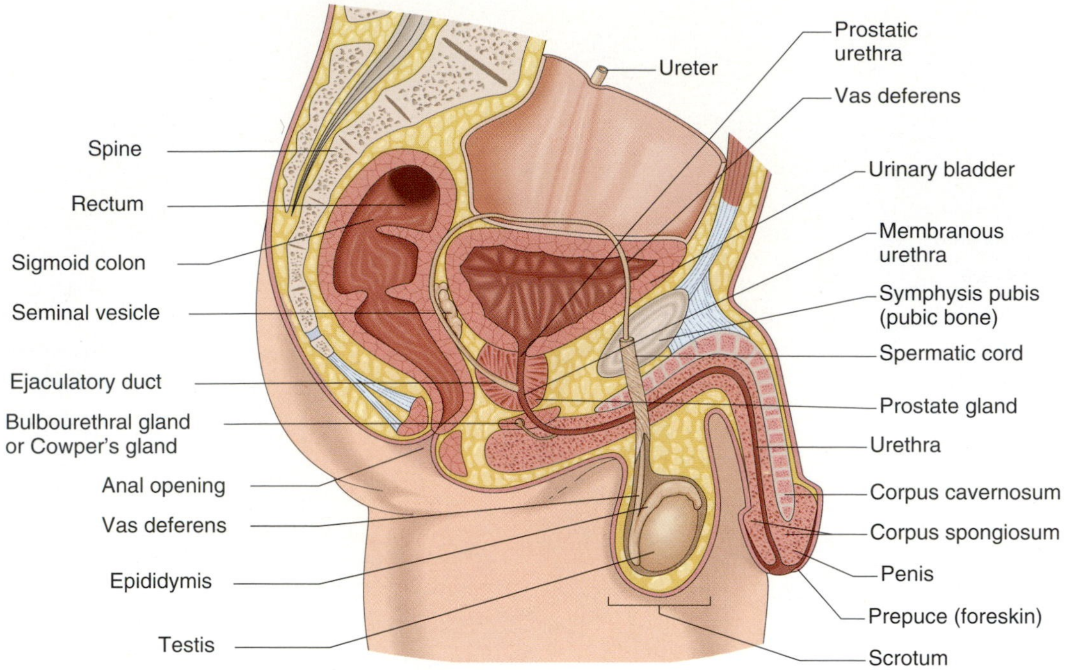
Spine
Rectum
Sigmoid colon
Seminal vesicle
Ejaculatory duct
Bulbourethral gland
or Cowper's gland
Anal opening
Vas deferens
Epididymis
Testis
Ureter
Prostatic
urethra
Vas deferens
Urinary bladder
Membranous
urethra
Symphysis pubis
(pubic bone)
Spermatic cord
Prostate gland
Urethra
Corpus cavernosum
Corpus spongiosum
Penis
Prepuce (foreskin)
Scrotum

Plate 7A Male Reproductive

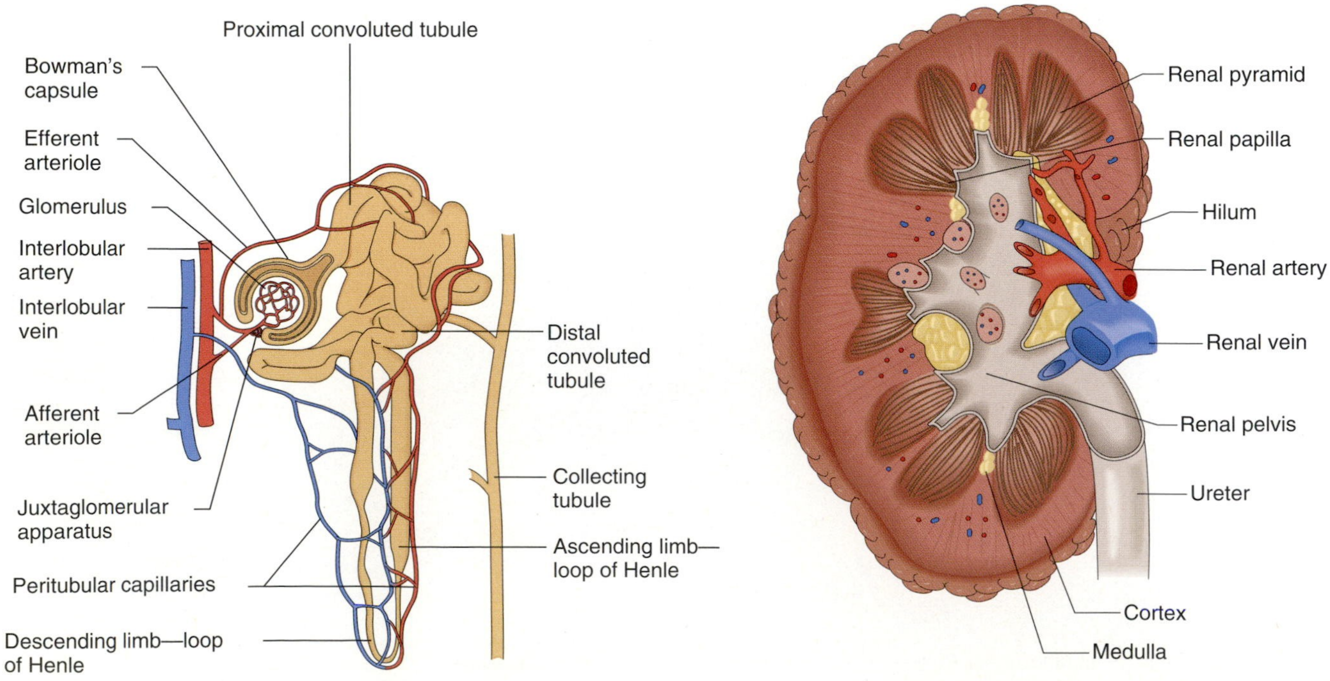
Proximal convoluted tubule
Bowman's
capsule
Efferent
arteriole
Glomerulus
Interlobular
artery
Interlobular
vein
Afferent
arteriole
Juxtaglomerular
apparatus
Peritubular capillaries
Descending limb—loop
of Henle
Distal
convoluted
tubule
Collecting
tubule
Ascending limb—
loop of Henle
Renal pyramid
Renal papilla
Hilum
Renal artery
Renal vein
Renal pelvis
Ureter
Cortex
Medulla

Plate 7B Nephron and Cross Section of Kidney

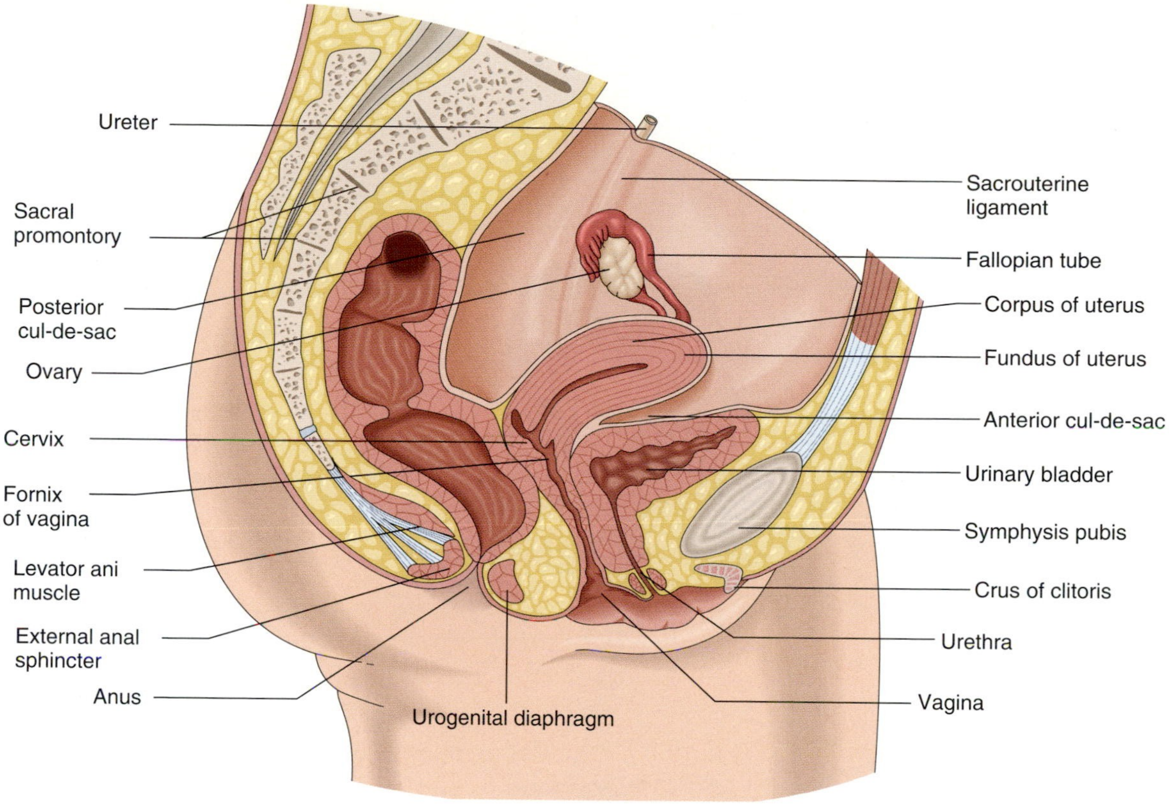

Plate 8A Female Reproductive

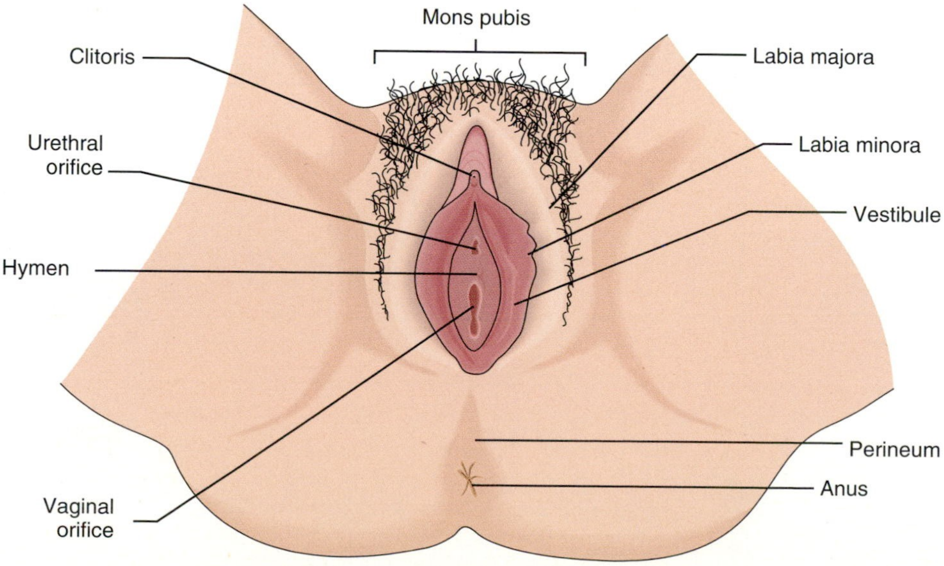

Plate 8B Female External Genitalia

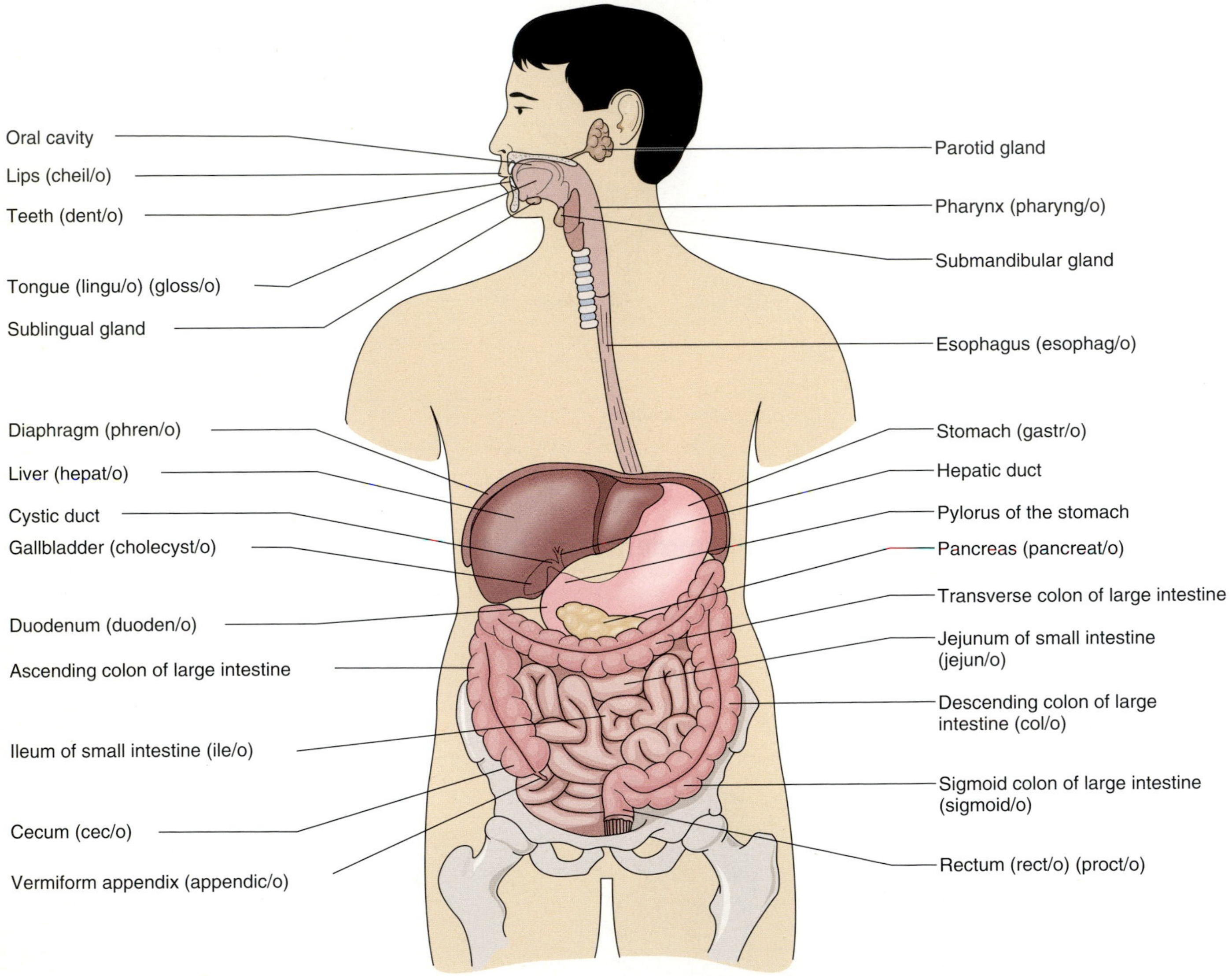
Oral cavity
Lips (cheil/o)
Teeth (dent/o)
Tongue (lingu/o) (gloss/o)
Sublingual gland
Diaphragm (phren/o)
Liver (hepat/o)
Cystic duct
Gallbladder (cholecyst/o)
Duodenum (duoden/o)
Ascending colon of large intestine
Ileum of small intestine (ile/o)
Cecum (cec/o)
Vermiform appendix (appendic/o)
Parotid gland
Pharynx (pharyng/o)
Submandibular gland
Esophagus (esophag/o)
Stomach (gastr/o)
Hepatic duct
Pylorus of the stomach
Pancreas (pancreat/o)
Transverse colon of large intestine
Jejunum of small intestine (jejun/o)
Descending colon of large intestine (col/o)
Sigmoid colon of large intestine (sigmoid/o)
Rectum (rect/o) (proct/o)

Plate 9 Digestive System

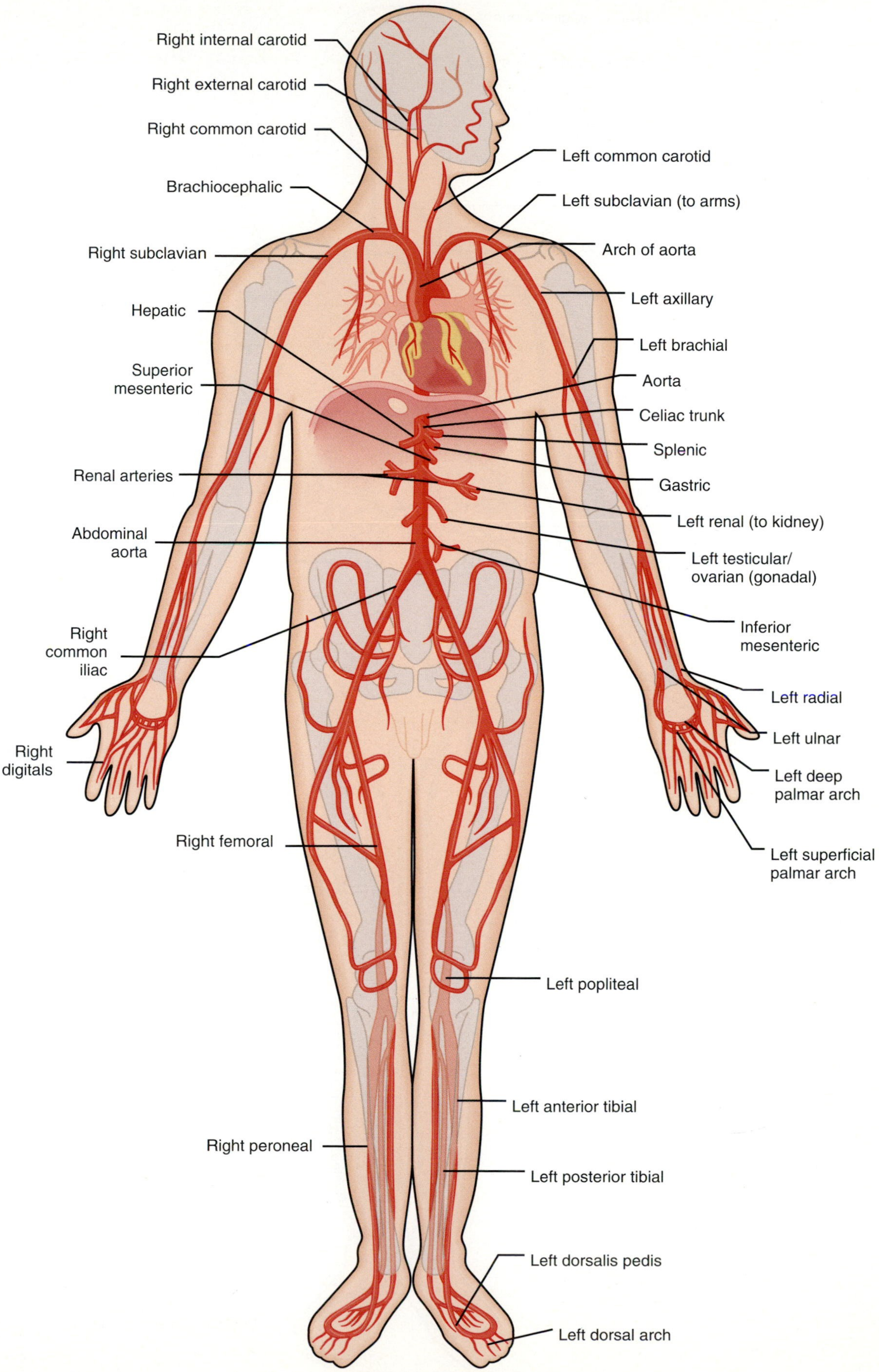
Right internal carotid
Right external carotid
Right common carotid
Brachiocephalic
Right subclavian
Hepatic
Superior mesenteric
Renal arteries
Abdominal aorta
Right common iliac
Right digitals
Right femoral
Right peroneal
Left common carotid
Left subclavian (to arms)
Arch of aorta
Left axillary
Left brachial
Aorta
Celiac trunk
Splenic
Gastric
Left renal (to kidney)
Left testicular/ ovarian (gonadal)
Inferior mesenteric
Left radial
Left ulnar
Left deep palmar arch
Left superficial palmar arch
Left popliteal
Left anterior tibial
Left posterior tibial
Left dorsalis pedis
Left dorsal arch

Plate 10A Arterial Distribution

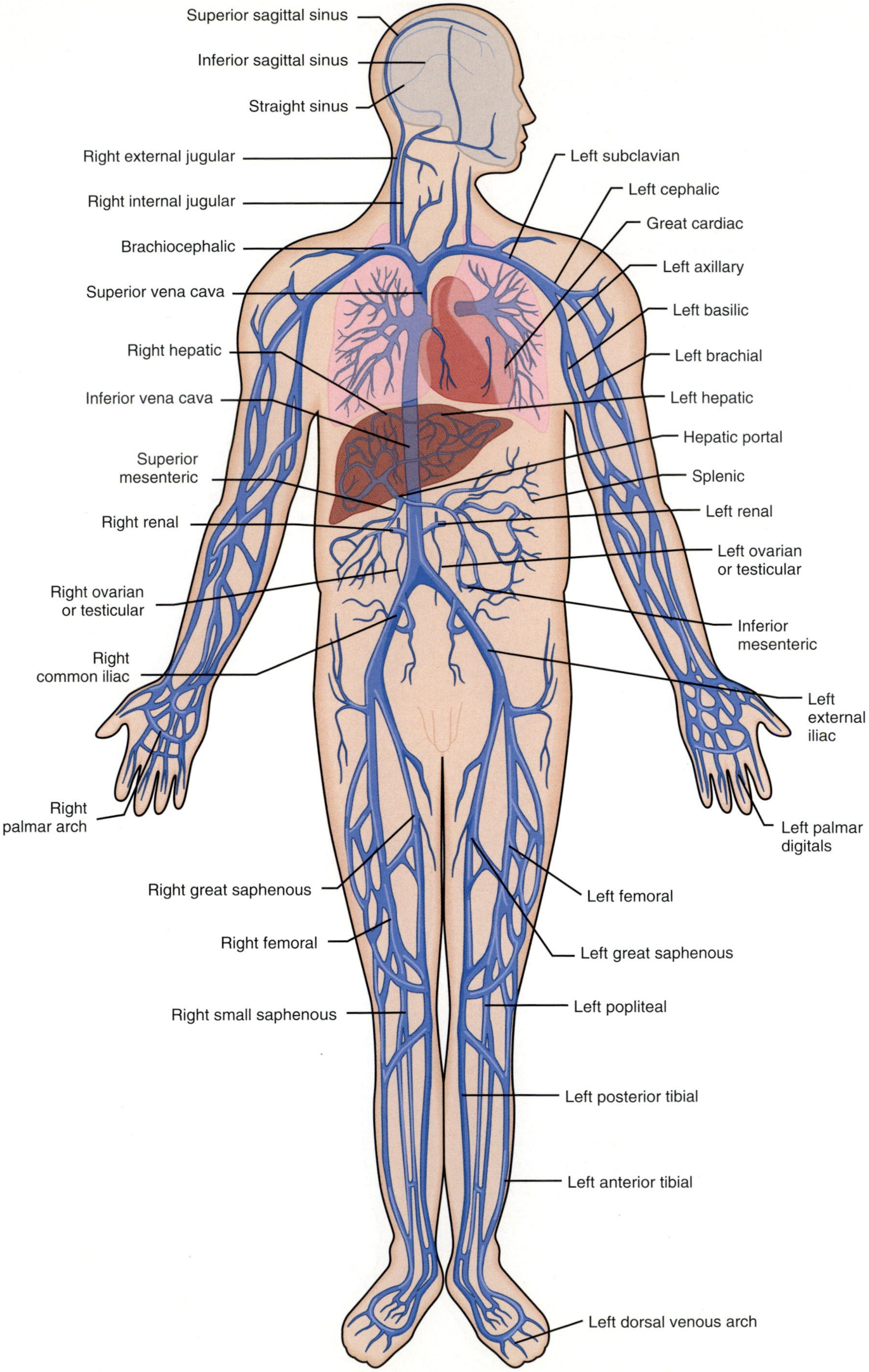
Superior sagittal sinus
Inferior sagittal sinus
Straight sinus
Right external jugular
Right internal jugular
Brachiocephalic
Superior vena cava
Right hepatic
Inferior vena cava
Superior mesenteric
Right renal
Right ovarian or testicular
Right common iliac
Right palmar arch
Right great saphenous
Right femoral
Right small saphenous
Left subclavian
Left cephalic
Great cardiac
Left axillary
Left basilic
Left brachial
Left hepatic
Hepatic portal
Splenic
Left renal
Left ovarian or testicular
Inferior mesenteric
Left external iliac
Left palmar digitals
Left femoral
Left great saphenous
Left popliteal
Left posterior tibial
Left anterior tibial
Left dorsal venous arch

Plate 10B Venous Distribution

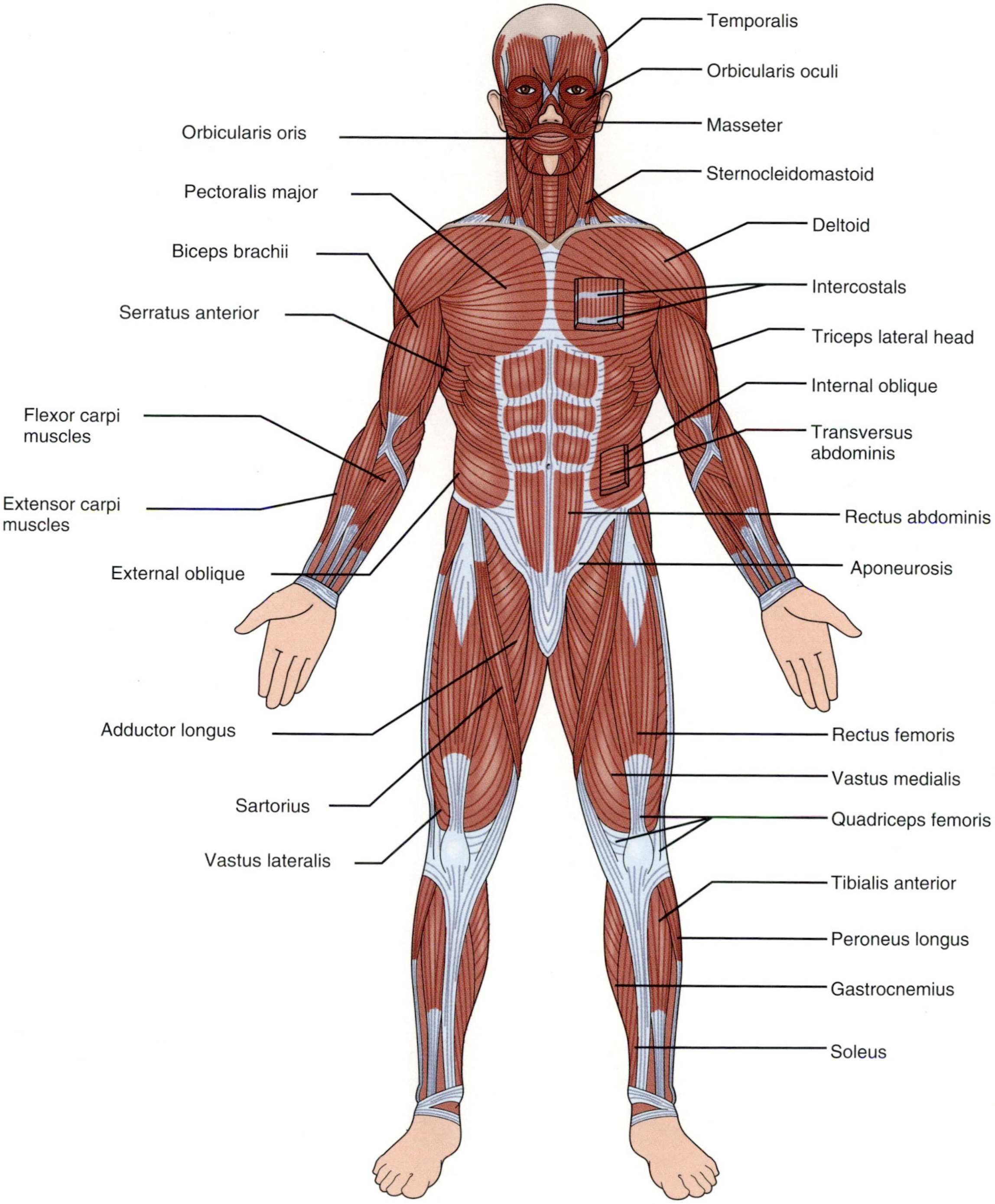
Temporalis
Orbicularis oculi
Masseter
Orbicularis oris
Sternocleidomastoid
Pectoralis major
Deltoid
Biceps brachii
Intercostals
Serratus anterior
Triceps lateral head
Internal oblique
Flexor carpi muscles
Transversus abdominis
Extensor carpi muscles
Rectus abdominis
External oblique
Aponeurosis
Adductor longus
Rectus femoris
Vastus medialis
Sartorius
Quadriceps femoris
Vastus lateralis
Tibialis anterior
Peroneus longus
Gastrocnemius
Soleus

Plate 11A Muscular System, Anterior

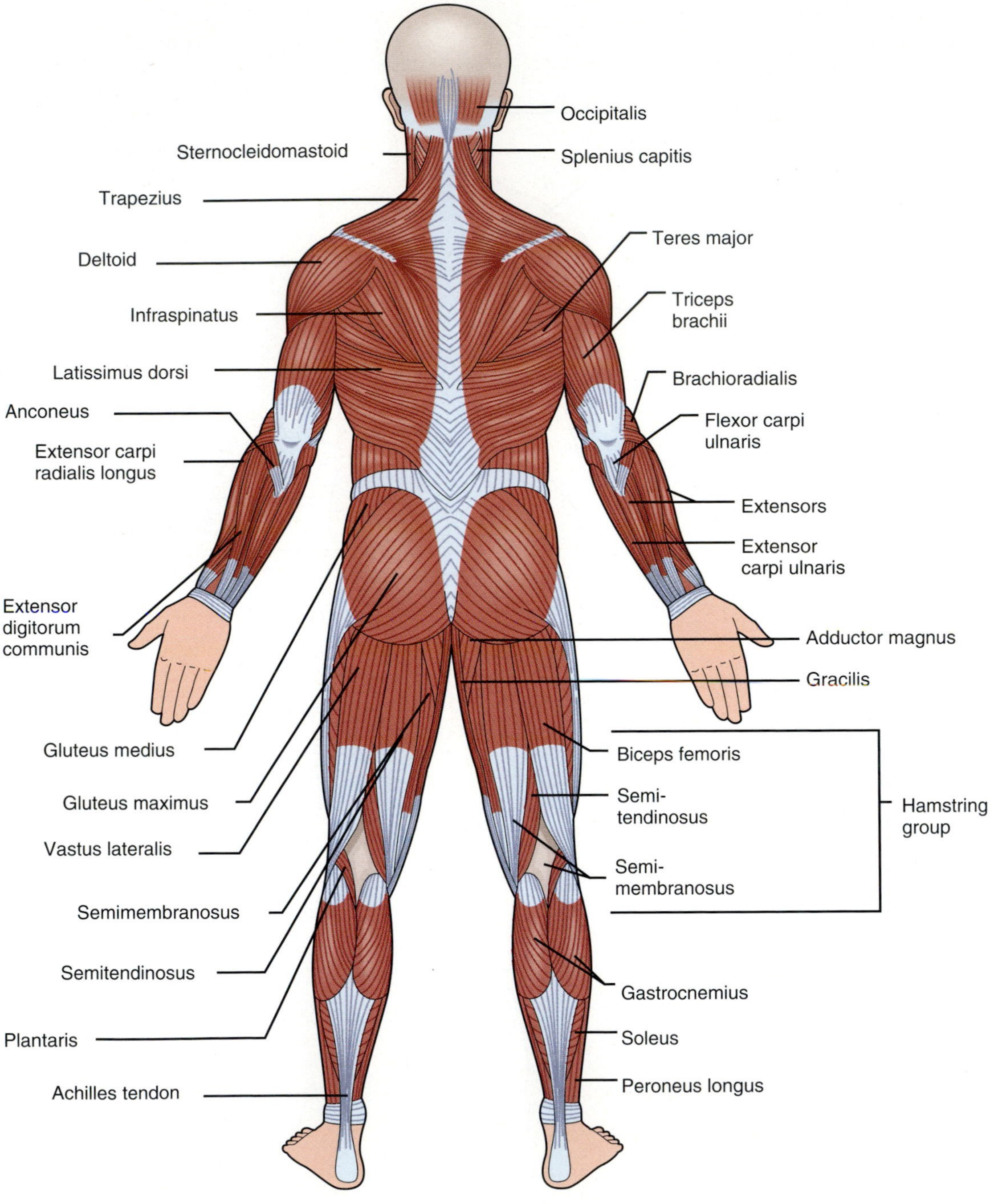
Occipitalis
Sternocleidomastoid
Splenius capitis
Trapezius
Teres major
Deltoid
Triceps brachii
Infraspinatus
Latissimus dorsi
Brachioradialis
Anconeus
Flexor carpi ulnaris
Extensor carpi radialis longus
Extensors
Extensor carpi ulnaris
Extensor digitorum communis
Adductor magnus
Gracilis
Gluteus medius
Biceps femoris
Gluteus maximus
Semi-tendinosus
Hamstring group
Vastus lateralis
Semi-membranosus
Semimembranosus
Semitendinosus
Gastrocnemius
Plantaris
Soleus
Achilles tendon
Peroneus longus

Plate 11B Muscular System, Posterior

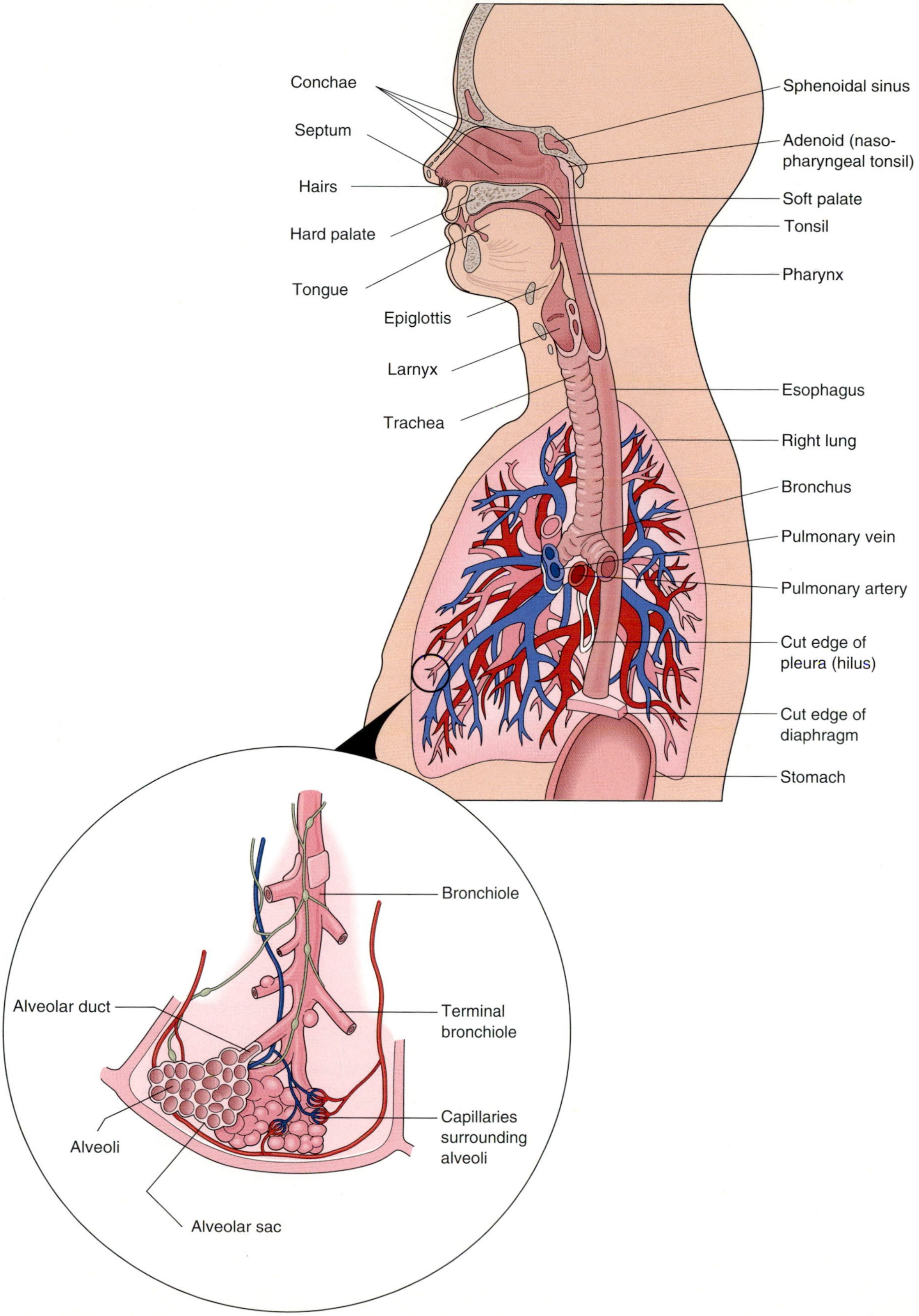
Conchae
Septum
Hairs
Hard palate
Tongue
Epiglottis
Larnyx
Trachea
Sphenoidal sinus
Adenoid (naso-pharyngeal tonsil)
Soft palate
Tonsil
Pharynx
Esophagus
Right lung
Bronchus
Pulmonary vein
Pulmonary artery
Cut edge of pleura (hilus)
Cut edge of diaphragm
Stomach
Bronchiole
Alveolar duct
Terminal bronchiole
Capillaries surrounding alveoli
Alveoli
Alveolar sac

Plate 12 Respiratory System

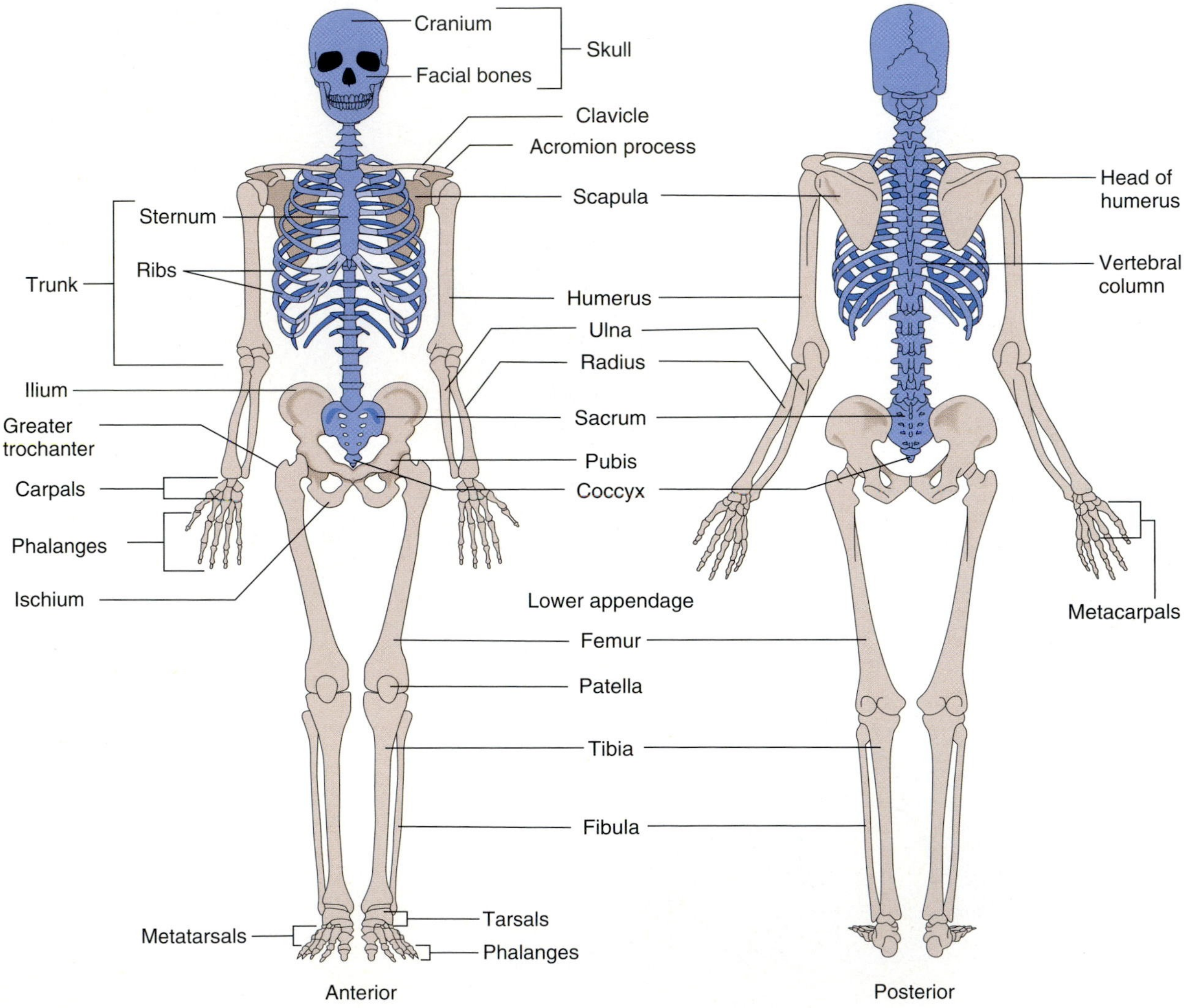
Cranium
Facial bones
Skull
Clavicle
Acromion process
Sternum
Scapula
Head of humerus
Trunk
Ribs
Vertebral column
Humerus
Ulna
Radius
Ilium
Greater trochanter
Sacrum
Pubis
Carpals
Coccyx
Phalanges
Ischium
Lower appendage
Metacarpals
Femur
Patella
Tibia
Fibula
Tarsals
Metatarsals
Phalanges
Anterior
Posterior

Plate 13 Skeletal System

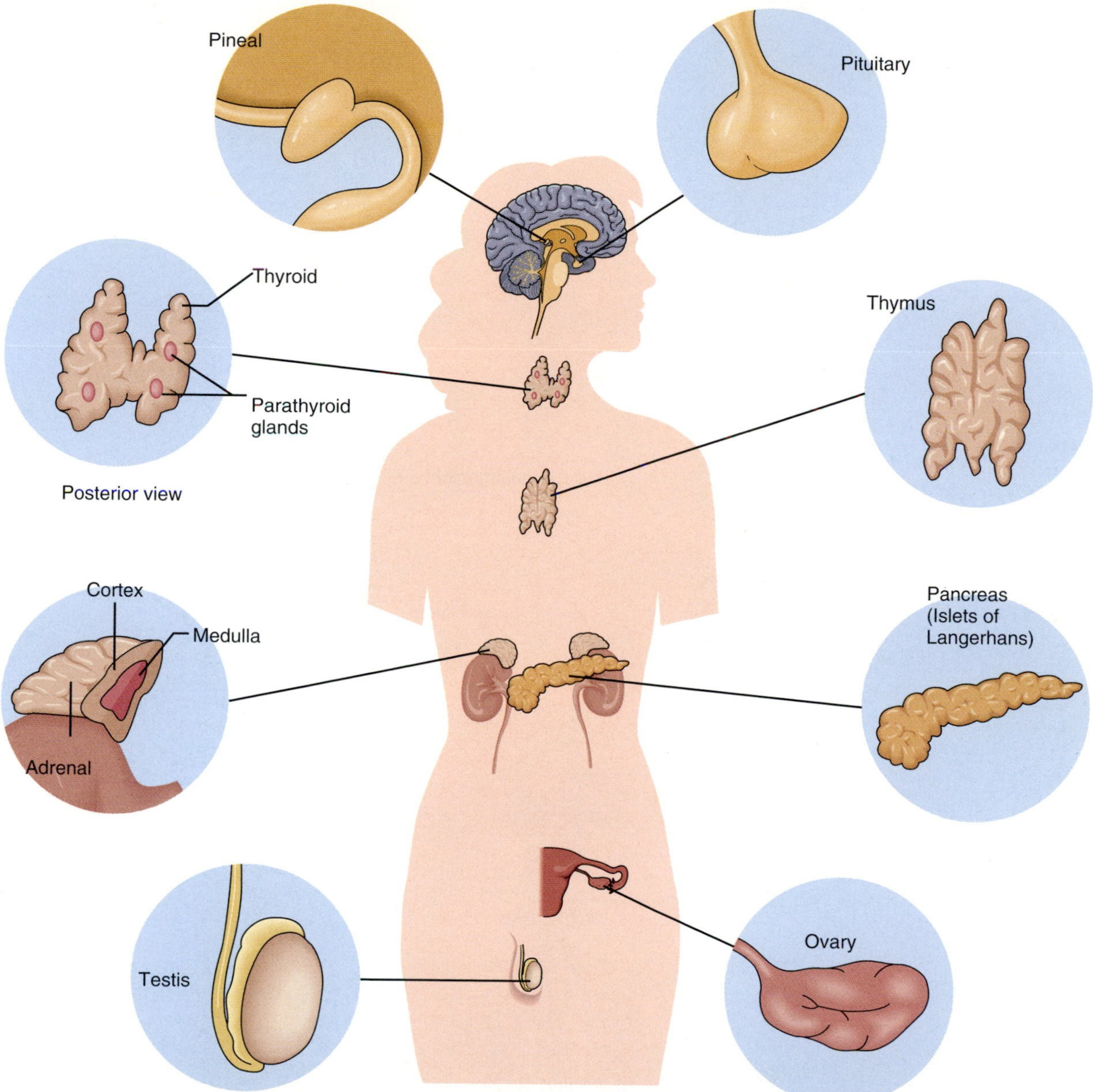

Plate 14 Endocrine System

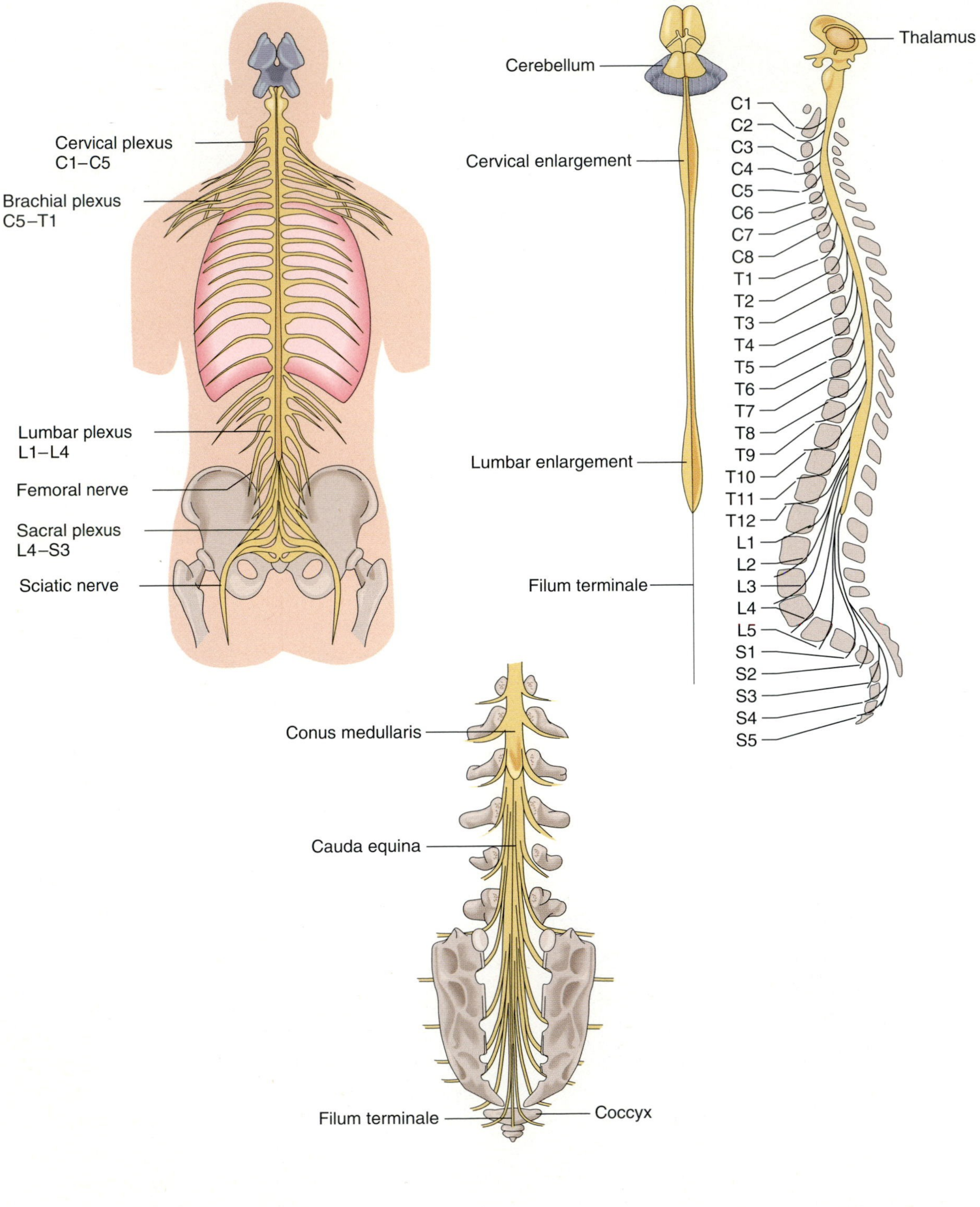
Cervical plexus
C1–C5
Brachial plexus
C5–T1
Lumbar plexus
L1–L4
Femoral nerve
Sacral plexus
L4–S3
Sciatic nerve
Cerebellum
Cervical enlargement
Lumbar enlargement
Filum terminale
Thalamus
C1
C2
C3
C4
C5
C6
C7
C8
T1
T2
T3
T4
T5
T6
T7
T8
T9
T10
T11
T12
L1
L2
L3
L4
L5
S1
S2
S3
S4
S5
Conus medullaris
Cauda equina
Filum terminale
Coccyx

Plate 15 Spinal Cord and Nerves

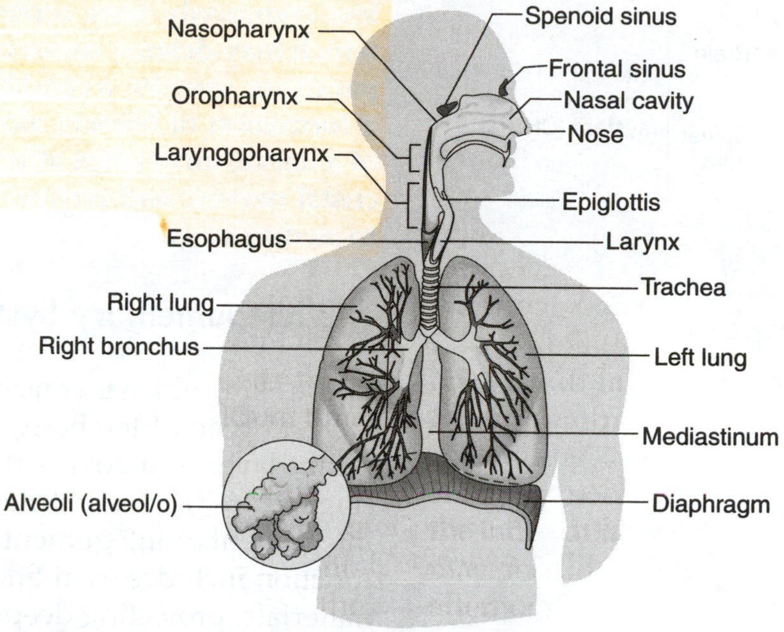

Figure 6-5 Structures of the respiratory system.

is carried to every cell. Carbon dioxide then returns to the alveoli and is eventually exhaled.

Common disorders of the respiratory system include:

- ❒ *asthma*—an allergic reaction in which the bronchioles swell making breathing difficult
- ❒ *bronchitis*—an inflammatory condition of the bronchi
- ❒ *common cold*—the most widespread of all communicable diseases, characterized by swollen and inflamed mucous membrane and discharge from the nose and throat
- ❒ *emphysema*—a condition that causes a swelling of the alveoli due to chronic bronchial obstruction, and which is common in heavy smokers
- ❒ *influenza*—a disease characterized by inflammation of the upper respiratory tract, with generalized aches and pains, and which is highly contagious
- ❒ *pleurisy*—an inflammation of the pleura
- ❒ *pneumonia*—an inflammation of the alveoli of the lung, which may be caused by bacteria or viruses
- ❒ *tuberculosis*—can be either acute or chronic, and is caused by the tubercle bacillus affecting the respiratory system

The Nervous System

The nervous system is our body's main communication system. It consists of three parts: the central nervous system, which is made up of the brain and the spinal cord; the peripheral nervous system, consisting of the nerves extending to the outlying parts of the body; and the autonomic nervous system, which controls all of our involuntary functions, such as the digestive system or the respiratory system (Figure 6-6). The nervous system also includes the sensory organs. These are the structures that make up our eyes and ears, our sense of taste, smell, touch, temperature, pain, pres-

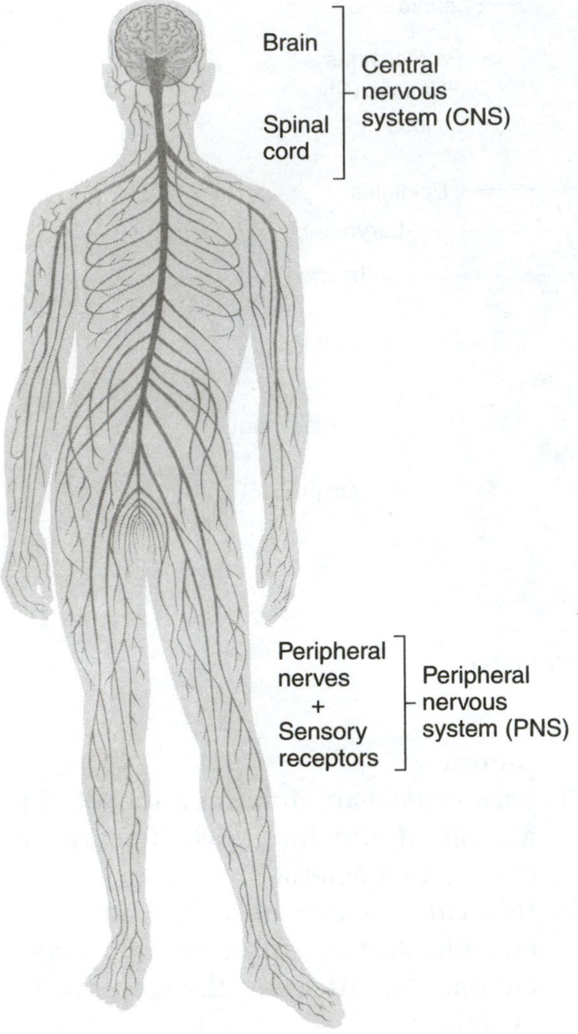

Figure 6-6 Structural organization of the central and peripheral nervous system.

sure, and balance.

Common disorders of the nervous system generally include **cerebrovascular accident (CVA),** often referred to as a stroke, in which there is a destruction of brain tissue as a result of hemorrhage from blood vessels of the brain; *epilepsy,* which is a chronic disorder with abnormality of brain functions, sometimes referred to as convulsive seizures; *meningitis,* an inflammatory condition involving the membrane covering the brain and the spinal cord; **paralysis,** which is a temporary or permanent loss of function, often accompanied by loss of sensation or voluntary motion; *poliomyelitis,* a less commonly seen acute viral disease which may destroy nerve cells and cause paralysis; *shingles,* a condition caused by a formation of blisters along the course of a nerve, most often affecting the intercostal nerves; and *vertigo,* often referred to as dizziness.

The Integumentary System

The skin, which is considered to be the largest organ of the body, is made up of a thin layer that covers the entire body (Figure 6-7). Sometimes called the integument or integumentary system, its function includes excreting excess waste materials, protecting deeper tissues, regulating body heat, and providing us with information about the environment, such as temperature, pain, or pressure, through its receptors. The integumentary system also has accessory organs. These organs include the hair, nails, sweat glands, and the oil glands.

Common disorders of the integumentary system include wounds, or lesions, and skin disease, such as athlete's foot, acne, and fever blisters.

The Urinary System

The primary function of the urinary system is the excretion of the body's waste products. Figure 6-8 shows the parts of the urinary system. The *kidneys* are a pair of bean-shaped organs located on the back of the abdominal wall. Their function is to filter waste materials from the blood. The *ureters* are tubes that extend from the kidneys to the *urinary bladder.* The urinary bladder is the sac in which urine is collected. The *urethra* is the tube from the urinary bladder that extends to the exterior, or outside, of the body.

The blood flows to the kidneys where waste products such as urea, uric acid,

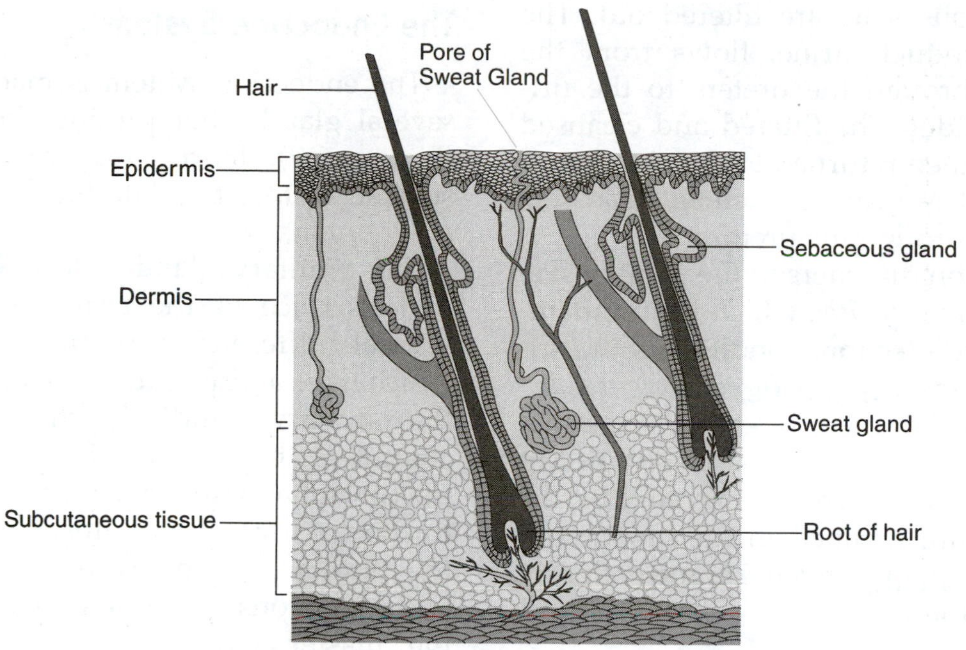

Figure 6-7 Layers of the skin.

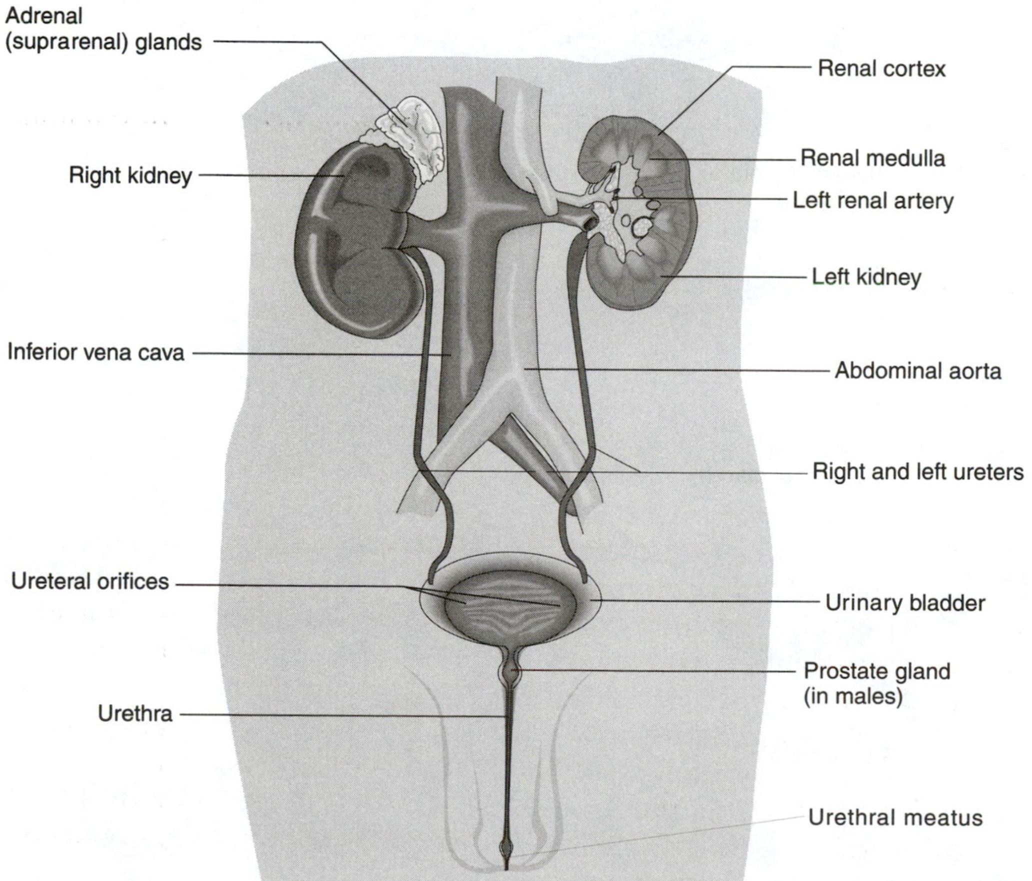

Figure 6-8 Anterior overview of the structures of the urinary system.

and various salts are filtered out. The waste product, urine, flows from the kidney through the ureters to the urinary bladder. The filtered and cleansed blood is then returned to the circulatory system. The urine is excreted from the bladder through the urethra.

Common disorders of the urinary system include *cystitis,* which is an inflammatory or infectious condition of the urinary bladder; **nephritis,** or *Bright's disease,* in which there is severe inflammation of the kidneys; *uremia,* a condition in which wastes normally excreted by the kidneys are retained in the blood; and **urinary calculi,** which are formation of kidney stones.

The Endocrine System

The endocrine system is made up of several glands that produce hormones (Figure 6-9). Hormones are chemical substances that regulate the function of other organs.

The pituitary gland is located at the under-service of the brain. It secretes several different hormones, each of which have a different function. Some of the pituitary gland's functions are the control of the activity of other glands, the control of body growth, and the contraction of involuntary muscles. Because the pituitary is involved in so many body functions, it is often referred to as the "master gland."

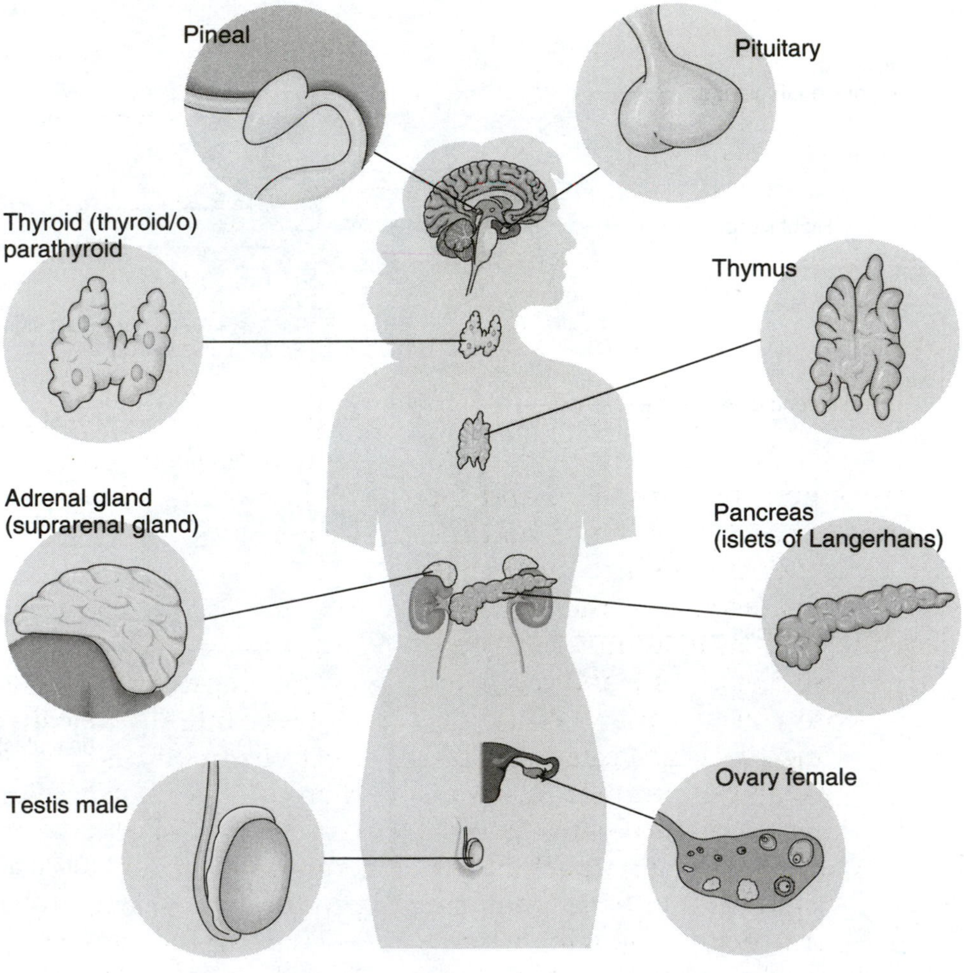

Figure 6-9 Structures of the endocrine system.

Acromegaly is a disease of adults that results from hyperactivity of the anterior pituitary. The bones of the face, hands, and feet widen. *Dwarfism,* a condition in which patients are abnormally small, and *giantism,* in which patients are abnormally large, may result from a deficiency or an excess of a hormone that controls body growth.

The *thyroid gland* is located just below the larynx in the neck. Its main function is to help control our growth and metabolism. The secretion of the thyroid gland is called thyroxine.

An enlargement of the thyroid gland is called a *goiter.* Goiters may result from a lack of iodine in the diet, which is necessary for the proper functioning of the thyroid. If there is an overexertion of thyroxine, an *exophthalmic goiter* can result. In the patient suffering from this disease, we often see the characteristic bulging eyes, a strained appearance of the face, intense nervousness, and a very rapid metabolic rate.

The other glands found in the endocrine system include the two pairs of *parathyroid* glands, which are embedded in the thyroid and control the use of calcium and phosphorus by the body, the two *adrenal* glands, located just above each kidney, responsible for controlling the release of energy in order for us to meet emergency situations and use of water and salt by the body, and the *islands of Langerhans,* which are small groups of cells located in the pancreas that secrete insulin. Insulin controls the rate of glucose metabolism and regulates blood glucose concentration. While the islands of Langerhans are located in the pancreas, they do not produce digestive juices and have no digestive function.

The sex glands are also part of the endocrine system. In the male, they are called the testes, and in the female, they are the *ovaries.* The testes produce hormones that regulation the production of sperm cells and the development of male secondary sex characteristics. The hormones produced by the ovaries regulate the development and activity of the female reproductive system. They are also responsible for the development of the female secondary sex characteristics and for body changes that occur during pregnancy.

Two glands that are least understood by most scientists are the thymus gland and the *pineal* gland. The thymus gland is located in the chest just behind the sternum. It produces hormones that stimulate the production of lymph tissue and lymphocytes. It also functions in immune reactions. However, its function is not well understood. We know that it is present at birth but begins to atrophy after about the age of sixteen. The pineal gland, which is located in the cranial cavity at about the middle of the brain, also provides us with little understanding of its function.

The disease most often associated with the endocrine system is called **diabetes mellitus,** which results from a lack of insulin being produced in the islands of Langerhans. Without enough insulin, the body is unable to use glucose. Patients with diabetes must control the disease by regulating their glucose intake. They do this by taking additional insulin at regular intervals.

The Reproductive System

The reproductive system includes both the internal and the external reproductive organs. Its purpose is to produce reproductive cells, called ovum in the female, and sperm, in the male, which unite in a process called fertilization, to produce a new human life.

The male reproductive system includes the scrotum, testes, penis, and prostate gland (Figure 6-10). The *scrotum* is a sac or pouch suspended between the thighs, which contains a pair of testes. The *testes* produce sperm cells and male sex hormones. The *penis* is the male organ of reproduction and urination, which is located in front of the scrotum. The *prostate gland* surrounds the neck of the gladder and the urethra and produces a fluid that helps sperm cells keep their motility.

The female reproductive system includes the ovaries, fallopian tubes, uterus, vagina, and the vulva (Figure 6-11). The *ovaries* produce egg cells, called ova or ovum, and female sex hormones. They are located in the upper part of the pelvic cavity. The *fallopian tubes* are ducts that lead from an area near the ovary to the uterus and carry the egg cells from the body cavity to the uterus. The *uterus* is the organ that contains and nourishes the embryo during pregnancy. The *vagina,* which is often referred to as the birth canal, is the muscular tube connecting the uterus with the exterior of the body. The *vulva* is the external part of the female reproductive system.

The union of the female's ovum with the male's sperm, is called **fertilization.** This union usually occurs in the fallopian tubes, with the fertilized egg continuing its passage down through the tube until it reaches the uterus. Six to eight days after fertilization takes place, the ovum becomes implanted in the uterine wall. The duration of pregnancy is about 40 weeks or 280 days. At the end of the pregnancy, hormones stimulate contractions of the uterine wall and birth occurs.

If an ovum is not fertilized by the

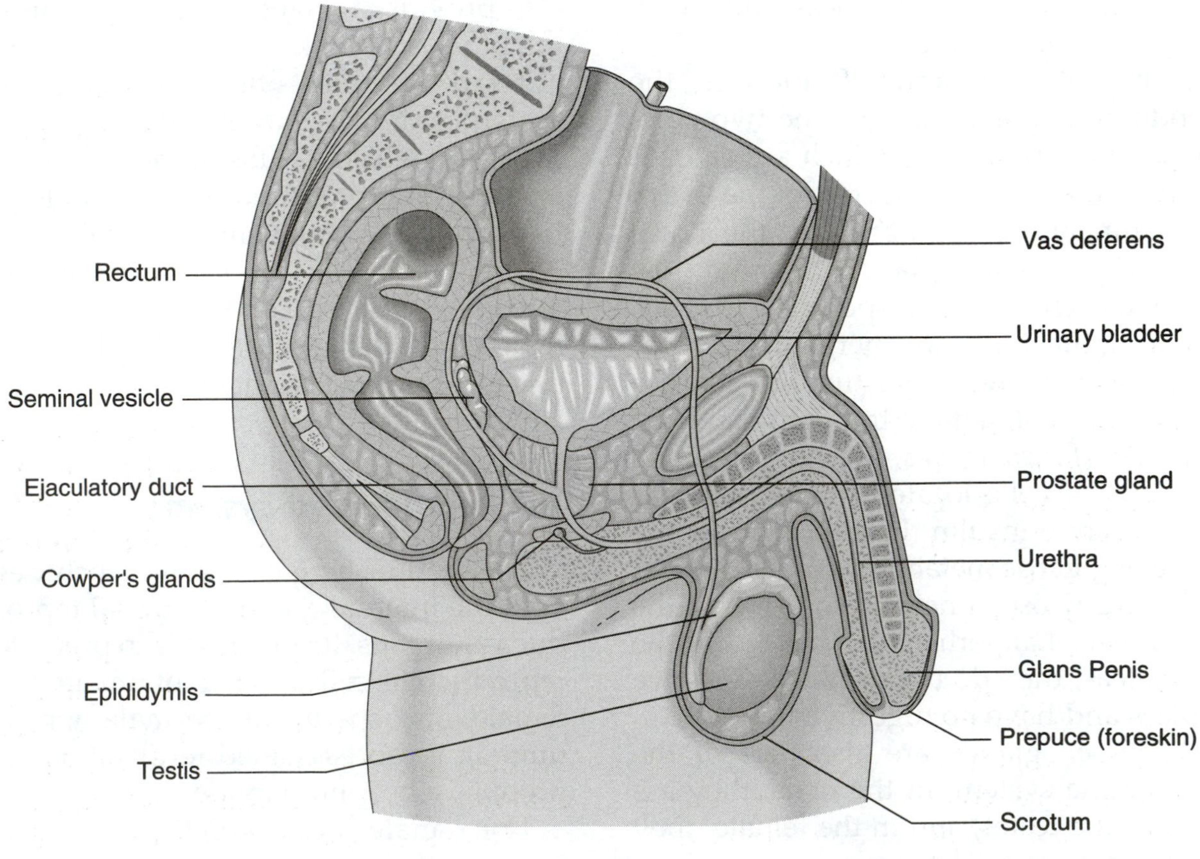

Figure 6-10 Cross section of the male reproductive organs.

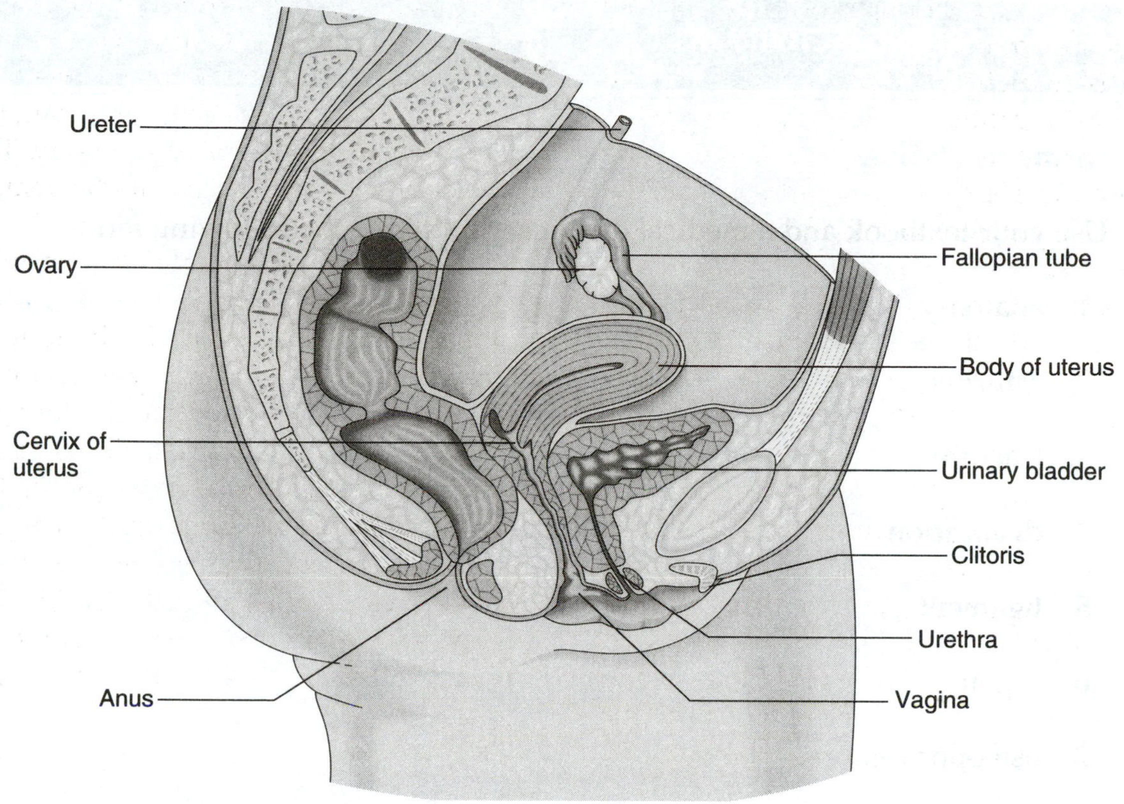

Figure 6-11 Cross section of the female reproductive organs.

sperm, a phenomenon known as *menstruation* occurs. It is the discharge of bloody fluid from the uterus at about twenty-eight-day intervals. Ova are produced at about the middle of this twenty-eight-day period. The uterine wall prepares for the implantation of a fertilized egg, however, when fertilization does not occur, the lining of the uterine wall sloughs off and is discharged. This loss of uterine lining leaves some areas bleeding, thus, blood is discharged from the uterus. The entire menstrual cycle is controlled by hormones.

There are many disorders of the reproductive system, however, the most commonly seen include **dysmenorrhea,** which is painful menstruation; *leukorrhea,* which is a vaginal discharge; **orchitis,** an inflammatory condition of the male's testes, which is often due to trauma, mumps, or other infections; *salpingitis,* which is an inflammatory condition of the fallopian tubes; and *sterility,* a less often seen condition in which either the male or the female may be unable to reproduce.

◆ SUMMARY

In this chapter, we talked briefly about the basic structure and function of the human body. We discussed the fact that there are nine systems of the human body, and each of these systems all have individual structures that function both independently and as part of a group in order to provide us with the necessary processes and functions required to live. We also talked about some of the more commonly seen disorders and medical conditions associated with each of these systems.

◆ ◆ LEARNING ACTIVITY 6-1

Terms to Define

Use your textbook and a medical dictionary to define the following terms:

1. anatomy
2. arthritis
3. fracture
4. dislocation
5. ligament
6. organ
7. osteoporosis
8. physiology
9. rickets
10. sprain
11. system
12. arthro
13. chondro
14. costa
15. cranio
16. osteo

◆ ◆ LEARNING ACTIVITY 6-2

Questions to Answer

Give complete answers to the following questions.

1. Give the purpose of the nervous system.
2. Name the three major divisions of the nervous system.
3. Describe all of the functions of the blood.
4. Name the two major phases of the circulatory systems and describe where each goes.
5. List the five parts of the circulatory system.
6. What organs make up the central nervous system?
7. Give two functions of the reproductive system.
8. Name the male reproductive organ and the types of cells it produces.
9. List the seven glands and the purpose of the hormones secreted by these glands.
10. What is the primary function of the lymphatic system?
11. Name the three regions of the brain and list the specific functions of each region.
12. In what three ways does food nourish the body?
13. What abnormal conditions may cause excessive fluid loses?
14. What are the symptoms of extreme fluid loss or dehydration?
15. Name the female reproductive organ and the type of cells it produces.
16. Define fertilization.
17. List the four components of blood.
18. What is the purpose of the red blood cells?
19. What is the purpose of the white blood cells?
20. How do platelets aid the body?

◆ ◆ LEARNING ACTIVITY 6-3

Terms Relating to Basic Anatomy and Physiology

Match the term to the definition.

a. bronchitis
b. cilia
c. inhalation
d. oxygenation
e. pharyngitis
f. pneumonia
g. tonsillitis

_________ 1. Tiny hairs in the lining of the nasal passages
_________ 2. Inflammation of the pharynx
_________ 3. Inflammation of the lungs caused by bacteria, viruses, or chemical irritants
_________ 4. Drawing air into the lungs
_________ 5. Inflammation of the bronchi
_________ 6. Combined with oxygenation
_________ 7. Inflammation of the tonsils

Match the term to the definition.

a. dehydration
b. digitalis
c. diuretic
d. edema
e. forced fluids
f. heart failure
g. kidney
h. incontinence
i. uremia
j. ureter
k. urinary bladder
l. void
m. urinal

_________ 1. Excessive accumulation of fluids in body tissue
_________ 2. Excessive loss of water from the body
_________ 3. Drug used to increase the output of urine
_________ 4. Excreting urine from the body
_________ 5. Tube connecting the kidney to the urinary bladder
_________ 6. Condition that occurs from failure of the heart to maintain adequate circulation
_________ 7. Organ that removes waste materials from the blood
_________ 8. High fluid intake
_________ 9. Inability to retain urine due to loss of sphincter control
_________ 10. Drug used to increase the force of heart contraction and slow the heartbeat
_________ 11. Failure of the kidney resulting in retention or urea and fluid in the tissues
_________ 12. Micturate
_________ 13. Organ that stores urine
_________ 14. Receptacle into which a patient voids

REVIEW QUESTIONS

1. A __________ is defined as an abnormal dilation or ballooning of a blood vessel.

2. A common bone injury in which there is a break in a bone is called a:
   a. dislocation
   b. fracture
   c. sprain

3. A disease of the musculoskeletal system in which there is an inflammation of bones at the joints with, accompanying pain and swelling of the joints, is called:
   a. dysentery
   b. atherosclerosis
   c. arthritis

4. What is the name of the structures responsible for holding bones together?

5. What structures make up the digestive system?

6. Blood vessels that carry blood away from the heart are called __________. Blood vessels that carry blood toward the heart are called __________.

7. Briefly explain the function of the respiratory system.

8. What is the medical term used to describe a heart attack?

9. Briefly explain the function of the urinary system.

10. Briefly explain the function of the nervous system.

7

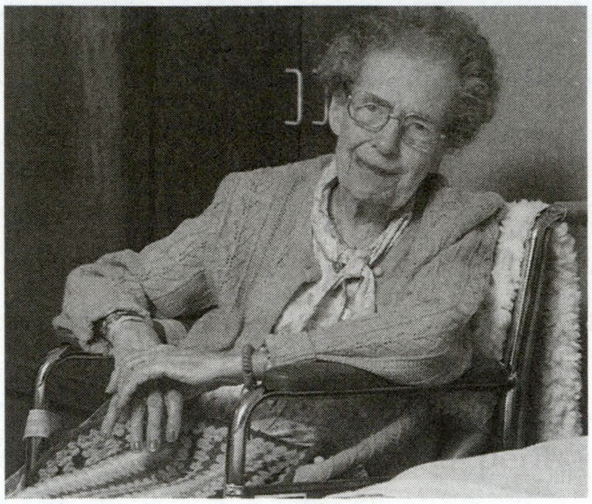

Applied Anatomy and Physiology of the Musculoskeletal System

OBJECTIVES

Upon completion of this chapter, you should be able to:

1. Briefly define the functions of the skeletal system.
2. Describe different types of bone tissue.
3. Discuss the functions of a long bone.
4. Identify the materials required for building bone.
5. Briefly describe the different types of bones.
6. Identify bones in both the axial and appendicular skeleton.
7. Discuss the role cartilage plays in the skeletal system.
8. Describe different types of joints and explain their movements.
9. Explain common disorders of bones, joints, and muscles.
10. Briefly define the functions of the muscular system.
11. Identify and briefly explain different types of muscles.
12. Explain how muscles contract.
13. Explain what is meant by the origin and the insertion of a muscle.

KEY TERMS

Articular cartilage
Articulation
Bursa
Cancellous bone tissue
Compact bone tissue
Contracture
Diaphysis
Endomysium
Endosteum
Epimysium
Epiphysis
Gout
Haversian canals
Kyphosis
Lordosis
Medullary cavity
Muscular dystrophy
Myasthenia gravis
Osteoarthritis
Osteoblast
Osteoclast
Osteocyte
Osteoporosis
Perimysium
Periosteum
Rheumatoid arthritis
Scoliosis
Sesamoid
Volkmann's canals

THE FRAMEWORK OF THE HUMAN BODY

The human body is often compared to a smooth-running machine, which has many intricate parts to it, all of which must work together in order to promote good health, growth, and life itself. As we have already discussed in Chapter 6, the body is a combination of organs and systems that are supported and protected by a framework of bones called the skeleton. The muscles working upon the skeleton provide us with all the basic movements that are needed as we work and play through each day of our lives.

THE SKELETAL SYSTEM

The human skeleton (Figure 7-1), considered the framework of our body, is made up of 206 bones in the body. These bones give form and shape to the various parts of our body. They also protect delicate organs, such as our brain and our

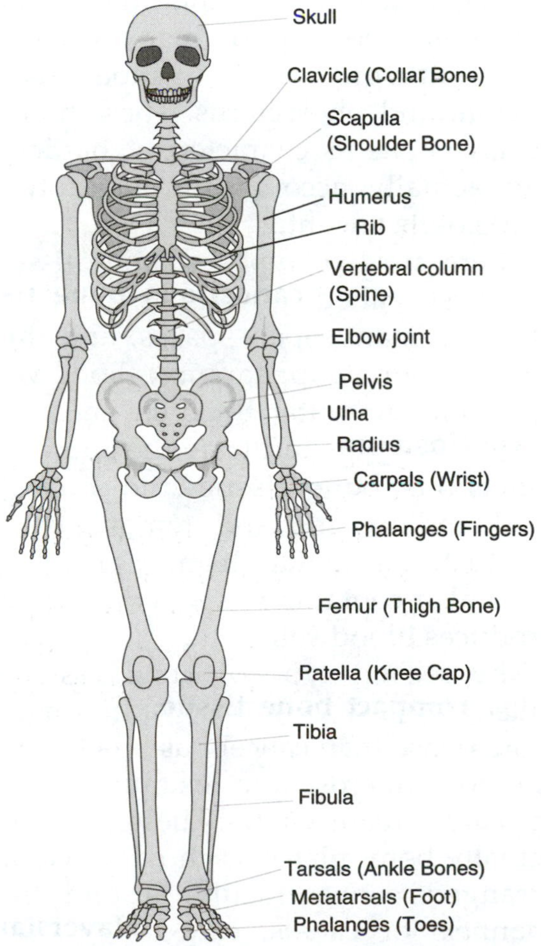

Figure 7-1 The skeletal system, also called the skeleton.

spinal cord. Bones also act as levers. Muscles are attached to the bones in order to enable movement. Bones also act as a storehouse for minerals by manufacturing some of the body's blood cells.

Functions of the Skeletal System

The human skeleton has five basic functions. These include providing support to the body, providing sites for muscles to attach, to make movement or locomotion possible, protection of body parts, producing blood cells, and storing fat and mineral salts, especially of calcium and phosphorus.

Structures of the Skeletal System

Bone is a type of connective tissue, which is made up of many collagen fibers impregnated with compounds of calcium and phosphorus. These minerals give bone its characteristic hardness and actually account for about two-thirds of its weight.

There are two types of bone tissue. The first, called **cancellous bone tissue,** has many open spaces, and thus gives a spongy appearance. Blood vessels from the outer bone cover, called the **periosteum,** infiltrate the spaces in cancellous bone tissue and provide food and oxygen and remove waste products of metabolism. Cancellous bone also contains red marrow, which produces blood cells.

The second type of bone tissue is called **compact bone tissue.** It is much more dense than cancellous bone tissue, and on microscopic examination it appears as many circles. These circles are actually bony plates, each of which are arranged concentrically around tiny channels or canals, called **Haversian canals.** These channels run longitudinally throughout the compact bone. There are also horizontal channels through compact bone, called **Volkmann's canals.** These microscopic channels extend from the periosteum to the Haversian canals and to the inner or medullary cavity of bones. Like the Haversian canals, they also contain minute blood vessels and nerves. Both the Haversian canals and the Volkmann's canals provide us with a means of transporting food, oxygen, and metabolic wastes, and a nerve supply throughout bone tissue.

Bone is considered living tissue and is made up of cells called **osteocytes.** There are two types of osteocytes. The first are called **osteoblasts.** These tiny structures, which actually form collagen fibers using calcium and phosphorus, are most frequently found in the periosteum and endosteum. The second type, called **osteoclasts,** are bone cells that destroy bone tissue.

Our bodies require many regulatory substances in order to build bone tissue. These include compounds of calcium and phosphorus, which are essential for bone production, vitamins A, C, and D, which are necessary for the proper absorption of mineral compounds, and the hormone *parahormone,* which is produced by the parathyroid glands and is required for the proper regulation of calcium and phosphorus levels in the blood. Deficiencies in any of these minerals, vitamins, and hormones can result in serious disorders of the skeletal system.

Structure of a Long Bone

Before we can actually discuss the different types of bones found in the human body, it is important that you first have a basic understanding of the gross structure of all bones. To better comprehend what each of these structures look like, let's look at a diagram of

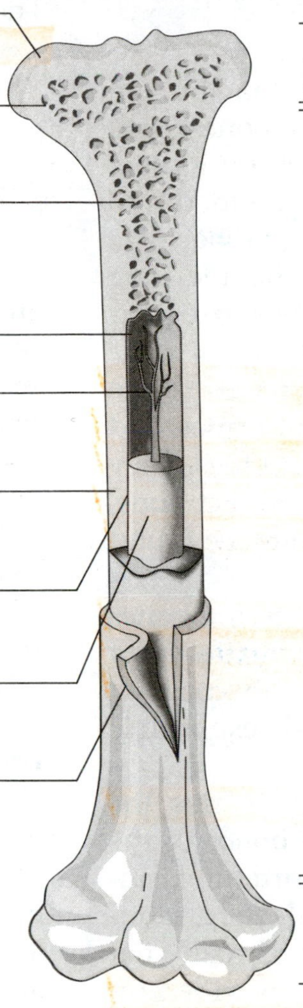

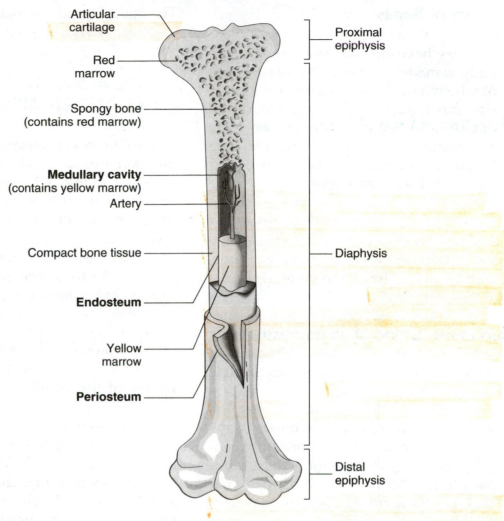

Figure 7-2 Anatomic features of a typical long bone.

a long bone (Figure 7-2).

The long, main portion or shaft of the bone is called the **diaphysis.** It appears hollow and cylindrical in shape, and is made up primarily of compact bone. The cylindrical shape of the bone provides it with the ability to accommodate maximum strength and support with minimum weight.

The ends of the long bones are called **epiphyses.** Their rounded shapes provide maximum space for muscle attachment, and their cancellous bone makeup and spongy appearance make the epiphyses more able to withstand shocks and jolts without harm.

The white, fibrous protective covering on the outer surface of the bone, which is well supplied with blood vessels, nerves, and lymph vessels, is called the **periosteum.** The periosteum is essential for bone growth and maintenance.

The hollow shaft of a long bone is called the **medullary cavity.** This cavity, which contains yellow bone marrow, is lined with the **endosteum,** which is primarily composed of osteoblasts with a few osteoclasts.

Articular cartilage covers the epiphyses in areas where the ends of separate bones meet in order to form a joint. This cartilage provides protection for the bone ends and helps to ensure smooth movement of the joints.

Types of Bones

As we have already stated, the human body is made up of over 200 bones, each of which have been modified for its specific function. They can be divided into five broad groups according to their size and shape. These groups include long bones, short bones, flat bones, irregular bones, and sesamoid bones.

Long bones include the bones of the upper and lower arm, the upper and lower leg, and the fingers and toes. They are mainly composed of compact bone, although cancellous bone may be found in the epiphyses.

Short bones, which include the bones of the wrist and ankle, are made up of cancellous bone covered with compact bone. These bones are most responsible for providing strength.

Flat bones, which include the ribs, the scapulae, and some of the bones of the skull, consist of an inner portion of cancellous bone with an outer layer of compact bone. Because of the broad, flat shape of these bones, they provide protection for vulnerable body parts and large areas of muscle attachment.

Irregular bones have unusual and specialized shapes. Their overall function is articulation, and their irregular shape makes it possible for them to fit smoothly in order to form joints. Some examples of irregular bones include the vertebrae of the spinal column, the bones of the inner ear, and some of the facial bones. Irregular bones are made up of inner cancellous bone covered with an outer layer of compact bone.

Sesamoid bones, which are small, rounded bones found next to joints, are covered with cartilage or ligaments. Their primary function is to help eliminate friction in joints and thus increase the efficiency of motion in hinge joints. The patella, or kneecap, is an example of a sesamoid bone.

◆ THE AXIAL AND APPENDICULAR SKELETONS

The human skeleton is usually grouped into the axial and appendicular skeletons (Table 7-1 and 7-2). The *axial skeleton* refers to bones which have been arranged around the long axis of the body. These include the bones of the skull, the vertebral column, the ribs, the sternum, the three small bones of the ear, and the hyoid bones.

◆ THE AXIAL SKELETON

Bones of the Skull

The bones of the skull include those of the *cranium*, which enclose and protect the brain, and the *facial* bones, which include the bones of the nose, cheeks, and the jaws. There are eight cranial bones and fourteen facial bones. The cranial bones include the *frontal, occipital, parietal, temporal, sphenoid,* and *ethmoid* bones (Figure 7-3). These bones form immovable or *synarthrotic* joints, and their surfaces are united by a thin, fibrous membrane, which gives greater protection from possible injury. In an infant, space between the cranial bones provides room for growth of the skull. These spaces are called *fontanels*, and are protected from injury by the fibrous membrane. Bone formation continues as the child grows and the fontanels close.

The Facial Bones

The facial bones include the *palatines*, which form the hard palate of the mouth

BONES OF THE SKULL				NUMBER OF BONES	
Cranium	frontal			1	
	occipital			1	
	parietal			2	
	temporal			2	
	sphenoid			1	
	ethmoid			1	(8)
Facial bones	turbinate			2	
Upper jaw	maxilla			2	
	nasal			2	
Cheek	zygomatic (malar)			2	
Lower jaw	mandible			1	
	lacrimal			2	
	palatine			2	
	vomer			1	(14)
Spinal column	vertebrae				
	cervical	1-7		7	
	thoracic	8-19		12	
	lumbar	20-24		5	
	sacral	25-29*		5	
	coccygeal	30-33**	1	(26; 30 in child)	
Chest (thorax)	ribs (12 pair)			24	
	sternum (including xiphoid process)			1	(25)
Inner ear bones	malleus			2	
	incus			2	
	stapes			2	(6)
Horseshoe-shaped bone	hyoid			1	(1)

*These fuse in adults to form the sacrum. **These fuse in adults to form the coccyx.

Table 7-1 The Axial Skeleton

	COMMON NAME	TECHNICAL NAME		NUMBER OF BONES	
Upper Extremities:	Shoulder girdle	clavicle		2	
		scapula		2	
	Upper arm	humerus		2	
	Lower arm	radius		2	
		ulna		2	
	Wrist	carpals		16	
	Hand	metacarpals		20	
	Fingers	phalanges		28	(64)
Lower Extremities:	Hip girdle	ilium	(these fuse in the adult to form		
	(pelvic girdle)	ischium	the innominate or hipbone)		
		pubis		2	
	Thigh	femur		2	
	Lower leg	tibia		2	
		fibula		2	
	Kneecap	patella		2	
	Ankle	tarsals		14	
	Foot	metatarsals		10	
	Toes	phalanges		28	(62)

Table 7-2 The Appendicular Skeleton

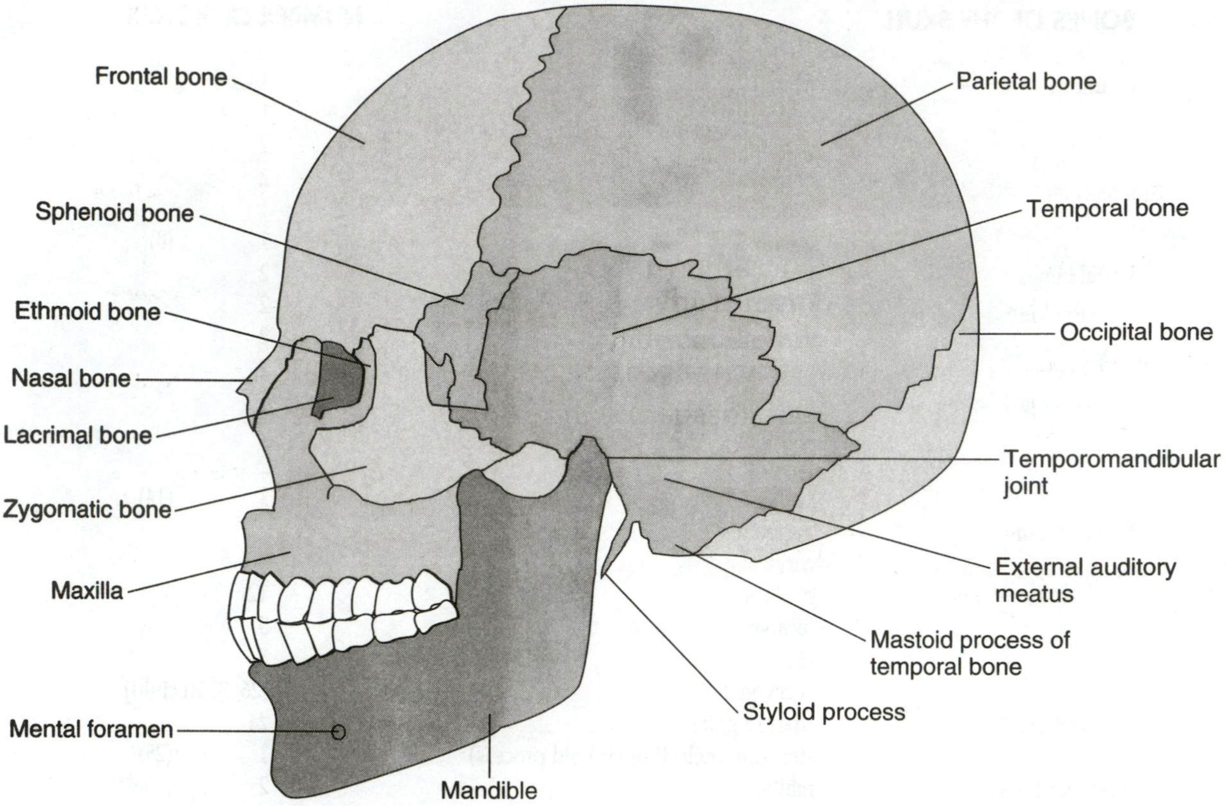

Figure 7-3 Lateral view of the skull.

and the lateral nasal wall, the *nasal bones,* the upper jaw or *maxillae,* the lower jaw or *mandible,* and the cheekbones, or *zygomatic (malar)* bones (Figure 7-4). The *lacrimal* bones, which are found at the inner side of the eye cavity, have a tiny groove that accommodates a portion of the tear or lacrimal duct. The *vomer* bone forms the lower and back portions of the nasal septum. And the *nasal conchae,* or *turbinate* bones, extend from the lateral wall of the nasal cavity.

The Spinal Column and Vertebrae

The vertebrae make up the spinal column (Figure 7-5). They protect the delicate nerves and structures that make up the spinal column, and help to make posture possible. In adults, there are twenty-six vertebrae, and in children, there are thirty-three. This difference is because in adulthood, several vertebrae fuse together. The vertebrae are numbered for convenience. The first seven are called *cervical* vertebrae, and are numbered C1 through C7. The next twelve are called the *thoracic* vertebrae, numbered T1 through T12. These provide dorsal attachment for the ribs. The next five are called the *lumbar* vertebrae, numbered L1 through L5, followed by five *sacral* vertebrae. The last vertebrae are called the *coccygeal* vertebrae. In children, there are four to five separate coccygeal vertebrae, which ultimately fuse together in adults to form the *coccyx.*

The Ribs

There are twelve pairs of ribs, which protect the delicate structures that make up our heart and lungs. These ribs attach

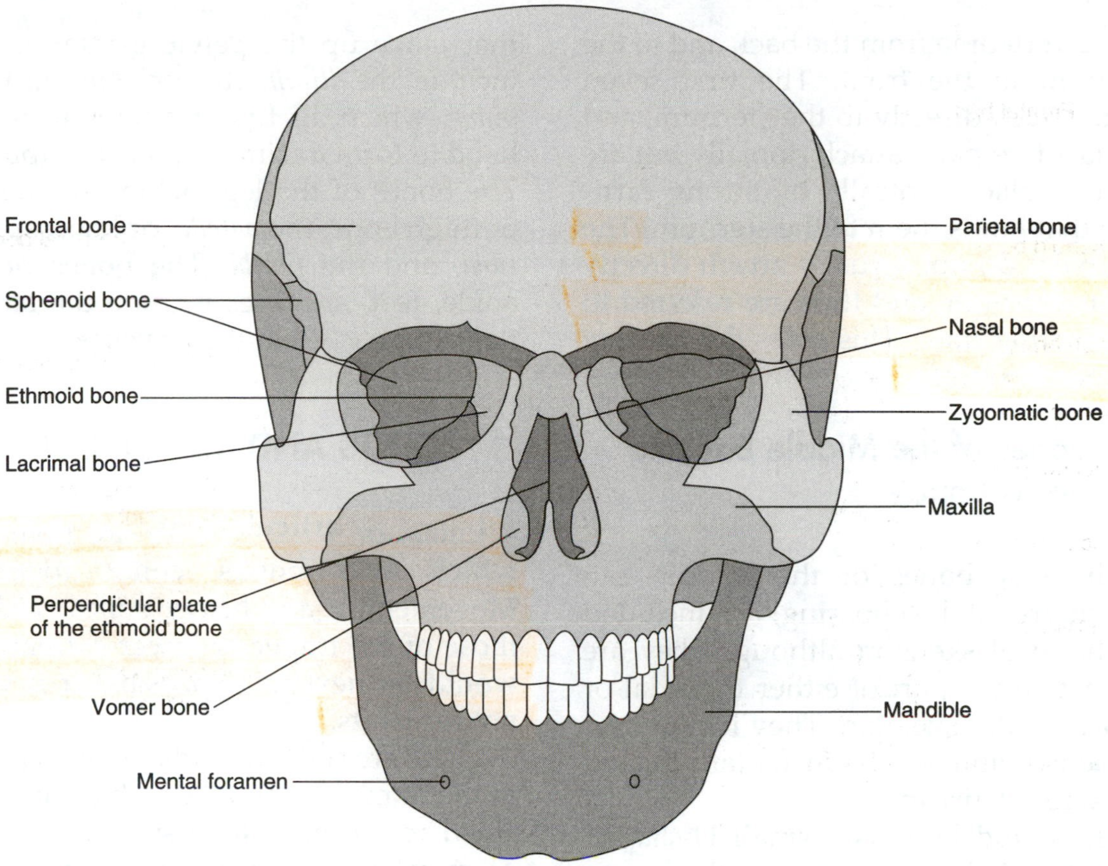

Figure 7-4 Anterior view of the skull.

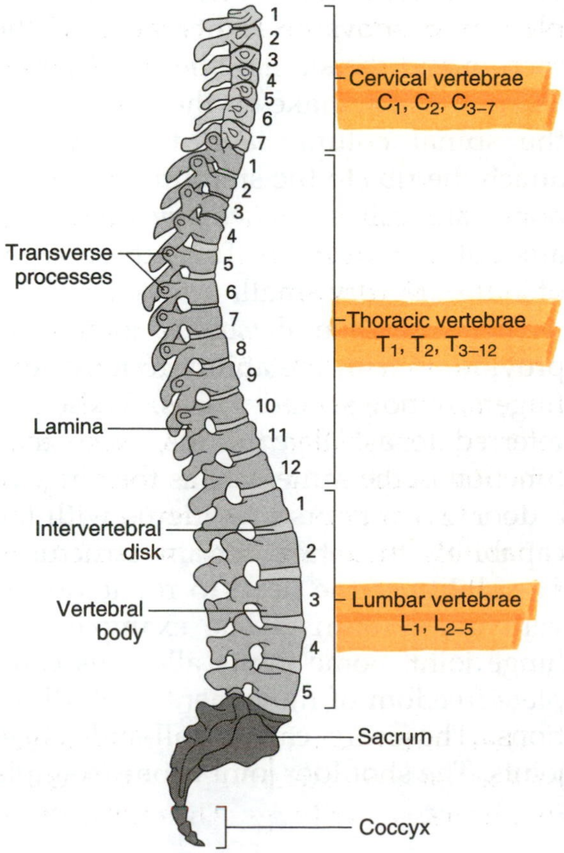

Figure 7-5 Lateral view of the spinal column.

to the vertebrae from the back and to the sternum in the front. The first seven pairs attach directly to the sternum, and the last five pairs attach dorsally but are held in place ventrally by strong cartilage that binds them to the sternum. The last pairs do not actually attach directly to the sternum, and thus are referred to as "floating ribs." This gives the rib cage greater flexibility.

The Bones of the Middle Ear and the Hyoid Bone

The tiny bones of the middle ear, which are vital to hearing, are included in the axial skeleton although they are not actually a part of either the axial or appendicular skeleton. They include the malleus (hammer, the incus (anvil), and the stapes (stirrup).

The hyoid bone is a small U-shaped bone that is located between the larynx and the mandible. It is quite unique in that it does not attach to any other bone, but rather is suspended from the styloid process of the temporal bone of the skull. It is very important because it provides an attachment for some of the muscles of the tongue.

◆ THE APPENDICULAR SKELETON

The appendicular skeleton includes all of the bones of the upper and lower extremities. This includes the bones of the shoulder girdle, the bones of the pelvic girdle, or hip, and the bones that make up the feet and toes.

The shoulder girdle consists of the *clavicle* and *scapula,* the *humerus* of the upper arm, the *radius* and *ulna* of the lower arm, the *carpals* of the wrist, the metacarpals of the hand, and the phalanges, or fingers, of the hand. The bones that make up the pelvic girdle, or hip, include the *ilium,* the *ischium,* and the *pubis,* which all fuse together in adulthood to form the innominate or hipbone. The bones of the leg include the femur, or thigh bone, the *patella,* or kneecap, the *tibia,* and the *fibula.* The bones of the ankle, feet, and toes include the *tarsals,* the *metatarsals* and the *phalanges.*

◆ JOINTS AND MOVEMENT

Joints, or **articulations,** are points at which two bones come together. Movement of any heavy bones, such as those of the upper or lower extremities, would be next to impossible if it were not for joints.

There are several kinds of joints found in the human body, all of which are classified according to their specific function or movement. Some are referred to as *immovable* because of their ability to provide stability and protection. Two examples of immovable joints include the sacrum and the skull. Other joints, such as those which make up the vertebrae of the spinal column and those which attach the ribs to the sternum, or breastbone, are called *partially movable.* The amount of movement from these types of joints are very small.

There are several *movable* joints that provide us with the ability to move our fingers, elbows, and knees. These are referred to as *hinged* joints, since they function in the same way as the hinge of a door. Pivot joints provide us with the capability to rotate certain structures. The ability of the head to rotate on the vertebral column is one example of a hinge joint. Some joints allow us complete freedom of movement in all directions. These are called ball-and-socket joints. The shoulder joint is one example of a ball-and-socket joint. And some joints have only one bony surface, thus allowing the bone to glide over another bony surface. These are called gliding joints. The wrist is an example of a gliding joint.

The type of movement at a specific joint is determined by the structure of the individual joint. And, as we have already stated, it would be impossible for us to maneuver or move any part of our body without the use of our joints.

There are several different types of movement that individual joints can accomplish. *Flexion,* for example, gives the joint the ability to decrease the size of an angle (Figure 7-6), while *extension* is just the opposite in that it allows the joint to straighten (Figure 7-7). A good example of flexion and extension is the movement of the elbow. While flexion brings the forearm close to the humerus and thus decreases the size of the angle, extension allows the arm to straighten.

Abduction is a motion that provides a bone with the ability to move away from the body (Figure 7-8), while *adduction* makes it possible to move the bone toward the body (Figure 7-9). If you move your foot away from the side of your body, that's an example of abduction; returning the foot to the side is adduction. *Rotation* is the movement that allows a bone to move on its own axis, such as your skull having the ability to move on the axis of the spinal column

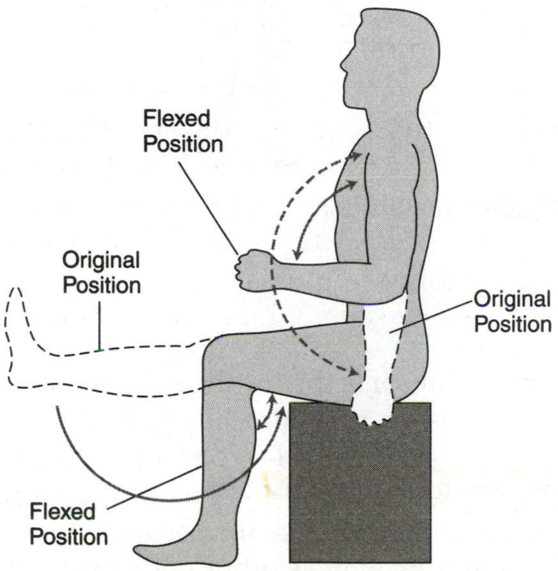

Figure 7-6 Flexion—bending a joint.

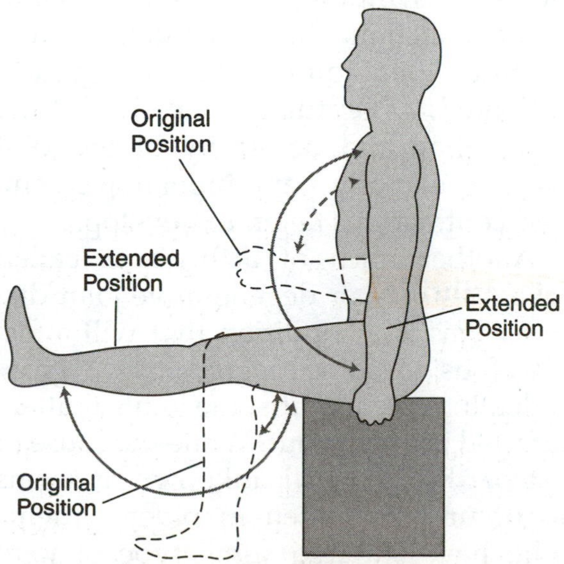

Figure 7-7 Extension—straightening a joint.

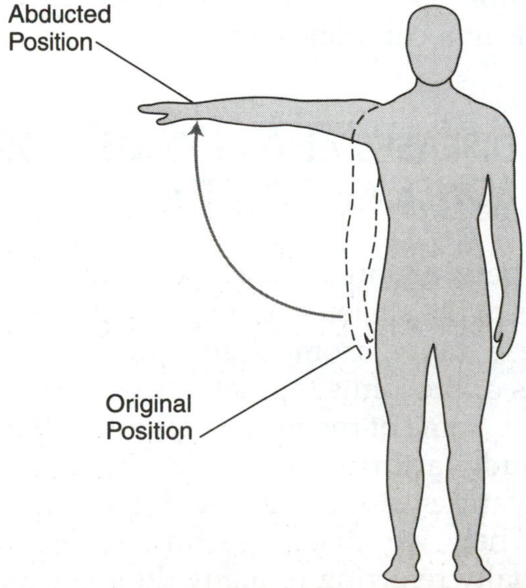

Figure 7-8 Abduction—moving an extremity away from the body.

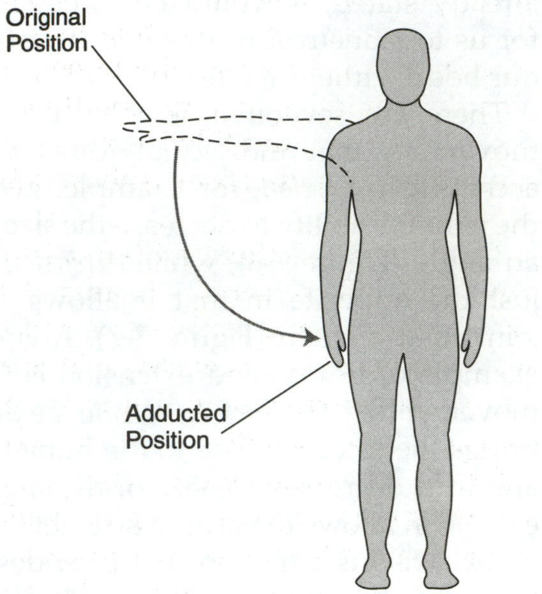

Figure 7-9 Adduction—moving an extremity back to the body.

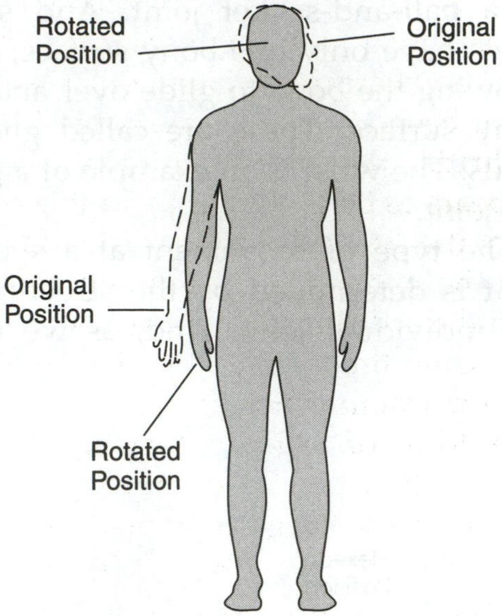

Figure 7-10 Rotation.

(Figure 7-10). Turning your head from side to side is an example of rotation. Finally, *circumduction,* which is the action of one end of a bone in a circle while the other end remains stationary, involves all of the movements of flexion and extension, abduction and adduction, and rotation. A good example of circumduction is moving your outstretched arms in a complete circle.

◆ DISEASES AND DISORDERS OF BONES AND JOINTS

There are many diseases and disorders of the skeletal system and the joints. These range from degenerative disorders of the joints to fractures of the bone itself. Some of the most common of these include arthritis, osteoporosis, rickets, curvatures of the spine, and gout.

When we discuss arthritis, we are actually referring to many different conditions of the skeletal system that may cause pain and deformity in the joints. In some forms of arthritis, the skin and connective tissue may also be affected.

There are several types of arthritis. **Rheumatoid arthritis** is one of the more serious types because it affects the bones and joints as well as other body systems, such as the lungs, muscles, skin, blood vessels, and the heart. The cause of rheumatoid arthritis is still unknown, but it has symptoms very similar to that of an infection. The structures located within the joint become greatly inflamed, eventually causing total destruction and deformity of the joint itself. Eventually, pain limits movement, and contractures begin to develop.

Another form of arthritis is called **osteoarthritis,** or degenerative joint disease. This is a condition that will affect all of us to some degree as we grow older. In osteoarthritis, the joints that are affected just wear out. While the cause of osteoarthritis is still unknown, it seems to occur more often in older patients who have suffered some type of joint trauma or in patients who are obese.

A third type of arthritis, which is caused by a bacterial infection, is called infectious arthritis. While other bacteria have been known to cause this form of arthritis, the most common offender appears to be gonococcus. In this condition, the patient's knee, wrist, and ankle are the joints most commonly affected, and the arthritis almost always occurs at the same time the patient has a genital gonorrheal infection.

A form of arthritis that affects over one million people each year, is **gout.** When present, gout generally affects only one joint, usually the big toe, and is characterized by crystal deposits in and around the affected point.

A disorder of the skeletal system that seems to be most commonly seen in elderly women and in those patients who have been confined to bed for long periods of time is **osteoporosis.** In this condition, there is a loss of mineral from the bone itself, thus causing the bones to become brittle and fracture more easily.

Two diseases that affect both the bone and the joints are *rickets,* which is a disease often affecting infants and children who do not have enough vitamin D in their diet, thus causing the bones not to harden properly and resulting in deformation and bending of the bones; and *bursitis,* an inflammatory condition of the **bursa,** or fluid-filled sacs in and around joints and tissues where friction would occur.

In addition to suffering from degenerative and inflammatory diseases of the skeletal system and joints, some patients may also experience some type of curvature of the spinal column. The most common of these include **kyphosis,** which refers to an exaggeration of the natural posterior curve, thus causing the patient to talk with a hunchbacked appearance; **scoliosis,** which is a side to side curvature of the spine; and **lordosis,** which is an exaggerated inward curvature of the lumbar region of the spinal column.

Fractures of the Skeletal System

No discussion of the disorders and injuries of the skeletal system would be complete without mentioning fractures (Figure 7-11). A fracture is a broken bone. It may be either closed (simple), or open (compound). An open fracture involves

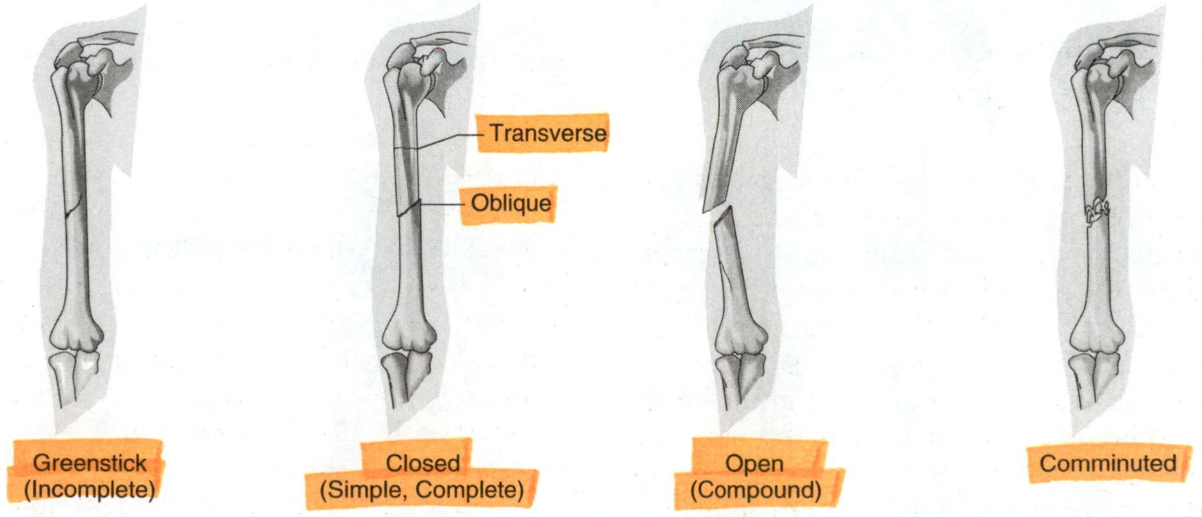

Figure 7-11 Types of fractures.

a break in the skin, as well as the bone, causing the bone ends to protrude through the skin. A closed fracture can be classified as a greenstick, complete, comminuted, or spiral. Greenstick fractures generally occur most often in children because their bones are much more flexible and tend to bend like a green stick rather than break. The greenstick fracture is incomplete. A complete fracture occurs when the two ends of the bone separate at the time of the break. A comminuted fracture is caused as a result of a complete fracture of the bone into more than two pieces. When this type of fracture occurs, surgery is generally indicated in order to reset the bone fragments. Spiral fractures, which are not often seen, generally result from twisting injuries, such as those suffered in skiing accidents.

Sprains and Dislocations

A sprain is an injury to the ligaments or connective tissue that supports a joint. A dislocation, on the other hand, is the actual separation of the bones that make up the joint. Many times, because of the severity of the trauma causing a joint to dislocate, a muscle strain or sprain may also occur with the dislocation. This type of dislocation is often characterized by an abnormal position and deformity of the affected joint.

◆ THE MUSCULAR SYSTEM

The muscular system has three basic functions (Figure 7-12). The first, and perhaps the single most important function, is to provide our body with its abil-

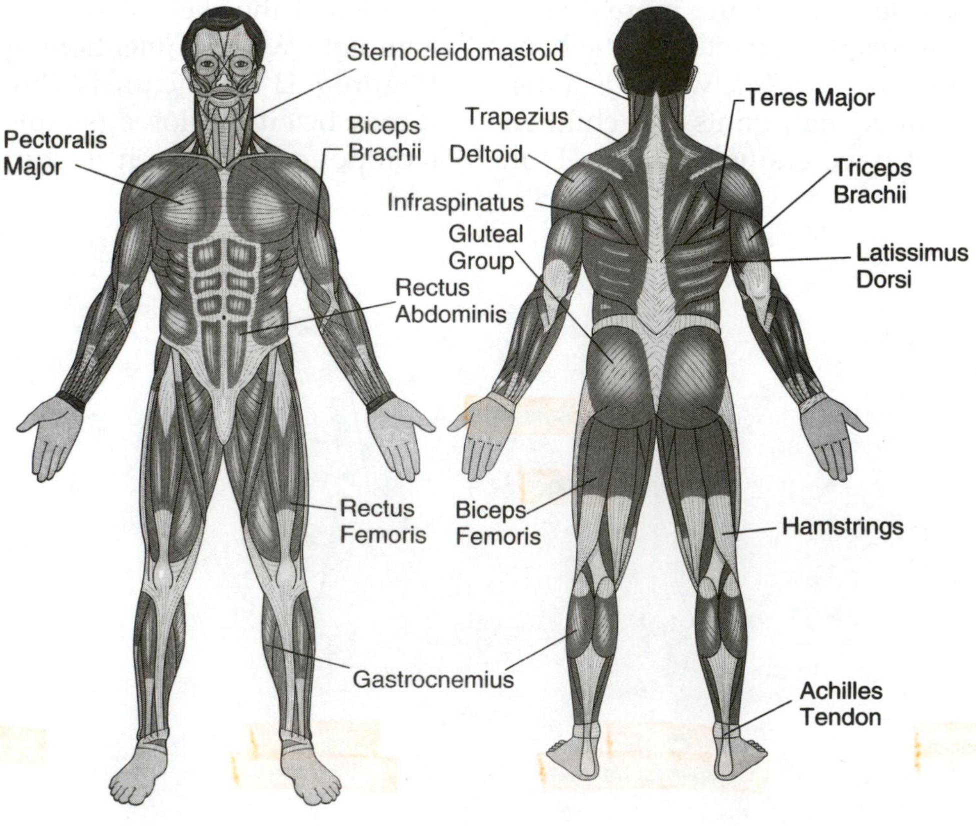

Figure 7-12 The muscular system.

ity to move. One only has to suffer the inability to be able to move, or to have limited motion, in order to realize just how important and relevant our muscles are to us. Another function of muscles is to maintain body positions or posture. This is how we are able to stand, sit, kneel, stoop, or assume any other posture. A third important function of the muscles is their ability to help maintain our body's temperature. Because of the size, or mass of muscles, they are able to produce large amounts of body heat that can later be transported throughout our body by means of circulating blood.

There are three types of muscle tissue (Figure 7-13). These include *skeletal* muscles, *smooth* muscles, and *cardiac* muscles. Skeletal muscles, along with the bones of the skeletal system, make it possible for us to move all the parts of our body. This includes not only our arms and legs, but also our internal organs, such as our diaphragm when we

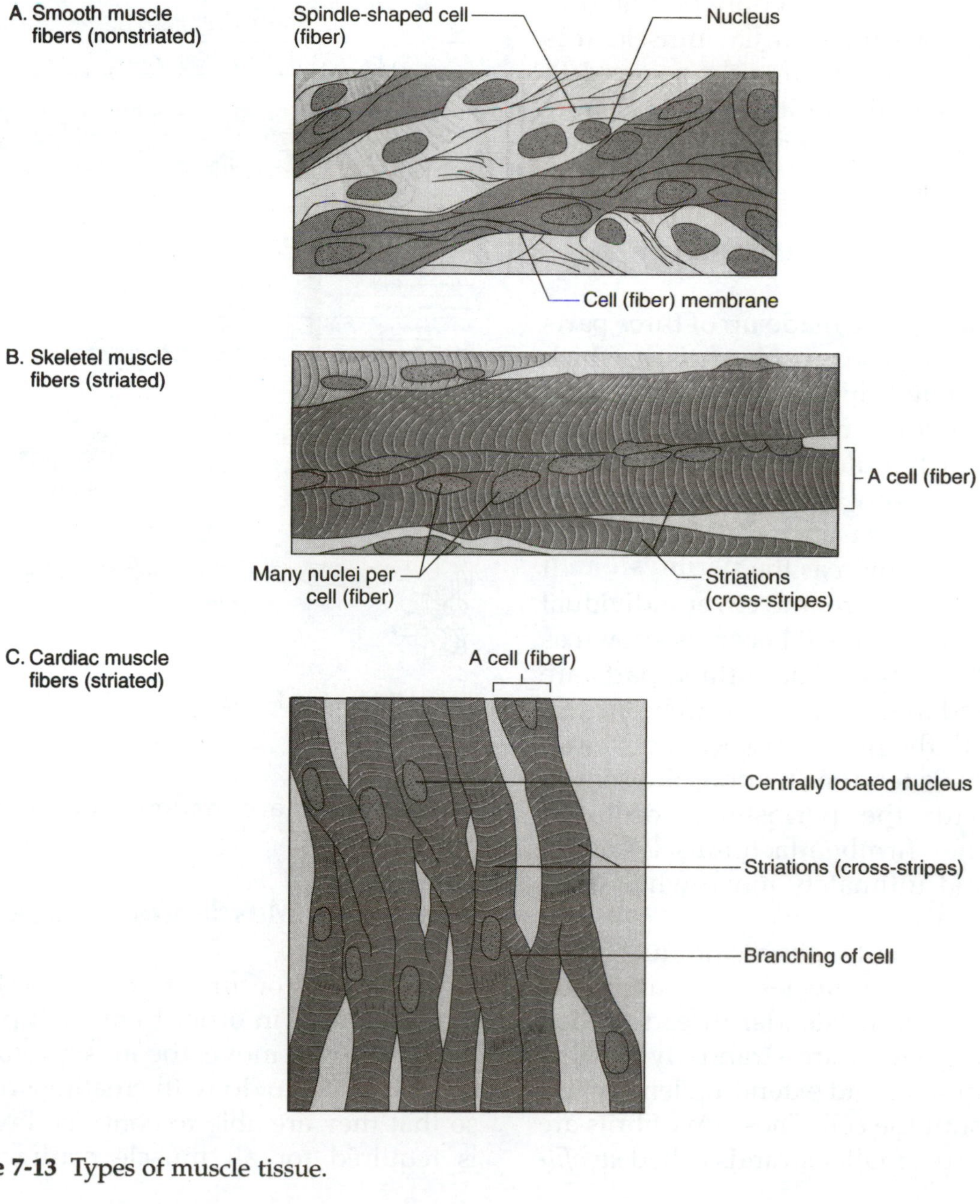

Figure 7-13 Types of muscle tissue.

breathe or the beating of our heart. Skeletal muscles, which are also called voluntary, and which attach themselves to bone, make up about 40 to 50 percent of our entire body weight.

Smooth muscles give our body its ability to control certain activities below our level of consciousness. For this reason, they are often referred to as *involuntary* muscles. Because internal organs or viscera are also controlled by smooth muscles, they may also be called *visceral* muscles.

The muscle that can only be found in the heart are called cardiac muscle. It is also an involuntary muscle, referred to as *striated* because of its physical characteristics, and often combines with other types of muscles.

Skeletal Muscle Structure

All muscles are made up of three parts (Figure 7-14). The outside surface, which is covered by a fibrous connective sheath and which folds inward in order to cover individual bundles of muscle fibers, is called the **epimysium.** Once the epimysium surrounds each individual bundle, it becomes known as the **perimysium.** It then extends in order to cover individual muscle cells, where it becomes known as the **endomysium.** These three parts are structured in such a way as to be continuous with the fibrous tissue that eventually forms a tendon. Tendons are continuous with the periosteum of bone, where they firmly attach muscles to the bones and ultimately move when muscles contract.

Skeletal muscle cells are unique in that they have many nuclei. They are made up of many long, slender threads, called *myofibrils,* which are strands lying next to one another and extending lengthwise throughout the cell. These myofibrils are made up of smaller strands called *myofilaments,* which are made up of bands of protein.

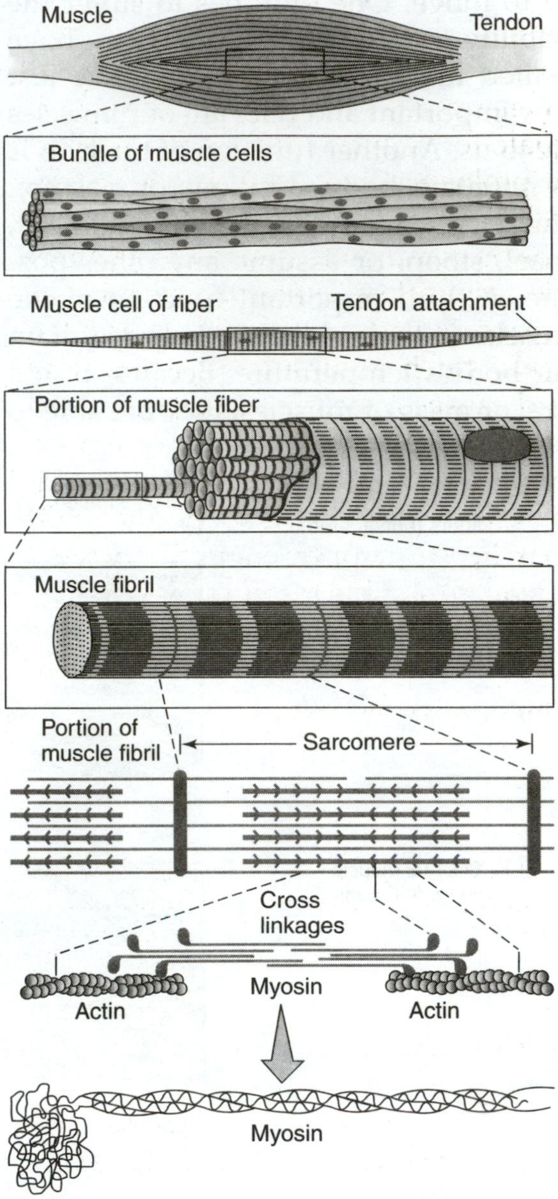

Figure 7-14 Muscle structure.

Energy and Muscle Contraction

While much occurs at the cellular level of the muscles in order to make it possible for them to move, the most profound changes have to do with creating energy so that they are able to contract. Energy is required for all muscle contraction.

This energy is supplied to the cells by aerobic respiration in which glucose combines with oxygen with the release of energy. If the oxygen supply is inadequate for cellular needs, as in strenuous or prolonged exercise, pyruvic acid provides energy without using free oxygen. This is commonly referred to as anaerobic respiration. When the pyruvic acid breaks down to release the energy, lactic acid, which accumulates in the tissues and causes a feeling of fatigue, is given off and released. What results is a process known as oxygen debt, a condition occurring because of the body's inability to supply enough oxygen for adequate aerobic respiration. When oxygen debt does occur, there may be muscle cramping or spasms following prolonged exercise.

Muscle Action

As we have already stated, movement is a major function of our muscular system. However, the only movement for which muscles are capable, is contraction followed by relaxation. Skeletal movement is accomplished by the pulling action on bones to which the muscles are attached.

All individual muscle cells contract when they are stimulated. And this stimulation is determined or affected, according to specific factors. These include oxygen and food supply, the number of fibers stimulated, and the extent to which activity is required.

In order for a muscle to be able to move, it must have two or more attachments. These attachments are generally to bones. The more fixed end or attachment of the muscle to bone is called its origin. The place of attachment of a muscle to a bone which it moves is called its insertion. Therefore, if you were to bend your elbow, you would be observing the origin of the *biceps brachii* at the scapula, which does not move, and the insertion at the *radius*, which does move.

Most of the muscles that make up our body are modified for their specific type of action. Terms used to describe these functions usually include the following:

- ❒ *flexor*—muscle that bends at a joint
- ❒ *extensor*—muscle that extends a part or increases the angle of a joint.
- ❒ *abductor*—muscle that moves a part away from the midline of the body
- ❒ *adductor*—muscle that moves a part toward the midline of a body
- ❒ *rotator*—muscle that revolves a part of its axis
- ❒ *sphincter*—circular muscle that closes an opening

◆ DISORDERS OF THE MUSCULAR SYSTEM

Like the bones which make up our body, muscles are also subject to many diseases and disorders. Two common degenerative disorders seen in the muscular system include **muscular dystrophy,** which is caused by a degeneration of the muscle cells that eventually causes the muscles to waste away and atrophy, and **myasthenia gravis,** a very poorly understood disease causing great muscle weakness and fatigue. In myasthenia gravis, the nerve impulses fail to initiate normal muscle contractions, eventually causing the patient to have the appearance of drooping eyelids and an inattentive appearance.

In addition to degenerative disorders, a muscle can become permanently shortened because of a formation of fibrous tissue replacing the muscle cells. If this occurs, a **contracture** develops. *Myalgia,* or muscle pain, is often seen in muscle cramps, and muscle spasms. Muscle cramps are painful, spasmodic muscle contractions of longer duration. A muscle spasm is a sudden, involuntary muscle contraction of a much shorter duration. If *myositis* occurs, there is a severe inflammation of the muscle tissue.

SUMMARY

In this chapter, we discussed the applied anatomy and physiology of the musculoskeletal system and the role these very important systems play in our everyday lives. We briefly discussed the function of both the bones and the muscles, as well as identified the various motions and movements of each of the individual structures that make up these two systems. We also discussed some of the most frequently seen disorders of the bones and muscles.

◆ ◆ LEARNING ACTIVITY 7-1

General Structure and the Skeleton

Give complete answers to these questions.

1. What is the basic structural unit of the body?
2. What is the name for a group of cells that carry out a certain function?
3. What is the name for a group of organs performing certain activities together?
4. List the functions of the skeleton.
5. Describe an articulation.
6. List three major types of joints.
7. Distinguish between cartilage and ligaments.
8. List four types of movable joints with an example of each.
9. Describe the spinal column.
10. What does the term *medial* mean?
11. What does the term *superior* mean?
12. *Dorsal* refers to which surface of the body?
13. Where would a *caudal* appendage be located?
14. If a foot is turned inward, what is the term used to describe it?
15. When the arms are moved away from the body, what term is used to describe the motion?
16. If the palm of the hand is turned to face forward, what term is used to describe this motion?
17. Which type of joint can perform all types of motions?
18. What does flexing a joint mean?

◆ ◆ LEARNING ACTIVITY 7-2

Questions to Answer on Muscles

Define these terms related to the muscular system.

1. muscular dystrophy
2. muscular atrophy
3. paralysis
4. strain
5. fibro
6. myo
7. tendon

Answer these questions.

8. What are the functions of muscles?
9. How are muscles attached to bones?
10. Name the three major types of muscles, and give the location of each within the body.
11. Tell where body paralysis occurs with paraplegia, quadriplegia, and hemiplegia.

◆ ◆ LEARNING ACTIVITY 7-3

The Skeletal System

Read the narrative, then write answers to the numbered questions. You should try to find answers at the health care facility, from classroom information, or from independent research.

Narrative

As Karen and Scott walk by the Emergency Room, they see Jimmy lying on a stretcher. "What are you doing here?" asks Scott. "Well," replied Jimmy, "I was rollerblading down University Drive when this guy in a Lexus slipped on the wet pavement and hooked my leg with his bumper. They tell me I have a compound fracture of my thigh bone, so it will have to be surgically repaired." Just then the emergency room aide comes in and tells Karen and Scott that Jimmy also has abrasions and multiple contusions. His dad has been called to come down and sign papers so Jimmy can have surgery. "That's really the pits," says Karen, "but since we're right here in the clinic, we'll keep in touch with you." As Karen and Scott walk out, Karen says,

(1) "I noticed that they put an antibiotic in Jimmy's IV. Why do you think they'd do that?"

"And Jimmy told me that he was given a tetanus booster, too?

(2) Do you know why that was necessary?" asks Scott.

Scott continues,

(3) "And what's the name of that bone that's broken?"

"I felt like a fool having to say "thigh bone." That sounds like a chicken! I'll bet he will be encouraged to drink milk while his fracture repairs itself, don't you?" asks Karen. Scott says,

(4) "What for? I don't know if he likes milk or not."

Scott asks, "Did you notice that before they did the surgical repair of the fracture, Jimmy was taken to Radiology for pictures of the broken bones?

(5) How do you suppose they positioned him for the pictures?"

Karen says, "After the surgery, I guess they will put a cast on that leg.

(6) I wonder what kind of cast they will use and how they will decide which will be best for him?"

"Yes," replies Scott, "and then they will probably get him some crutches and teach him how to walk with them.

(7) Which gait do you think he'll use?"

Karen asks,

(8) "Why do they always try to get patients with fractures to exercise?"

Later, as Jimmy is in Physical Therapy learning how to walk with crutches, he sees a man who lost a leg just below the knee in an industrial accident. He thinks to himself,

(9) "What kinds of prostheses are available for this man, and how would one decide which kind to use?"

Jimmy has had a lot of quiet time to think about the accident. Even though he will recover completely, he has been pretty uncomfortable, even miserable, as he waits for his leg to heal. Not only that, he can't rollerblade or drive a car. So he's been thinking.

(10) "How could this collision have been prevented? What safety measures did I neglect, and what could the driver of the Lexus have done to prevent this accident?"

REVIEW QUESTIONS

1. A __________ refers to a joint that is slightly movable.

2. Briefly explain the difference between cancellous bone tissue and compact bone tissue.

3. An osteoblast refers to:
   a. bone cells that form bone
   b. bone cells that destroy bone tissue
   c. a bone cell

4. What is the name of the long, main portion, or shaft, of a bone?

5. A sac or cavity found between bones in joints or between tendons and bones is called:
   a. bursa
   b. cartilage
   c. endosteum

6. __________ refers to the place of attachment of a muscle to a bone which it moves, while __________ pertains to the more fixed end or attachment of a bone.

7. What is the name of the fibrous connective sheath that surrounds individual bundles of muscle fibers?

8. True or false: An immovable joint is called a synarthrosis.

9. What is the name given to small rounded bones found next to joints, which function to help eliminate friction and increase efficiency in hinge joints?
   a. zygomatic
   b. ethmoid
   c. sesamoid

10. What is the name of the white, fibrous protective covering on the outer surface of bone?

SECTION III

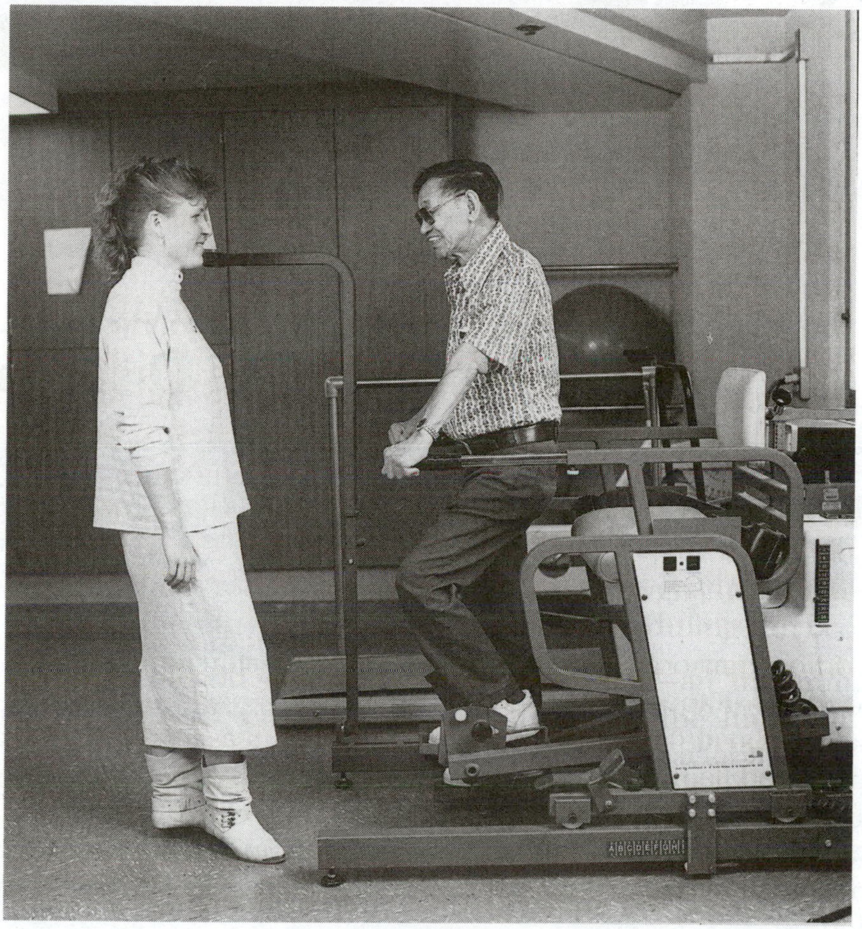

MEDICAL DISORDERS AND PHYSICAL THERAPY

8

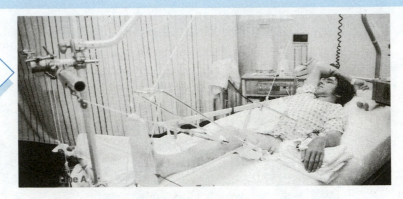

Using Physical Therapy to Treat Common Medical Disorders

OBJECTIVES

Upon completion of this chapter, you should be able to:

1. Define the role of physical therapy in caring for patients with special medical conditions.
2. Discuss the role of the physical therapy aide in assisting with treatment of patients diagnosed with common musculoskeletal and neurological disorders.
3. Discuss the role of the physical therapy aide in assisting with treatment of patients diagnosed with common cardiovascular and respiratory disorders.
4. Discuss the role of the physical therapy aide in assisting a patient with an amputation.
5. Explain the role of the physical therapy aide in assisting patients with burns and common dermatologic conditions.
6. Discuss the role of the physical therapy aide in assisting patients diagnosed with common medical conditions of the eyes, ears, nose, and throat.
7. Discuss the role of the physical therapy aide in assisting patients diagnosed with common genitourinary disorders.

KEY TERMS

Bursitis
Guillain-Barre Syndrome
Lumbago
Multiple sclerosis
Muscular dystrophy
Sciatica

The role of the physical therapy aide in assisting patients diagnosed with various types of medical conditions is one that often requires specific knowledge and understanding of some of the most basic physical therapy modalities. Much of the care prescribed by physicians often involves the introduction of physical therapy as a means of treating the patient. While most people believe that physical therapy is only useful in treating patients diagnosed with musculoskeletal conditions, many health care providers and physical therapists agree that the hands-on techniques and modalities used in physical therapy are frequently beneficial, and often essential, in meeting the needs of patients suffering from medical dysfunctions and disorders of many of our other body systems.

TREATING COMMON MUSCULOSKELETAL DISORDERS

There are many physical therapy modalities that are beneficial in treating patients diagnosed with a musculoskeletal disorder. However, before a decision can be made as to the type of therapy that can be employed in order to help these patients, it is extremely important that the physician perform a complete evaluation of the patient's pain, its type and location, and its severity.

The presence of a patient's pain is what is often considered to be a subjective decision, meaning that much of the information as to its type, location, and severity is generally made by the patient. Therefore, in order to ascertain an accurate evaluation of the pain, the doctor or physical therapist will frequently use certain factors to judge the presence, location, duration, and severity of the patient's pain and discomfort. These factors often include an assessment of the following conditions:

- *pain occurring after a patient rests and then improves with movement*—this is usually a sign of osteoarthritic joints and sometimes mild sprains and strains
- *pain occurring upon weight bearing*—this may be a sign of "static" deficiency or overstraining of the lower extremities
- *pain occurring immediately after an injury*—this is often equated with the presence of a fracture or a major tear of a muscle, ligament, or tissue
- *pain occurring after an interval*—this usually means the presence of a minor strain or sprain
- *pain occurring upon movement of a joint and ceasing when the joint is at rest*—this is usually a sign of an acute joint disorder or injury, or sometimes of a sprain or strain
- *pain radiating along the distribution of a nerve*—this usually suggests the presence of a lesion or impingement on the nerve by contracted muscles
- *pain occurring while a person is working or after work*—this is usually an indication that the injury was sustained

during the person's work time or as part of his or her occupation

Treating Arthritis and Rheumatic Conditions

Because of the many physical therapy modalities available to the physician, he or she is sometimes at a loss in determining what to prescribe for patients suffering from arthritis or rheumatic conditions. Therefore, in most cases, the physician often employs the following plan of treatment:

- *for subacutely inflamed joints*—application of moist heat or very mild infrared heat approximately thirty minutes two to three times per day
- *for acute stage arthritis*—no massage or exercise is prescribed during the acute stages of arthritis, except when the involved joint is moved through a full range of motion two to three times each day
- *for subacute and chronic stages of arthritis*—in these stages, physical therapy is generally administered at least once a day in the form of heat, massage, and graded exercises; heat may be applied through moist heat, infrared lamps, warm paraffin applications, warm tub baths, or diathermy

Assisting with the Administration of Heat Modalities

In the acute stage, heat is rarely used as a treatment for arthritic and rheumatic conditions. Therefore, during this phase of treatment, you may be called upon to assist the patient in keeping him or her comfortable by ensuring adequate rest and using various types of splints for immobility of the affected joint(s). Medication may also be prescribed during this period. In the nonacute phase of arthritic or rheumatic conditions, however, various forms of heat are often used to provide comfort and treatment for the affected joints. These generally include the following:

- *paraffin baths*—these are particularly helpful in the treatment of hands and fingers
- *infrared heat*—this is often considered the most convenient form of heat; treatments are usually by way of an infrared lamp, kept approximately eighteen inches away from the part being treated, for a period of thirty to forty-five minutes, administered two to three times a day
- *electric heating pad*—may be used by the patient, provided that the part being treated is wrapped in a towel to prevent burns; treatment may be two to three times a day for a period of up to forty-five minutes
- *hot tub baths*—should be taken prior to the patient beginning any form of therapeutic exercises; frequently used for treatment of hand, forearm and feet; temperature of water should not exceed 102°F, and bath should not last longer than twenty minutes

Assisting with Administration of Massage

Massage, which is often preceded by some form of heat, is usually started soon after the acute inflammatory process in the joint has subsided. This is noted by a diminished redness, swelling, and tenderness at the affected area. Use gentle strokes, followed later by deeper stroking motions, kneading, and friction of the surrounding muscles. Superficial, or very light stroking, may also be started over the affected joint. Massage should never cause the patient pain. Remember, it is usually better to give too little than too much, and unless contraindicated, every patient with nonacute rheumatoid arthritis should have this form of treatment at least ten to fifteen minutes at least twice a day.

Assisting with Range of Motion Exercises

The purpose of assisting the patient with range of motion exercises is to first strengthen the muscles that are needed to maintain good bone position within a joint, and second, to help increase joint motion. This can only be accomplished by putting a joint through its full range of motion up to the point in which a patient can tolerate the pain. An affected joint should be carried through its full range of motion at least several times a day.

All types of exercises can be used in the treatment of arthritis. These range from passive exercises, to active exercises, to active resistive. If a joint is exercised too much, however, the condition may become aggravated. If it is moved too little, motion can become limited. Therefore, to guide the patient between these two extremes, there are two points of information, or rules, which you can observe when assisting the patient with range of motion exercises. First, always remember that any exercise that produces pain during the same or the following day should be reduced in frequency or stopped altogether. Second, any exercise that is painful only at the time it is being administered, or for an hour or two afterwards, is always considered beneficial.

Range of Motion Exercises for the Hand and Wrist

The sequence for assisting the patient in performing range of motion exercises for the hand and wrist, includes the following:

1. Have the patient make a fist; then instruct the patient to stretch the fingers as straight as possible. If the fingers remain bent, rest the hand palm down on a table. The other hand should be held firmly on top of the affected hand. The forearm of the affected arm is then raised in an effort to flatten the bent fingers. The fingers should then be spread apart.
2. The patient should then touch the top of each finger to the end of the thumb, making as round a circle as possible.
3. Bend the wrist forward and backward as far as possible, and move the fingers toward the thumb. Turn the wrist slowly back and forth as though turning a doorknob.

Range of Motion Exercise for the Elbow

The sequence for assisting the patient to perform range of motion on the elbow, includes the following:

1. Lying on the back, with the upper arm resting on the bed or table, instruct the patient to bring the fingers to the top of the shoulder.
2. Then, with the palm turned upward, the hand should be brought down to the bed or table, while at the same time straightening the elbow.

Range of Motion Exercise for the Shoulder

The sequence for assisting the patient to perform range of motion on the shoulder, includes the following:

1. Standing with the arms resting at the sides and the palms pointed toward the body, instruct the patient to raise the arm sideways as far as possible away from the body, and then return; then raise the arm forward, upward, and as far back as it will go, and then return.
2. Lying on the back with the legs straight and arm at the sides, the patient is then told to raise the arms forward, upward, and back as far as they will go; the arm is then swung out to the side and around the back to the side of the body.

Range of Motion Exercise for the Ankle

The sequence for assisting the patient to perform range of motion on the ankle, includes the following:

1. Have the patient bend the foot up and down slowly, and then alternately turn it in and out.
2. Sitting on the edge of the bed or table, the foot should then be moved through a circular motion.

Range of Motion Exercise for the Knee

The sequence for assisting the patient to perform range of motion of the knee, includes the following:

1. Lying on his or her back, with the leg straight, have the patient contract the muscles of the entire leg, tightening the kneecap and flattening the knee down on the surface of the bed or table.
2. Then, have the patient come to a sitting position, with the legs hanging over the edge of the bed or table and above the floor. Instruct the patient to then straighten the legs and lower them again, alternating between the left and the right leg.
3. Then, still in a sitting position, with the legs straight, the patient raises the knee off the bed or table, sliding the foot back and thus bending and straightening the leg alternating between the left and the right.
4. The sequence is completed by having the patient lie on his or her back and ride a bicycle.

Range of Motion Exercise for the Hip

The sequence for assisting the patient to perform range of motion of the hip, includes the following:

1. Have the patient lie on his back with the legs held straight. The legs should then be moved approximately fifteen inches to the side, and then back.
2. While still on the back, the patient should then raise and lower the legs slowly, with the knees first straight, and then bent.
3. Then, lying face down and with the knee kept straight, the leg is moved backward.

Treating Low Back Pain

Unfortunately low back pain, or what is frequently referred to as **lumbago,** is a very common condition suffered by patients of all sizes and all ages. Because of the increase of this pathology, there is a very good possibility that at some point in your career you may be required to assist in the treatment of a patient suffering from some form of lower back pain. It is for that reason that it is important for you to have an understanding of some of the differential characteristics associated with this condition. Some of the more common of these include:

- localized or generalized low back pain is often considered the chief symptom associated with lumbosacral and sacroiliac strain
- patients with a history of having been aware of something snapping or slipping in the back suggests a periosteal or ligamentous tear
- back pain felt upon awakening, but which rapidly seems to improve after the patient becomes involved in the day's activities, is often characteristic of mild or chronic arthritis of the spine
- recurring attacks of low lumbar backache with sciatica felt in the back of the leg is usually the result of a defective intervertebral disk; in most instances, the pain appears to be intensified by sneezing or coughing during periods of acute pain
- pain that is definitely localized, but which does not seem to radiate, often occurs when there is a fracture or abscess of the vertebrae
- pain that seems to disappear during the night and then increases during the following day or evening as a backache is often associated with poor body posture

Assisting the Patient with Back Pain

Patients suffering from back pain are often most comfortable if they sleep on a very firm mattress, lying in a supine position. Additional support to the lower back is also helpful. This may include taping, the use of a binder, or a pillow placed under the knees while the hips are flexed.

Moist hot packs administered for twenty minutes, at least three or four times a day, as well as infrared heat therapy, may also be used to treat the patient suffering from back pain. The heat should not be applied continuously, and neither should a heating pad be used all the time or all night since prolonged application of heat tends to increase congestion, thereby defeating its purpose.

In acute cases, massage should not be attempted, however, it may be used later as the acute stage begins to subside. Very light massage that gradually becomes deeper may be indicated; the type used will greatly depend on the degree of acuteness of the symptoms.

In some cases, you may use corrective exercises for treating back pain, but only after the acute stage is ceased and the patient has become ambulatory, or after the symptoms have become milder. Since there are many different back exercises that may be prescribed, it is often up to the physical therapist to instruct the patient in the type of exercises that would best be suited for treating a particular condition. The following exercises are designed to strengthen the stomach muscles and stretch the contracted back muscles. The patient should begin by doing each exercise at least ten times a day, and then increase by one each day until he or she is doing each exercise up to twenty times a day. Remember, too, some pain during the performance of exercises is acceptable, however, if the pain lasts for several days, the number of times the exercises should be done should be reduced.

Therapeutic Exercises for Lower Back Pain

To assist the patient in performing therapeutic exercises that will help in the treatment of lower back pain, you can instruct the patient to:

- lie on the back with a rolled blanket or small pillow under the knees; then, with the hands held up beside the head, tilt the pelvis to flatten the lower back on the table by pulling up and in with the lower abdominal muscles; hold the back flat and breathe in and out easily, relaxing the upper abdominal muscles
- with the patient lying on his or her back, the knees should be bent, with the feet placed flat on the table; with the hands up beside the head, the pelvis is tilted to flatten the lower back on the table; the legs are then straightened as much as possible with the back held flat; keeping the back flat, the knees should then return to a bent position, sliding one leg back at a time
- sit with the legs extended forward, placing a rolled blanket under the knees to allow slight knee bend; then pull in with the abdominal muscles, keeping the pelvis tilted back, and reach forward toward the toes, bending the lower back
- sit with the knees straight, and then reach forward toward the toes; then have the patient try to bend at the hip joints by tilting the pelvis forward
- lie on the abdomen and contract the buttocks (gluteal muscles)
- lie on the abdomen and grasp the top of the bed with the hands; then raise one thigh, and then both thighs at the same time
- lying on the abdomen, grasp the side of the bed with the hands; then raise one knee and cross it over the opposite one by rotating the lower part of the back; keeping the chest and shoulders flat, the other knee is then moved in the same manner
- lying on the back, draw one knee up to the chest and bring it up tight with the hands; then, without allowing the knee to straighten out, return it slowly to its original position; repeat with the other knee
- lying on the back and drawing one knee to the chest, straighten the knee, pointing the leg upward as far as possible; flex the knee and return it to its original position; alternate with the opposite leg, repeating the cycle eight to ten times.

Treating Lumbosacral Strain

Strains on the back are usually caused by less severe injuries than those resulting in sprains. Therefore, the signs and symptoms are often less pronounced. However, failure on the part of the patient or the patient's doctor to recognize a strain and then to treat it as a possible troublemaker can often result in the patient suffering from a prolonged disability.

A firm binder is often applied to a patient who has suffered a lumbosacral strain. Heat, massage, and daily graduated active exercises may also be administered. Between treatments, the patient should have a hot bath daily, followed by at least thirty minutes of rest before going out of doors. If the symptoms appear to grow worse, or if they are prolonged for more than a week, it would be wise for the patient to have a few extra days of rest and receive the treatment prescribed for a back sprain.

Treating Back Sprains

Any sudden twist or fall when one is in a strained position, often results in back sprain. This can be a result of slipping while straining to lift a heavy object, or not lifting the object properly. A back sprain can also be caused by suddenly having a weight thrown upon you. A back sprain can cause tearing of the ligaments and muscle attachments about the back, minute hemorrhages, ecchymoses, and often, swelling at the site of the sprain.

When a back sprain occurs, the patient often feels pain immediately, causing the person to cease his or her daily activities; however, after a few hours, the pain may subside and the person will return to these activities. Continued use of the back can aggravate the condition, and the next morning, or a day or two later, the pain can become so severe that the patient cannot even get out of bed or stand.

In order to provide the patient with the proper treatment, it is extremely important that the sprain be diagnosed early and the patient be placed on bed rest. Most often, these sprains are in the lower back, usually in the lumbosacral or sacroiliac area. They may not appear sufficiently serious to cause much concern, but allowing the patient to be up and about or to assume faulty posture in order to relieve his or her discomfort will only prolong the condition.

Treatment for back sprain generally starts with rest, heat, and massage during the first week, followed by daily graduated exercise to help restore function. Strapping may also be applied for two to seven days after the patient has become ambulatory, but if at all possible, it should be avoided because it makes proper massage next to impossible. If the patient does not respond to these treatments, he or she should be seen by an orthopedist. However, lack of response does not necessarily mean that physical therapy is contraindicated for sprains of the back.

Treating Bursitis

Bursitis, which is inflammation of the bursa, can usually be relieved by the application of physical therapy. The affected part should be placed at rest, with an ice bag applied to the affected area. In some cases, infrared heat given for thirty minutes twice a day, may also be administered. As the pain diminishes, careful massage and relaxed motion can also be employed. Later on, you may begin to assist the patient with active range of exercises.

Treating Cervical Disorders

There are many pathological conditions that can arise in the cervical region of the spine. Of these, the most common include whiplash injuries, arthritic changes such as those resulting from osteoarthritic, rheumatic, or traumatic origin, muscular and ligamentous strains, and vertical disk injuries caused by the compression or irritation of one or more cervical nerves at the site of a protruding disk.

The patient with an acute cervical disorder is often hospitalized, put into traction, and given such treatments as the physician prescribes. Cervical traction, which has been used for many years for the treatment of neck injuries, may be applied continuously or intermittently. When applied correctly, continuous traction assures a certain amount of immobilization of the cervical spine, straightens it, and enlarges the intervertebral opening, or foramina, to relieve compressive or irritative forces upon the nerve roots, thus relieving muscle spasm. Heat, in the form of hot packs, is also useful in treating patients with a cervical disorder, as is massage in relieving muscle spasms. In some cases, the physician may also inject a local anesthetic or prescribe certain medications for the relief of pain.

Treating Degenerative Joint Disease (Osteoarthritis)

In caring for a patient diagnosed with degenerative joint disease, you must understand that rest is by far the most important part of the physical therapy program. Rest may be local or general, depending upon the parts of the body involved. Since overuse of affected joints is thought to bring about the symptoms and may also be a factor in producing further damage in osteoarthritis, complete bed rest may appear more rational; however, this is not really very practical for most patients, and is probably not necessary. When a patient suffers an acute or severe exacerbation of the symptoms, particularly in the knees, hips, or spine, absolute bed rest for a few days may be the most rapid means of relieving the pain. Other physical therapy modalities that are frequently used in the treatment of degenerative joint disease often include the application of heat, massage, and therapeutic exercise.

◆ TREATING COMMON NEUROLOGIC DISORDERS

While there are many different types of neurological disorders, the application of physical therapy can be much more beneficial to some more than others. Some of the more common disorders that can be treated with the use of therapeutic modalities include cerebral vascular accident, or stroke, **Guillain-Barre Syndrome, multiple sclerosis, muscular dystrophy,** Parkinson's disease, and protrusion of an intervertebral disk.

Treating a Patient Who Has Suffered a Cerebral Vascular Accident

The patient who has had a cerebral vascular accident, or stroke, resulting in hemiplegia, is often treated with physical therapy in order to prevent or correct deformity, to improve his or her motor function, and to help in the development of the ability to carry out the basic activities of daily living to the extent that he or she can, at least partially, take care of personal needs.

Treatment for a patient who has suffered a stroke is usually initiated as soon as possible. In most cases, it can be started within the first week following the stroke. Numerous modalities and techniques, which can be used alone or in combination, are available and helpful to the physician in the management of the hemiplegic patient. The more common of these include heat, stimulating massage, movement re-education, therapeutic exercises, and training in the use of such assistive devices as a walker, braces, crutches, and canes.

Preventing Deformity in the Stroke Patient

There are four simple procedures that that be carried out during the acute stage following the stroke and while the patient may still be bedridden. All of these will help prevent some of the deformities commonly seen in the hemiplegic patient. The four procedures include:

- placing a small pillow in the axilla on the affected side to prevent adduction of that arm toward the shoulder
- using a footboard or applying a posterior leg splint to the affected leg to prevent toe drop and shortening of the Achilles tendon
- placing sandbags along the lateral surface of the affected leg to help prevent outward rotation of the leg
- assisting the patient to practice quadriceps range of motion exercises to help maintain and improve muscle strength needed for ambulation

Assisting the Patient with Range of Motion Exercises

Exercise is a very important part of the treatment in hemiplegia. The type of exercise used will, of course, depend greatly on the condition of the patient's affected extremities. Various types of movement can be used, such as active and passive, assistive and resistive, as well as muscle re-education.

When assisting the patient, it is always a good idea to start with the two of you looking in front of a mirror while you are demonstrating an exercise, and then allowing the patient to always perform the exercise before the mirror. While the patient is performing the exercise, it is important to watch closely and observe that the patient is not becoming too fatigued, out of breath, or dizzy. Also, you can allow the patient to use his or her unaffected limb to assist the affected one only when motion is impossible without assistance.

Slow, passive movements of the affected extremities and your encouragement of active movements of all extremities should be started as soon as possible after the most acute stage of illness is over. Special attention should also be given to the upper extremities. The following is a list of suggestions for active exercises that will help the patient to prevent the development of contractures and deformities following a stroke:

- flexing the fingers and touching the thumb with each finger; extending and spreading the fingers; making a fist
- flexing and extending the wrist, and then flexing the elbow, trying to touch the shoulder; extending the arm and bringing it to the side
- using the unaffected hand to lift the affected one to the head, and then to the opposite side and back
- flexing, extending, and spreading the toes, dorsiflexing the feet, and flexing and extending the knees
- grasping and holding of different sizes and shapes, then lifting them with the fingers; using a large pencil to draw large circles on a piece of paper
- assisting the patient to attempt to walk by practicing to raise and swing the affected leg while supporting him or herself; a walker can be used for support while doing this exercise

Assisting the Patient with Re-education for Walking

With proper training, many hemiplegic patients can be taught to walk again. However, the degree to which a person's normal gait can be restored greatly depends upon the amount of residual function retained by the quadricep muscle on the affected side. If the patient is able, there are certain steps that you can initiate in order to help in the re-education of a patient's ability to ambulate or walk. These steps include the following:

- ❐ getting the patient out of bed and into a standing position as soon as possible in order to help prevent loss of the sense of balance and muscle atrophy
- ❐ if necessary, fitting the affected ankle with a brace in order to prevent plantar fixation and supination of the foot leading to foot drop, and to give the patient confidence in weight bearing
- ❐ using two chairs or the parallel bars for support, having the patient practice weight bearing on the involved leg
- ❐ instructing the patient in the technique involved in the reciprocal gait, which is the normal gait for walking and that involves moving one leg and the opposite arm forward at the same time, and then the other leg and its opposite arm
- ❐ teaching the patient to raise his or her foot from the floor by flexing the hip and knee, extending the affected leg forward at the knee, and then extending the hip until the foot touches the ground, heel first

Assisting the Stroke Patient to Regain Arm, Hand, and General Body Control

The reestablishment of arm and hand movement for a hemiplegic patient should always begin with passive exercises to the shoulder and stretching. This helps to prevent flexion deformities at the elbow, wrist, fingers, and thumb. As soon as some voluntary movement of the arm becomes possible, the next step is to introduce functional activities, which are usually assisted through the implementation of occupational therapy activities.

When assisting the patient to regain control of his or her body, it is important to understand that this always begins with teaching the patient how to move in bed so that his or her position can be changed from supine to prone and from supine to sitting. The patient must also learn how to use the unaffected leg to move or raise the paralyzed leg and how to swing both legs laterally so as to bring them over the side of the bed preparatory to standing.

The hemiplegic patient will also need instruction in how to get in and out of a wheelchair and how to propel it by using the unaffected arm and leg. Some wheelchairs are equipped with a one-arm drive mechanism, which is particularly useful for patients with unilateral paralysis. Also, the patient who can learn how to walk without the aid of a cane, crutch, or brace needs to learn how to cope with different floor surfaces, both indoors and ground surfaces outdoors. He or she must also learn how to stand up unassisted, sit down, climb stairs, step up and down a curb, and cross a street.

Treating a Patient with Guillain-Barre Syndrome

Guillain-Barre Syndrome is a term that has been given to a condition often seen in patients with viral encephalitis. It is a disorder that is characterized by the absence of fever, pain or tenderness in the muscles, motor weakness, and the interruption or lack of motor reflexes.

Treatment in the acute stage of Guillian-Barre Syndrome usually consists first of an evaluation of the patient's condition, followed by a utilization of passive range of motion exercises, breathing exercises, correct positioning in bed, and application of heat. In the later stages of the syndrome, rehabilitation is generally based upon an evaluation of the patient's needs and the results of tests of muscle strength. The therapeutic modalities and activities initiated at that point usually include range of motion exercises, activities to develop functional skills, re-education of the affected muscle groups, standing and balancing, ambulation and gait training, functional activities in order to improve strength, dexterity, range of motion of the upper extremities, and instruction in the performance of the activities of daily living.

Treating the Patient Diagnosed with Multiple Sclerosis

Multiple sclerosis is a highly complex, chronic, progressive neurological disease that is caused by changes in the white matter of the brain and spinal cord. It is often classified as being either *acute,* with a sudden onset, *chronic remittent,* which is characterized by extensive involvement and by exacerbations and remissions that are almost complete and last over a long period of time, and *chronic progressive,* which is accompanied by symptoms that persist and are without periods of remission. Unfortunately, multiple sclerosis can be accompanied by many varied symptoms, and the number and degree to which the patient experiences them is usually different with each individual person.

Signs and Symptoms of Multiple Sclerosis

In most cases, the signs and symptoms of multiple sclerosis usually develop slowly and over a period of time, although occasionally they may appear quite suddenly and be acute in nature. In most instances, there is complete recovery from the first symptoms. This period of recovery, however, is actually a *remission* that can vary in length from days to years. Unfortunately, when the symptoms are the result of a large lesion that causes ataxia, paraplegia, or mental deterioration, they tend to become permanent.

The most common symptoms of multiple sclerosis are diplopia, nystagmus, intention tremor, ataxia, weakness, slurred speech, and spasticity. When the cerebellus is involved, the patient often exhibits spasticity of one or both legs along with ataxia and tremor. Emotional disturbances may also accompany multiple sclerosis. When this happens, the patient may become euphoric, depressed or emotionally unstable and experience personality changes and loss of memory.

Sadly, the prognosis for patients diagnosed with multiple sclerosis is often unfavorable. The course of the disease varies greatly, but survival is usually estimated between five to twenty years. The outlook for patients with one or a few symptoms is often more favorable than for those with a combination of symptoms, especially if the cerebellus in involved. And death is usually the result or complication or conditions resulting from the patient's lowered resistance to infection.

Assisting in the Treatment of Multiple Sclerosis

The goal in treating patients with multiple sclerosis evolves around retraining the patient to ambulate, helping to maintaining a high level of physical and mental activity, and facilitating family management of the patient in the more advanced stages of the disease. Many patients are able to continue with their work, home life, and social activities for a number of years after the onset of the disease. Therefore, your main objective in treating someone with multiple sclerosis should be to help that person to do as much as possible for him or herself for as long as possible. The use of assistive devices will often prolong the patient's ability to do something on his or her own. And it is often more psychologically sound and beneficial for these patients to continue their regular activities within the limits imposed by their condition than for them to give up and assume the attitude of being a complete invalid.

Treating the Patient Diagnosed with Muscular Dystrophy

Muscular dystrophy is an inborn abnormality of muscle that is characterized by dysfunction and eventual deterioration. While there are numerous types of dystrophies, regardless of the type, the disease has an insidious onset with the chief symptoms being weakness, tightness and atrophy of muscles, and absence of deep tendon reflexes.

Tightness of muscles in the upper extremities occurs primarily in the pronators of the forearm, the wrist and finger flexors, and the scapulo-humeral flexors and adductors. Tightness in the lower extremities usually occurs early and affects the gastrocnemius, coleus, hamstring muscles, the iliotibial band, and the hip flexors. Contractures also occur early and are severe, usually because the muscle itself is the site of the pathological lesion. Deformities caused by these contractures are the main reason for early loss of the person's ability to walk.

Assisting in the Treatment of Muscular Dystrophy

Patients diagnosed with muscular dystrophy are encouraged to remain ambulatory for as long as possible, and exercises that help to increase flexibility of the muscles are generally started early. When indicated, the patient is also taught breathing exercises. The patient should also be encouraged to do strengthening exercises, however, it is important that he or she not exercise to the point of fatigue. Massage may also be implemented, since it often delays the development of contractures.

Braces and assistive and ambulatory devices are hardly ever used if the patient can manage without them, however, if contractures do not respond to physical therapy modalities, supportive splints or braces may be necessary and may defer the eventual need for a wheelchair.

Since the use of prolonged physical therapy may not be necessary, the patient is frequently placed on a program of home care early on in his or her treatment, and then seen by a physical therapist on a regular check-up basis. For this reason, most therapists believe that the patient should receive early and adequate instruction in procedures for carrying out their activities of daily living.

Treating the Patient Diagnosed with Parkinson's Disease

Unfortunately, for the patient diagnosed with Parkinson's disease, physical therapy can only offer temporary symptomatic relief and improvement. Such improvement, however, is often considered quite beneficial. Muscular rigidity can be lessened by an active range of motion exercises, and under the proper supervision and encouragement of the physical therapy department, some bedridden patients may be taught to walk again, improve their posture, and ultimately, become more independent. Active exercises that are graded to the patient's tolerance can also be useful in combating atrophy. And in the event that limitation of motion occurs, causing the patient to experience pain upon movement, heat may also be used.

Treating the Patient with a Protrusion of an Intervertebral Disk

During the time in which diagnostic studies are performed in order to determine the possible need for surgery, the application of physical therapy is often useful in most cases in which there is a suspicion of a protrusion of an intervertebral disk. Treatment usually includes complete bed rest on a firm mattress, traction to the legs or head, or sometimes both, and the use of heat and sedative massage at the painful areas. Mild diathermy of short duration and infrared heat may also be used. Frequently, symptoms of a protrusion of an intervertebral disk are relieved by these treatments within a short period of time, after which gradual mobilization may be initiated along with the use of various exercises for muscles in the abdominal, gluteal, and lumbar regions. Patients should also be taught how to prevent further excessive back strain when stooping and sitting down and during other bodily movements.

Treating the Patient with Sciatica

Sciatica is one of the most common neurological disorders that can be treated by physical therapy. The three types most frequently encountered include subacute and chronic sciatica associated with rheumatism and arthritis, true neuritic sciatica, and sciatica that is associated with prolapse of an intervertebral disk.

During the acute stage of this disorder, the patient is often put on bed rest, with a fracture board placed between a firm mattress and the spring. The affected leg may be partially flexed by placing a pillow under the knee and a small, firmer pillow placed under the lumbar area. Heat may also be applied to the lower gluteal region and lower back, but should be discontinued if it causes an increase in pain. Diathermy is sometimes used, but only in low intensity. Ultrasound therapy has also proved to be very beneficial.

Once the acute pain has subsided, massage and postural exercises can be used while the patient is still on bed rest. And before the patient is allowed up and able to get out of bed, he or she should be fitted with a lower back support and taught to maintain the correct posture. If one leg is shorter than the other, a heel lift may also be required.

◆ TREATING COMMON CARDIOVASCULAR AND RESPIRATORY DISORDERS

Heat is both a therapeutic modality and a powerful vasodilator that acts directly upon the blood vessels. In sufficient doses, it can increase the temperature of the blood. When it is applied to any part of the body, heat can also increase the temperature of the tissues, thus aiding in the body's metabolism.

The application of heat is often used in the treatment of many cardiovascular and respiratory disorders. Of these, those you may encounter most frequently include peripheral vascular disorders, emphysema, asthma, and chronic bronchitis.

Treatment of Patients with Peripheral Vascular Disorders

In peripheral vascular disease, circulation of the extremities should be increased by warming the patient's trunk and thighs or opposite normal extremities. Electric heating pads and hot water bottles should never be used or applied directly to the affected extremities. Thermostatically controlled heating is the safest. Hot soaks may also be used in the treatment of such peripheral vascular disorders as gangrene and decubitus ulcers, however, the water should never be warmer than 102 to 105 degrees Fahrenheit. The use of cold therapy has also recently been regarded as a recommended means of safeguarding the patient against or minimizing the result of gangrene resulting from arterial occlusion.

In addition to heat and cold therapy, other treatments may be used for peripheral circulatory disturbances. Once such modality is the introduction and use of the *Buerger-Allen exercise.* Consisting of three stages and lasting about ten minutes in duration, the exercise is usually performed three to six times at each session, with the session repeated at least two to four times a day.

In the first stage of the exercise, the patient lies on his or her back, with a watch in sight, and resting the legs on an inclined plane that is raised to an angle of 45 degrees. The legs are kept raised until the feet are thoroughly blanched. Usually this takes up to two minutes. In the second stage, the patient sits with his or her legs hanging over the edge of the bed or treatment table, and puts the feet and toes through a series of motions. The ankles are flexed downward, and then upward; the feet are rocked inward, and then outward; the toes are spread and then closed again. As the patient performs the movements, the feet should start becoming flushed, until eventually, the entire foot to the tips of the toes are a strong pink color. This usually takes from one to three minutes. If the toes begin to look cyanotic or the patient complains of pain in them, the feet should be elevated immediately.

In the third and final stage of the exercise, the patient lies supine, with the legs horizontal and the patient is wrapped in a woolen blanket warmed by a hot water bottle or electric heating pad, for approximately five minutes. In this way, the reactionary flush achieved by the exercises in stages I and II is maintained.

Treating Respiratory Disorders

Of the many respiratory disorders treated in today's health care facilities, those that can benefit most from physical therapy include emphysema, asthma, and chronic bronchitis.

Assisting the Patient with Emphysema

Emphysema is a fairly common lung condition that is characterized by an abnormal enlargement of the alveolar spaces in the lungs and destructive changes in the alveolar walls, resulting in the collection of air in the interstices of the connective tissue and the intra-alveolar tissue of the lungs. These changes often cause an impairment in the most vital aspect of breathing; that is, the ability of the lungs to exchange air efficiently. Emphysema may occur at any age and is most often seen in people who are heavy smokers.

The goal of physical therapy in the treatment of emphysema is to help the patient to breathe more efficiently without the aid of a nebulizer or other breathing apparatus. Properly executed, exercises can be used to help strengthen muscles that will help more oxygen into the patient's lungs and thus reduce dyspnea. Postural drainage can also be used to help remove obstructions in the bronchial tubes.

Some exercises can also be helpful in the treatment of emphysema. They include the arm-lift breathing exercise, exercises to help increase the strength of abdominal muscles and of lateral chest muscles used in breathing, handclapping, and exercises to correct posture.

Arm-Lift Exercise

This exercise can be done in the standing position or when the patient is lying down. Its goal is to help increase the exchange of air in the lungs. In the standing position, the patient breathes in slowly through the nose while, at the same time, raising the arms forward and upward until they are fully extended over the head. After the patient takes in as much air as is needed, the arms are slowly lowered while exhaling, using one-third more time than was used to inhale.

Exercise to Strengthen Chest Muscles

This exercise helps to strengthen not only the lateral chest muscles used in breathing, but also the abdominal and other chest muscles. With the patient lying flat on the bed or table, the knees are flexed and the feet are placed firmly on the mattress or table surface, and the trunk is raised while twisting it either to the right or to the left. The hands may be held either behind the head or raised forward to the right or left. The exercise should be repeated at least five times with the patient twisting to the right and then five more times twisting to the left.

Handclapping Exercise

For the handclapping exercise, the patient should be standing erect. While maintaining good posture, the hands are then brought forward and clasped, with the arms being thrown backward as far as they can at shoulder height. The sequence is completed by bringing the arms forward again and then repeating the entire procedure.

Assisting the Patient with Asthma

Asthma is a respiratory disorder that is characterized by recurrent attacks of dyspnea during which expiration is particularly labored. These attacks are often the result of a spasm of the smooth muscle of the bronchi, as well as swelling of the mucous lining causing an increase in the secretion of mucus.

In most cases of asthma, the ability to use the diaphragm in breathing and to expand the basal areas of the lungs have been compromised or lost. In addition, the chest is often tense and the neck muscles in vigorous action, making it almost impossible to practice diaphragmatic breathing. Therefore, the patient has to be taught how to relax and keep the upper thorax still and to use the diaphragm in breathing.

Exercise to Correct Posture

In some cases, it may be necessary to correct the patient's posture before he or she can receive the maximum benefit from some of the breathing exercises. To accomplish this, the patient should stand with the shoulders erect and the chest thrust forward. Breathing is then done slowly through the nose, gradually increasing the amount of air being inhaled. The air is then expelled slowly while the chin is kept up and the correct posture maintained.

Assisting the Patient with Chronic Bronchitis

Chronic bronchitis is a respiratory condition that is characterized by chronic inflammation of the lining of the larger and medium-sized bronchi, usually occurring as a result of an infection. It is most common in middle-aged and older people, especially those living in industrial areas or in cold, damp climates and those with low resistance. It may also be caused by irritations arising from some chemicals, gases, dust, and smoke.

The main goal in treating a patient with chronic bronchitis is to increase his or her ability to take in oxygen. It is also important to raise the resistance of the bronchial tree to infection. The various exercises that are used in the treatment of emphysema and asthma can also be used in treating chronic bronchitis.

◆ TREATING COMMON DISORDERS OF THE EYES, EARS, NOSE, AND THROAT

Many of the most common disorders of the eyes, ears, nose, and throat can be helped by physical therapy modalities. Although some of the treatments used may be considered by some to be old-fashioned, they are both helpful and useful in the treatment of many of these conditions.

Treating Conditions Affecting the Eye

Two of the most common conditions affecting the eye for which physical therapy can be helpful in treatment are acute conjunctivitis and chronic meibomitis. Patients who are diagnosed with acute conjunctivitis can use a cold compress applied to their eye for the first twenty-four hours, followed by moist or dry heat. For patients with chronic meibomitis, massaging of the lids is often very helpful.

Treating Conditions Affecting the Ear

There are two common disorders that can benefit from use of physical therapy modalities. The first is called eczema of the auricle, in which there is a scaly appearance to the outside of the ear. This is easily treated with the application of ultraviolet irradiation. Chronic otitis media, which is a chronic inflammation of the middle ear, may also be treated with ultraviolet irradiation, as well as with short wave diathermy.

Treating Conditions Affecting the Nose

The most common disorder of the nose for which physical therapy can be useful is *sinusitis,* which is an inflammation of the nasal sinuses. Hot, moist towels can be applied over the sinuses, with an infrared lamp pointed directly at the towels. Diathermy may also be used if there is drainage, however, it should only be applied at low intensity for no longer than twenty to twenty-five minutes, using the air-spaced technique or a special sinus applicator.

Treating Conditions Affecting the Throat

There are three conditions of the throat that can most benefit from the application of physical therapy. They include laryngitis, or inflammation of the larynx, pharyngitis, or inflammation of the pharynx, and tonsillitis, which is inflammation of the tonsils. In the acute stage of laryngitis, heat treatments, in the form of infrared irradiation or hot compresses, may be helpful, as in diathermy with the electrodes placed on each side of the neck. Cold compresses are also sometimes used. Patients suffering from pharyngitis may be treated with infrared heat, diathermy, and hot compresses. Ultraviolet irradiation may also be used in the region of the inflamed pharynx. For patients diagnosed with tonsillitis, the application of hot compresses, infrared heat to the neck, and short-wave diathermy, with the electrodes placed on either side of the neck, may also be useful.

◆ TREATING COMMON DERMATOLOGIC DISORDERS

Physicians frequently use certain physical therapy modalities in treating common skin disorders before they refer their patients to a dermatologist. One such modality is ultraviolet heat, which is often used in the treatment of such skin disorders as acne vulgaris, alopecia areata, boils and carbuncles, eczema seborrheicum, lupus vulgaris, neurodermatitis, and psoriasis. The application of ultraviolet heat and radiation is also quite beneficial in the treatment of decubitus ulcers and in some infected wounds.

Patients suffering from an excessive buildup of scar tissue may also benefit from physical therapy. In some cases, the scarring may only involve the skin, while in other cases, it may extend into deeper tissues surrounding the joints, tendons, and nerves. Forceful manipulation of scar tissue only results in tearing and further scarring. Therefore, treatment for these patients usually involves the application of hot moist packs, ultrasonic therapy, friction type massage, and active exercises and stretching. In severe cases, scarring may require surgical intervention.

◆ USING PHYSICAL THERAPY TO TREAT BURNS

One of the most serious complications of burns is the development of deformities caused by the contraction of scar tissue. During the healing of burns that have destroyed the entire thickness of the skin, fibrous tissue must form in order to compensate for the loss caused by the burn. Once formed, this interlacing of collagen fibers undergoes a period of active contraction, and the forces exerted in this vital process are considerable. The overwhelming value of physical therapy in the treatment of burns is that it minimizes the process by which fibrosis takes place.

The degree of scarring that develops following a burn greatly depends upon the force and effectiveness of the treatment and medication, as well as the responses by the patient to the healing process. In all cases, treatment should begin as soon as possible after the injury.

When using physical therapy to treat burns, the following modalities have proved most useful:

❒ *dry heat*—various sources can be used to help relieve pain

- *massage*—helps to stimulate the blood supply to the burned area, reduces the amount of scar tissue that develops, loosens scars and overcomes a tendency for them to retract or contract, and helps to restore function of the involved joints
- *whirlpool bath, paraffin baths, and Hubbard tub baths*—helps to increase movement and motion of the affected body parts
- *ultraviolet irradiation*—helps to improve the patient's general condition by stimulating healing, overcoming low-grade infections, and preparing the burned area for eventual plastic surgery
- *dry cold*—helps in overcoming traumatic and postoperative swelling

◆ USING PHYSICAL THERAPY IN THE TREATMENT OF AMPUTATION

Following surgery, patients who have had a limb amputated are usually referred to a physician specializing in orthopedics. However, there are many physical therapy modalities that can be used before this person is ready to be fitted for his or her prosthesis.

When physical therapy is used as a treatment in caring for patients who have sustained an amputation, the main goal of the treatment is to prepare the stump for early and efficient use of a prosthesis. The modalities used for such a task generally include heat, massage, and therapeutic exercise. Whirlpool baths are considered the preferred source of heat, since they improve circulation and relieve pain that has been caused by the persistent edema and excessive buildup of periosteal connective tissue. Massage is usually administered at a later time, after it has been determined that there is no possibility of infection. Early therapeutic exercise of the remaining part of the limb results in reduction of edema and is usually good preparation for the use of an artificial limb.

◆ USING PHYSICAL THERAPY IN THE TREATMENT OF GENITOURINARY DISORDERS

While there are many urinary tract infections and disorders that can be helped by the early use of physical therapy modalities, those that seem to benefit from it most include prostatic disorders, cystitis, some disorders of the kidney, and spasms occurring in the ureters. For most of these conditions, physical therapy treatments often include the use of diathermy and infrared heat.

Assisting the Patient with a Prostatic Disorder

For patients suffering from an acute inflammation of the prostate, local heating by means of diathermy, hot irrigations, or hot sitz baths are very helpful and frequently used in conjunction with medications.

Assisting the Patient with Cystitis

Patients diagnosed with an inflammation of the urinary bladder, or cystitis often experience pain and spasms that can be greatly relieved by heat-producing methods, such as hot sitz baths, hot packs to the suprapubic area, infrared heat to both the suprapubic and perineal regions, and diathermy applied by a special electrode. While the application of physical therapy is especially helpful before the symptoms are relieved by antibiotics, it is often continued throughout the entire period of the infection.

Assisting the Patient with a Kidney Disorder

Heat applied locally to the renal area by means of warm baths, hot packs, infrared lamps, or diathermy may be a very effective measure in relieving the patient of the often dull ache and colicky pain associated with kidney disorders. Mild massage is also helpful in relieving painful muscle spasm, as is diathermy which it is used as an adjunct to other methods in the treatment of oliguria or anuria resulting from crystallization of sulfa drugs within the kidney's tubules.

Assisting the Patient Suffering from Spasms in the Ureter

When a spasm occurs in the ureter as a result of the formation of a calculus (stone) or trauma from instrumental examination of the ureter, the local application of infrared heat or diathermy is often used to help produce relaxation of the ureter.

SUMMARY

In this chapter, we discussed the role of physical therapy aide in using various therapeutic modalities to help treat patients diagnosed with special medical conditions and disorders. In our discussion, we talked about the many types of therapeutic treatments used to care for patients diagnosed with musculoskeletal, neurological, cardiovascular, and respiratory disorders. We also discussed the usefulness of physical therapy as a modality for treating patients with amputations, burns and skin conditions, disorders of the eyes, ears, nose, and throat, and genitourinary disorders.

◆ ◆ LEARNING ACTIVITY 8-1

Common Disorders

Describe each disorder or injury listed below:

1. osteoarthritis
2. gout
3. bursitis
4. sprain
5. dislocation

Give complete answers to these questions.

1. List and describe two major types of fractures.
2. List and describe four types of closed fractures.
3. What is hypertension?
4. What is an embolism?
5. Describe what occurs in arteriosclerosis.

REVIEW QUESTIONS

1. A neurologic condition that is highly complex, chronic, and progressive, and in which changes in the white matter of the brain and spinal cord occur, is called:
   a. multiple sclerosis
   b. muscular dystrophy
   c. radiculitis

2. A neurologic condition that is caused by irritation of the spinal nerve roots, and which is manifested by pain and by alterations in perception of sensation or in muscle function, is called:
   a. multiple sclerosis
   b. muscular dystrophy
   c. radiculitis

3. What is the name of the medical condition that is frequently seen in patients with viral encephalitis?

4. __________ is a term used to describe painful and labored breathing.

5. __________ is a pathological condition that is usually caused by direct trauma to the coccyx and that often results in a sprain of the sacrococcygeal ligaments.

6. A term often used to denote an acutely painful back, is __________.

7. An inflammation of the muscles characterized by aching pain in the affected muscles is called:
   a. bursitis
   b. myositis
   c. polyneuritis

8. What is another name for tennis elbow?

9. __________ is a term used to denote a group of nonspecific illnesses characterized by pain, tenderness, and stiffness of the joints, muscles, or adjacent structures.

10. A term that refers to any condition of a joint in which direct trauma has been directed onto it, resulting in a disturbance in the synovial membrane, is called __________.

SECTION IV

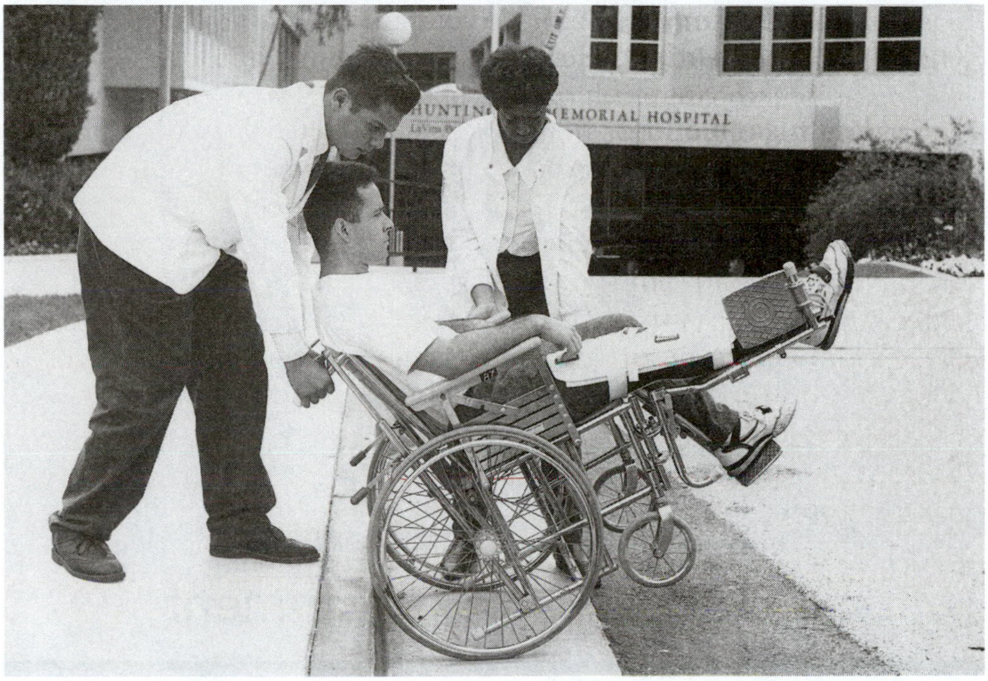

PATIENT PREPARATION

9

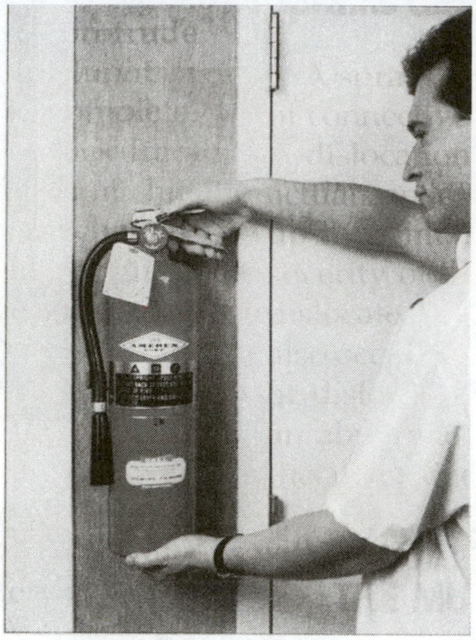

Safety in the Working Environment

OBJECTIVES

Upon completion of this chapter, you should be able to:

1. Define the term environment as it relates to the medical area.
2. Discuss the purpose for keeping the medical environment safe.
3. Explain how to manage the medical external environment.
4. Discuss the role temperature, humidity, ventilation control, light regulation, color, noise control, neatness and order, control of odors, and providing for the patient's privacy play in managing the health care environment.
5. Discuss the physical therapy aide's role in providing a safe environment.
6. Discuss how to prevent accidents in the heath care environment.
7. Identify patients at risk of having accidents.
8. Describe how to prevent falls in the health care environment.
9. Discuss how to prevent burns in the health care environment.
10. Explain the importance of practicing good body alignment and movement in the working environment.
11. Describe how the physical therapy aide can practice good body alignment and movement.
12. Discuss the concept of asepsis and infection control.
13. Explain how medical asepsis is carried out through proper handwashing.
14. Demonstrate correct handwashing technique.
15. Discuss how microorganisms grow and spread.

KEY TERMS

- Abduction
- Adduction
- Balance
- Body alignment
- Body mechanics
- Environment
- External environment
- Gravity
- Hospital clean
- Humidity
- Hyperextension
- Infection control
- Medical asepsis
- Microorganisms
- Safety
- Temperature
- Ventilation

The term **environment** is a word frequently used to describe any condition that affects the life or development of a person in his surroundings. In health care, we often use the term *therapeutic environment* to describe both those factors that influence the patient's **external environment,** and those that make up the internal composition of the body. All health care workers, including the physical therapy aide, are expected to practice those techniques and skills that provide the patient with a safe and environmentally sound atmosphere (Figure 9-1).

In the physical therapy area, the aide is concerned with two tasks—carrying out the skills and techniques necessary to assist the patient in achieving a greater degree of health and providing those skills and techniques in a proper and acceptable way. To do so, constitutes providing a safe environment, practicing proper aseptic techniques, and using good body mechanics.

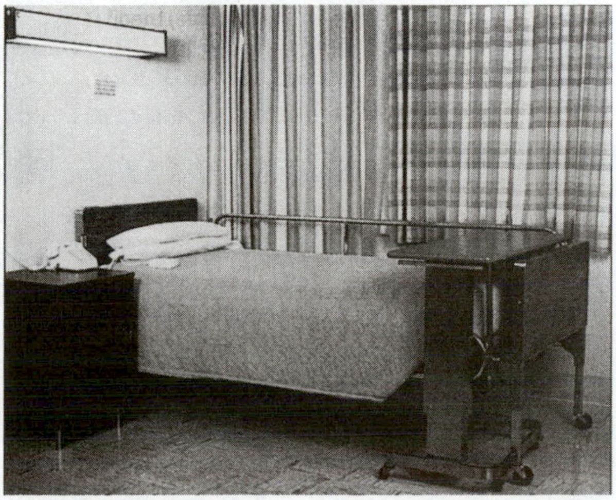

Figure 9-1 The patient's unit becomes his home.

MANAGING THE EXTERNAL ENVIRONMENT

In today's modern health care setting, many people share the responsibility of maintaining and managing the external environment. This includes engineers, who maintain temperature through control of heating, cooling, and ventilation; housekeeping personnel, who provide cleanliness and a pleasant appearance; and the health care team, who provides safety, privacy, neatness, and order for the patient's well-being.

There are several specific external environmental factors of concern to the members of the physical therapy team. These include the regulation of temperature, humidity control, ventilation, light, use of color, control of noise, neatness and order, elimination of noxious odors, safety, and privacy.

Regulation of Temperature

Temperature affects our comfort and even our disposition. A range between 68 and 72 degrees Fahrenheit is generally maintained in most air-conditioned facilities.

Some air-conditioned facilities have individual controls in treatment rooms to allow for flexibility in temperature control. When this is not available, fans, coolers, and heaters may sometimes be used.

Humidity Control

Humidity is the amount of moisture in the air, and a range of 30 to 50 percent is normally comfortable. Very low humidity dries the respiratory passages. As the temperature increases, air can hold more water. At 50 degrees Fahrenheit, saturated air holds approximately 4.2 grains of water per cubic foot of air. At 90 degrees Fahrenheit, nearly three times as much water is retained.

There is no simple method of decreasing humidity; it has become a technical problem for air-conditioning experts and is accomplished only by modern engineering methods. However, a vaporizer or humidifier can sometimes be used around patients in order to increase the humidity in some respiratory conditions.

Ventilation Control

Ventilation refers to the movement of air; stale air can be oppressive. The use of fans increases comfort because the air is in motion even though the temperature and humidity remain unchanged. In most health care settings, air-conditioning is used for ventilation and temperature control. Windows are not used for these purposes and should not be open.

Light Regulation

Lighting contributes to a patient's well-being; however, some illness, such as those seen in disorders of the nervous system, cause *"photophobia"* in which light is painful to the eyes.

A sunny room is cheerful and can improve a patient's spirits. Therefore, it is important to provide adequate lighting in all patient areas. This means a light that is bright enough to see without *glare* and to avoid eye strain. Good light is *soft* and *diffused.* It does not make sharp shadows. Overhead fluorescent lighting is generally effective (Figure 9-2).

Use of Color

In the patient environment, some

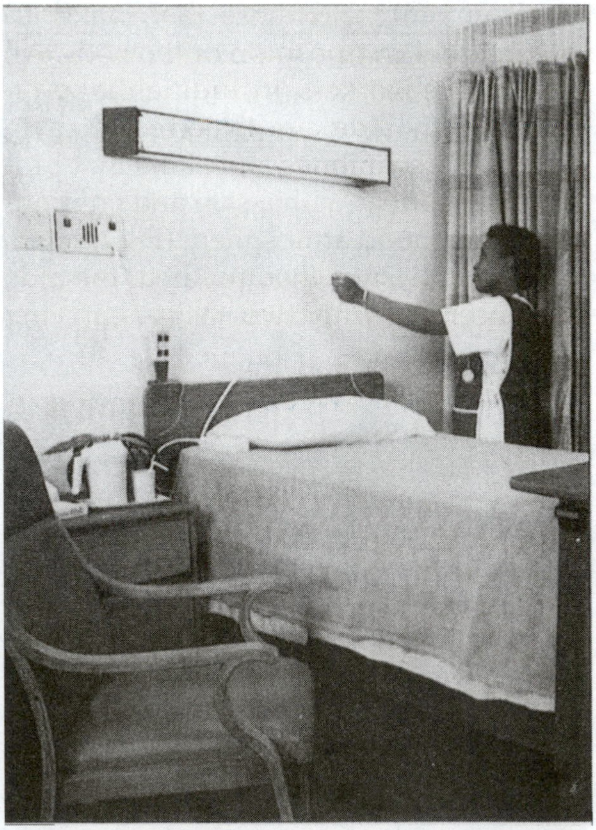

Figure 9-2 The best lighting is indirect lighting; the over-bed light.

bright colors stimulate while others sooth. The location of the source of light influences color. Decorators are aware of this, and colors in patient treatment rooms are usually subdued pastels.

Noise Control

Noise is a negative environmental factor, and it can affect one's health. People who are careless or thoughtless about talking and laughing cause unnecessary noise. Voices carry loudly in corridors, which seldom have drapes or other sound-absorbing materials. Equipment and machinery, such as those that are rolled down hallways, are often noisy. Dropping equipment causes startling noises, therefore, many health care facilities and physical therapy offices use carpeting or resilient floor materials and sound-absorbing ceilings in an effort to decrease noise. This still does not reduce the major source of noise—people. Skill in human relations, involving both tolerance and courtesy in dealing with others, is very important for all members of the health care team including the physical therapy aide. By practicing these lifelong skills, you can help reduce "people noise" for all of your patients.

Neatness and Order

Some people seem to thrive on living in clutter while others are offended if a picture hangs even slightly crooked. Therefore, it is important that the office and the individual treatment rooms be kept in sufficient order to be safe. This can easily be accomplished by tidying up and removing used items after every patient, and by doing your part as a member of the health care team in seeing to the office being kept neat and orderly.

Prevention and Control of Odors

Odors can be pleasant or unpleasant. Unfortunately, unpleasant smells have a tendency to permeate in some health care settings. In order to avoid odors from existing in the facility, all members of the staff should follow good prevention techniques. This includes disposing of refuse properly, removing items, such as wilted flowers and stagnant water, from bases, and avoiding being a source of odors yourself.

Good ventilation and cleanliness are far more effective in controlling odors than scented air sprays and other masking devices. **Hospital clean** should be a reality as well as an expression. Prompt and proper disposal and scrupulous cleanliness can decrease odors.

Providing Privacy

Privacy is essential for the patient's well-being. Always remember to knock gently and identify yourself before entering when the door to a treatment room is closed. Closing the curtain around the patient's cubicle can spare embarrassment to the patient, the physical therapist, and yourself.

Hospital workers, including those working in the physical therapy department, become accustomed to situations and functions that would be embarrassing to the nonmedical person. A discreet withdrawal from the room provides privacy for the shy patient to perform such functions as undressing for a treatment.

Remember, lack of privacy, like noise, is a frequent source of patient irritation. The thoughtful aide can do much to decrease these irritations.

PROVIDING A SAFE ENVIRONMENT

Providing a safe environment is everyone's responsibility. Remember that **safety** is necessary in preventing accidents and in reducing the possibility of lawsuits. Various types of accidents occur in environments where patients are seen. The most common are falls, burns, cuts or bruises, altercations with others, loss of personal possessions, such as money, choking, and electrical shock. The alert physical therapy aide is always on the lookout for safety hazards and corrects them so that accidents can be prevented.

Patients at Risk of Having Accidents

Some patients are more likely to have an accident than others. Those that are more at risk include confused and elderly patients and those taking certain types of medications. Their safety is your concern. Elderly patients often need special attention. They may be forgetful or have decreased sensory perceptions such as dimmed vision or decreased hearing that deprives them of some of their "danger warning" capabilities.

Another group of patients at risk are children. They have a tendency to climb, touch, taste, and eagerly explore their environments. They need special protection to prevent their curiosity from causing injury.

Preventing Falls

Falls are particularly hazardous in health care settings. Many falls can be prevented by removing foreign objects from the floor that might cause a patient to trip. Handrails and grab bars should also be installed in bathrooms and in corridors to assist weak or debilitated patients.

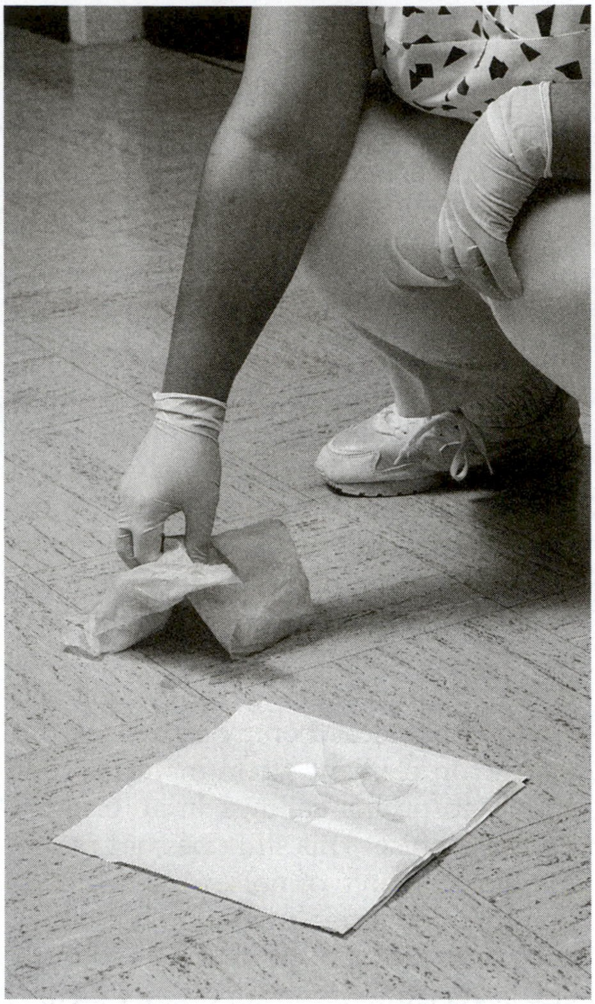

Figure 9-3 Small pieces of glass may be picked up carefully with several thicknesses of damp paper towels.

If you see a spill, mop it up immediately and post a Slippery When Wet sign when it is being mopped. Usually only one side of the floor is mopped at a time, allowing half to remain dry for use (Figure 9-3).

Another way to prevent falls from occurring is to provide assistance to patients who have poor vision or difficulty seeing. It is especially important that scatter rugs and clutter be removed and that furniture remain in customary locations.

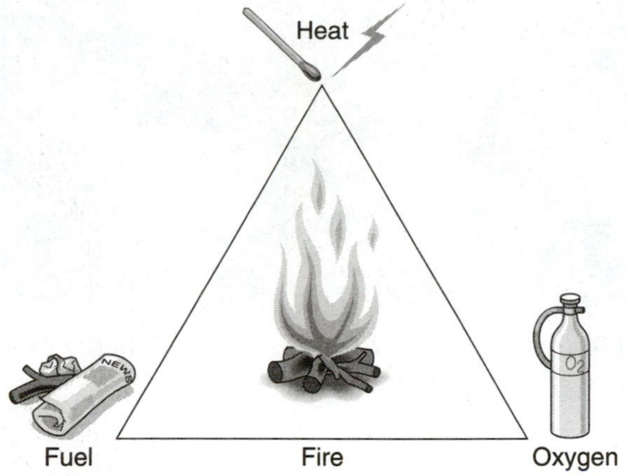

Figure 9-4A The fire triangle represents the elements needed for combustion (burning).

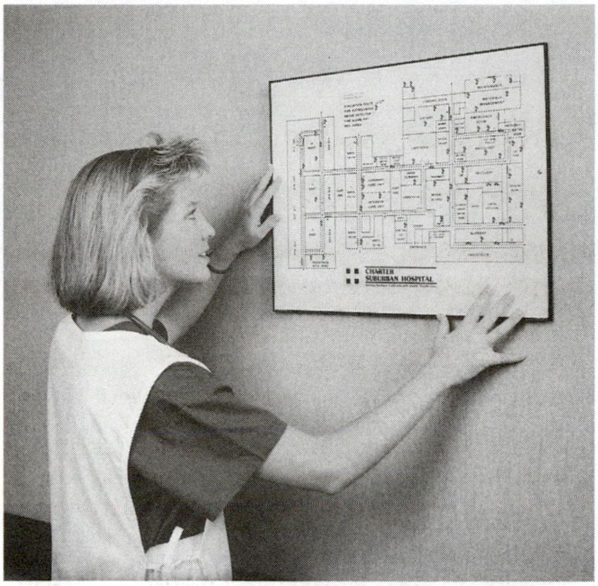

Figure 9-4B All personnel should know the escape plan in the event of a fire.

Preventing Burns

The alert aide looks out for safety hazards and corrects them so that burns can be prevented. Testing the temperature of solutions used for soaks or packs and heating devices is necessary to prevent burns. Remember that some patients may have debilitating diseases, such as diabetes, paralysis, or others that cause impaired circulation, and the patient may not even be aware that she has been burned.

Inspection of all electrical plugs, cords, and equipment before use can prevent accidents. Oily rags and other combustible materials usually are stored in metal containers that have tight lids. Oxygen tanks and other gas containers under pressure should be secured with straps or by other means to prevent falling (Figure 9-4A thru E).

Another way in which to prevent fires from occurring is to only allow smoking in designated places. If oxygen is used or kept close by, a No Smoking sign should be placed in full view for all patients and workers.

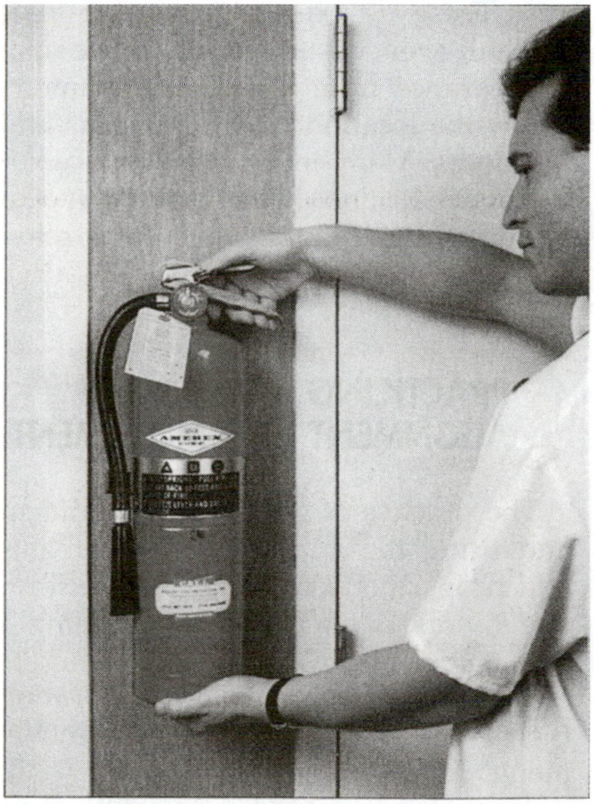

Figure 9-4C All personnel should know the escape plan in the event of a fire and should know where fire extinguishers are located.

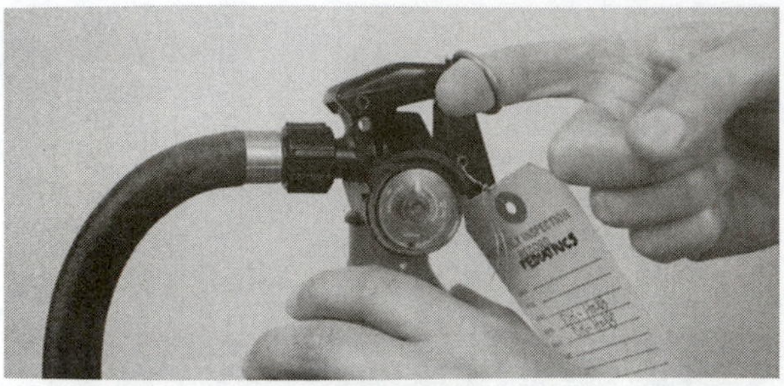

Figure 9-4D Use of the fire extinguisher. Remove pin.

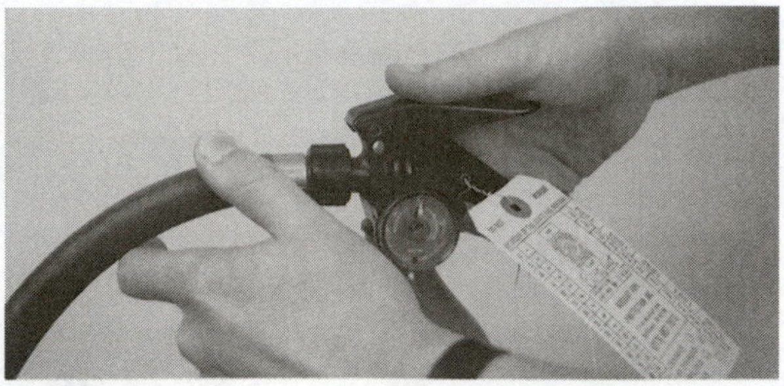

Figure 9-4E Use of the fire extinguisher continued. Push top handle down.

Fire in a hospital or health care setting is always a possibility; therefore, it is important to know the rules for fire safety. Generally, the agency's fire regulations will be taught in the first few days of employment. Many local fire departments hold regular fire safety classes for employees in health agencies in their area. These are required in most states if a health agency is to receive its fire safety clearance from the fire department. Know the location of extinguishers and fire doors. Many institutions have occasional fire drills. Always make sure you know what to do in case of a fire or other disaster.

◆ PRACTICING GOOD BODY ALIGNMENT AND MOVEMENT

The practice of good body alignment and using the appropriate movements and proper body mechanics to perform one's work is also part of providing a safe environment. Health care workers are very active people. In performing their work, they use a variety of movements as they reach, push, carry, lift, pull, stoop, sit, stand, and walk. Your activities as a physical therapy aide will require that you, too, use these movements as you reach for supplies from a shelf, lift and carry objects, push wheelchairs or stretchers, stoop to pick up objects from the floor, or walk, stand, or assist in ambulating a patient.

All of us have been performing these movements most of our lives, so why do we single them out for consideration now? What is the point? The answer is that with knowledge of proper body alignment and movement your work may be easier, you may prevent injury to yourself and your patient, and you will present a more attractive appearance as you work. You should always be conscious that you are using proper body alignment for yourself and the patient. This includes knowing how to balance yourself correctly in order to avoid strain or injury to yourself (Figure 9-5).

One of the most common injuries to physical therapy workers is severe muscle strain, usually of the lower back, although it may occur in the shoulders or the abdomen. Low back strain is painful and generally takes a long time to heal. It often requires hospitalization, bed rest, or traction and it is costly in lost salary and medical fees. It is also very preventable. Low back strain and other muscle strains are caused by improper body alignment, loss of balance, and poor body movements.

Your employer and your coworkers would much rather prefer you to be a health worker than a patient with an injury that could have been prevented. The knowledge and use of proper body

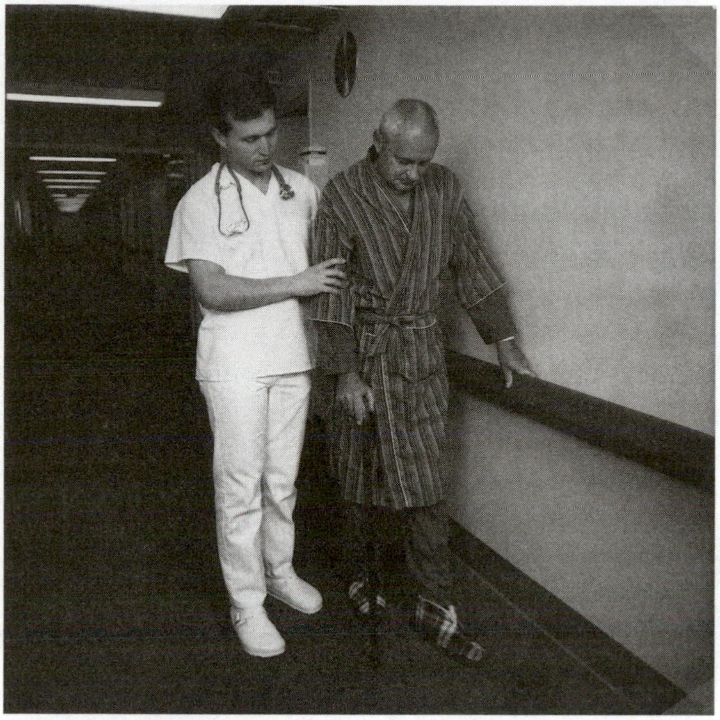

Figure 9-5 The proper standing position allows the physical therapy aide to move safely in any direction as needed.

alignment, balance, and movement will help you to prevent injury to yourself.

Body Alignment and Balance

Alignment is defined as the proper relationship of the body segments to one another. When the segments are properly aligned, it is easier to maintain body **balance.** Balanced posture means a body that is stable, steady, and not likely to tip or fall.

The main portions of the body, that is the pelvis, thorax, and the head, are supported by structures below them that are often very small such as the small bones in the feet and in the vertebrae. To maintain the proper relationship and balance of these anatomical parts, the ligaments and muscles must be used effectively (Figures 9-6A and B).

The force of gravity affects balance because it is constantly pulling the body toward the earth. Therefore, in order for proper balance to exist, there must be a center for the **gravity,** a base of support, and a line of gravity.

Center of gravity refers to an area located in the pelvis about the level of the second sacral vertebrae. The exact location may vary slightly, depending on body structure. A base of support provides a stable stance for keeping the body from toppling over, as well as stability in movements such as lifting, pushing, or pulling.

Line of gravity pertains to an imaginary line that falls in the frontal plane of the body, that is, one which passes behind the ear downward just behind the center of the hip joint and then downward slightly in front of the knee and ankle joint. Individual variations may occur according to skeletal build and the curvature of a person's spine.

When a person stands in an erect posture so that the line of gravity falls as stated above, body balance is preserved

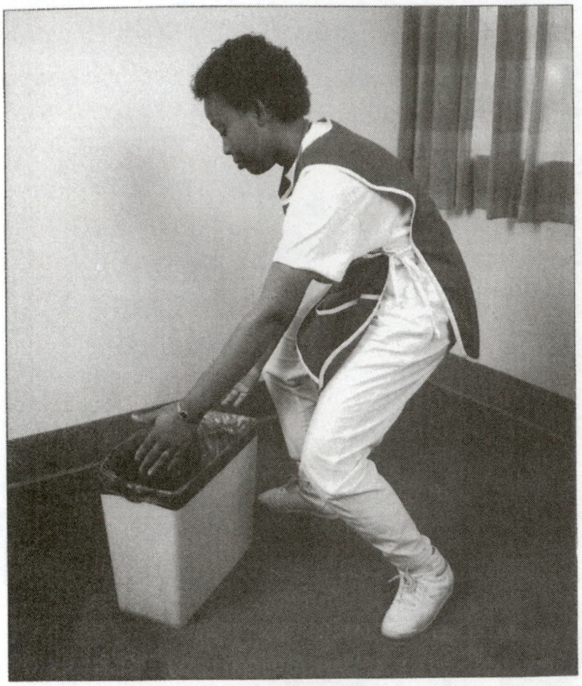

Figure 9-6A Bend at the knees and hips and stand close to the object. Keep the back straight and lift using the muscles in the arms and legs.

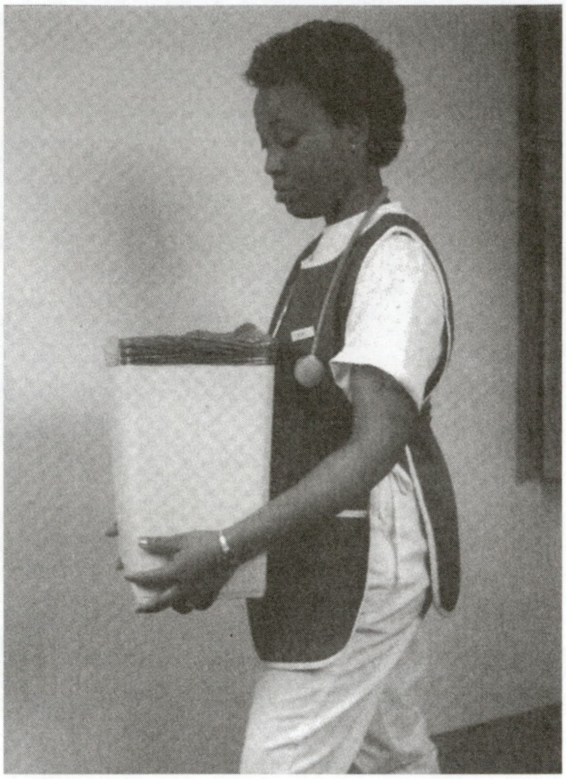

Figure 9-6B Hold the object close to the body.

and there is minimal resistance needed to overcome the force of gravity. If the posture is out of alignment, the body weight distribution is shifted, the balance is upset, the muscles no longer work together, and the gravitational pull is increased.

Body Movement

As we discussed in Chapter 6, the joints of our body allow movement when the muscles contract and pull on bones. Various terms are used to describe these movements, they include the movements of flexion, extension, hyperextension, abduction, and adduction.

If you hold your arm out straight, the elbow joint forms a straight line, or a 180-degree angle. By bending the elbow joint, you decrease the angle. This is called *flexion. Extension* is the joint movement opposite to flexion. When you straighten the arm that is bent at the elbow, or the leg that is bent at the knee, you are increasing the angle at the joint and extending the arm or leg.

Some joints allow for increasing the angle more than 180-degrees or beyond a straight line. This is called **hyperextension.** You hyperextend your neck each time you raise your chin and tilt your head backward. The knee joint also allows the movement of hyperextension. You can feel this movement if you stand normally with the knee joint nearly straight and then force the knee joint nearly straighter until the joint is locked or rigid.

Abduction is another term used to describe certain joint movements. Abduct means to move away from the midline of the body. The opposite movement of abduction is **adduction,** the movement to bring the part back toward the midline of the body.

The major body movements are flexion, extension, adduction, and abduction. The muscles that produce these movements are called flexors, extensors, adductors, and abductors.

Checking for Good Body Alignment

Before beginning any body movement, you should always align the balance your body properly in order to prevent strain and injury. To do this, you can use some basic checkpoints. First, always remember to start from a good base of support. Make sure you distribute your weight evenly on both feet, and keep your knees slightly flexed. Remember to tuck in your buttocks and keep the abdomen up and in. Raise your rib cage up, and, finally, always keep your head erect.

When performing a task, always remember to work at a comfortable height, to keep the work close to your body, to use smooth, coordinated movements, and to "set" or prepare the muscles for action. If you are required to reach for an object or to assist a patient, start by checking for good body alignment, stand on a footstool, if needed, with your feet apart. Always advance one foot forward in the direction of the reach, look and reach in front of you rather than overhead, and stabilize your body by setting your muscles. Remember to lower the object with smooth, coordinated movements, and, before stepping off the stool, remember to look down.

◆ ASEPSIS AND INFECTION CONTROL

Practicing safety in the working environment includes many factors. As we have already discussed, it includes maintaining the external environment, avoiding accidents, and practicing good body movements. Providing a safe atmosphere for both you and the patient also includes the practice of good medical asepsis and infection control.

It cannot be emphasized enough that one of the most important tasks you have in the health care field is providing a healthy environment for both your patients and yourself. A clean, dry, well-lit and airy atmosphere goes a long way toward preventing the growth of germs or killing those that already exist.

One of the simplest methods we have to prevent the spread of germs and disease is the use of proper handwashing techniques. It is a safety skill not only for you personally but also for your patient and your coworkers. You will wash your hands before and after doing any procedures that involve direct or indirect contact with a patient, after contact with waste materials, before handling any food or food receptacles, and at any other times when your hands are soiled.

Handwashing for Asepsis: Understanding the Germ Theory

As you enter your career in health care and particularly in the field of physical therapy, you need to develop an understanding of how germs cause disease and how health care workers use principles of medical asepsis to carry out one of the most important patient goals—that of protecting the patient from infection. **Medical asepsis** includes the techniques and skills used to render any medical setting free of disease-causing microorganisms, although nonharmful microorganisms may still be present. The most crucial of these skills, and one of the most effective actions in preventing the spread of infection, is handwashing

PROCEDURE #5: Completing the Two-Minute Handwash for Medical Asepsis

To complete a two-minute handwash, make sure you have: soap dispenser, waste container, paper towels.

1. Remove all jewelry.
2. Approach the sink; stand in a comfortable position, leaning slightly toward the sink, and maintain good body alignment; avoid contaminating your clothing by touching the sink.
3. Turn on the water with a dry paper towel and keep it running continuously throughout the procedure.
4. Adjust the temperature of the water.
5. Wet your hands with water by holding your hands down toward the sink, lower than your elbows; the water will then drain down the wrists to the fingertips and carry the bacteria away.
6. Apply soap or detergent.
7. Wash your hands. This usually takes about 30 seconds for the palms, 10 seconds for the backs of the hands, and 10 seconds for the fingers. Wash the palms using a rotary or circular motion and friction.
8. Rinse well. Hold your hands with fingers pointing downward and avoid touching any portion of the sink with your hands.
9. Wash your wrists and forearms with soap, spending 10 to 15 seconds per each wrist and forearm.
10. Rinse your arms and hands, remembering to drain in a downward motion.
11. Repeat steps 5 through 9.
12. Inspect your knuckles.
13. Clean your fingernails using an orange stick or a curved end of a flat toothpick.
14. Dry your hands well.
15. Turn off the running water; use a paper towel to turn off the hand faucet; and discard it into the wastebasket after finishing.
16. Apply lotion as desired.
17. Leave the sink area neat and clean.

Our everyday world is filled with **microorganisms,** which are extremely small bits of plant or animal life too small to be seen with the naked eye. They can be seen and studied with the use of a microscope. Only a small number of microorganisms are harmful to the human body and capable of causing disease. These are referred to as germs, or *pathogenic* organisms. Bacteria are one-celled microorganisms; some are pathogenic and cause infections, whereas others are *nonpathogenic.*

People come in contact with microorganisms and germs constantly, but the body's defenses are strong enough to protect us from diseases most of the time. Microorganisms consist of protein, have a certain amount of weight, and are unable to move about on their own. Because of their size, they are picked up and carried by the slightest air current, and they settle on any convenient surface. Because they have weight, they drift lower and lower until they settle on a surface, so the heaviest concentration of microorganisms will be present on solid objects.

Microorganisms are found on all skin surfaces. Large numbers are found within the body, especially in the air passages of the respiratory tract, in the mouth, and along the entire length of the digestive tract. Normal, harmless residents of the intestinal tract include *Escherichia coli (E. coli)* (Figure 9-7). These organisms may cause an infection if introduced into a different part of the body, such as the urinary bladder, or into an open wound. The skin is an effective barrier against pathogenic organisms, and it protects the delicate organs within the body. Vigorous washing removes most of the microorganisms on the surface of the skin that are picked up when we come in contact with objects, but it cannot remove all of those that reside in the grooves and crevices that are present in the outer layers of skin. Additional protection against microorganisms is provided by the immune system of the body.

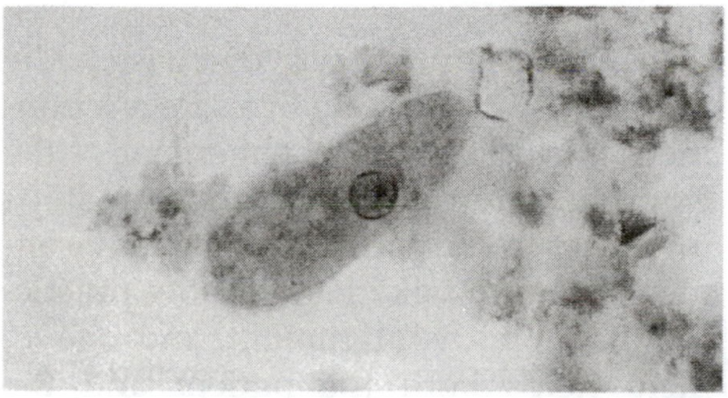

Figure 9-7A Intestinal protozoa *Escherichia coli (Courtesy of the Centers for Disease Control and Prevention, Atlanta, GA).*

Infections are caused by germs that invade the tissues of the body and set up a chemical reaction that causes the tissues to react in the symptoms associated with the disease. Generally, an infection can develop if the body is exposed to a large number of pathogenic organisms or if it is attacked by germs that are very strong and virulent. Infections can also be caused if the individual has a low resistance.

Through the use of medical asepsis, health care workers can provide a safe environment for patients who are particularly susceptible to infections. Medical asepsis includes various actions and skills that reduce the number of pathogenic organisms present in the immediate vicinity. It is necessary to reduce the number of all microorganisms in order to lower the number of pathogens; this is done by frequent handwashing, cleaning dirty or soiled surfaces, disposing of highly contaminated items, and using sterile equipment and supplies.

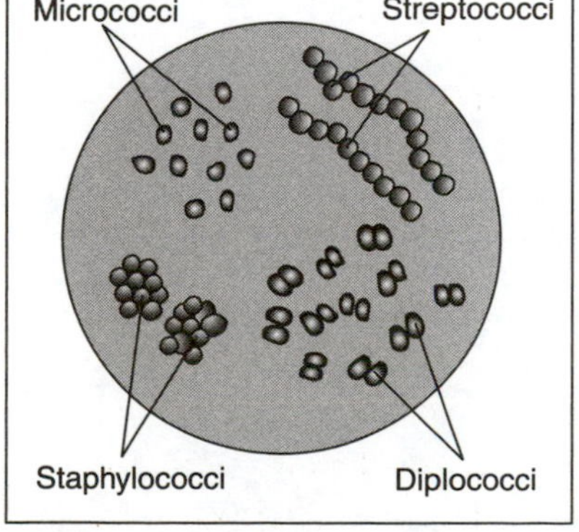

Figure 9-7B Kinds of cocci.

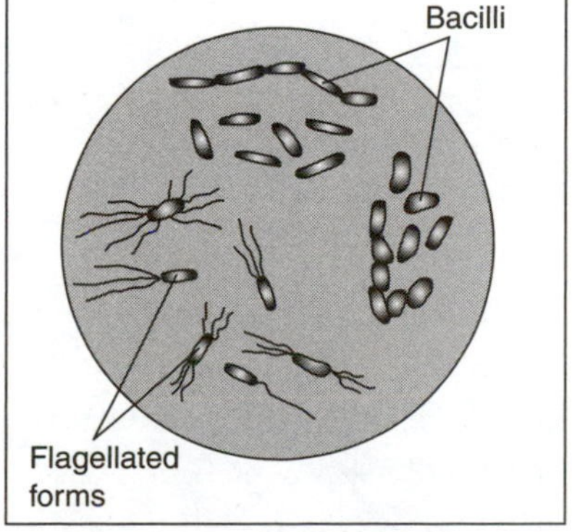

Figure 9-7C Kinds of bacilli.

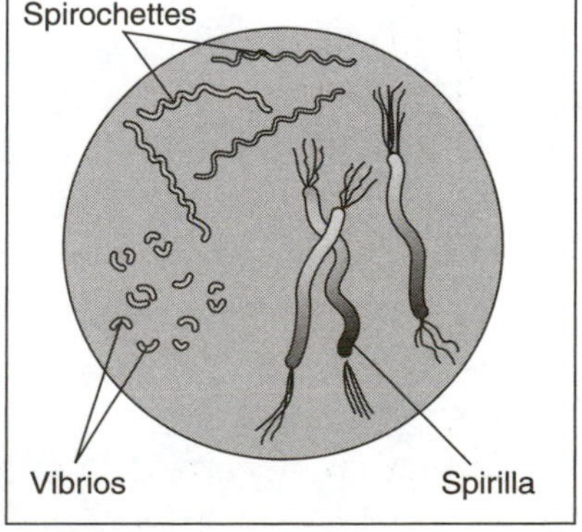

Figure 9-7D Spiral forms.

How Microorganisms Grow and Spread

Because microorganisms are living organisms, they need certain environmental conditions in order to help them live and grow. These include moisture, food, oxygen, temperature, and darkness.

Microorganisms are incapable of moving by themselves, so they must rely on other vehicles for transportation from one site to another. For an infection to occur, the pathogens have to be able to escape from the reservoir or host where they have been allowed to multiply and then be transmitted to another host. They can be carried by human, animal, or insect carriers; on objects, such as furniture, clothing, and medical equipment; by air currents produced by winds, drafts, sneezing, or coughing; and in foods, such as water, milk, and other ingestible materials.

The most common method of transporting microorganisms is by direct contact with an infected person, contaminated materials, or supplies. They are carried on the hands or skin to another susceptible person. In the health care environment, microorganisms are generally spread from worker to worker, from equipment to patient or worker, from patient to patient, and from worker to patient.

◆ PERFORMING PROPER HANDWASHING

In order to provide a safe environment for the patient and to reduce the number of microorganisms as well as the total number of pathogens, you should wash your hands frequently when providing care. Hands should be washed before and after providing care, after touching contaminated materials or equipment, after going to the bathroom, and before handling food. In addition to washing your hands frequently, you should also follow the appropriate steps for completing a two-minute handwash for medical asepsis. Refer to Procedure 5.

◆ SUMMARY

In this chapter, we discussed the importance of working in a safe environment, including the management of the external environment and the steps involved in providing a safe environment. We also talked about how practicing good body alignment and movement helps both the patient and the health care worker maintain a safe working environment. Finally, we discussed asepsis and infection control, and the importance of following good handwashing techniques in order to keep the environment safe and free of disease.

◆ ◆ LEARNING ACTIVITY 9-1

Safety First

Fill in the blanks to the following questions.

1. Clear floors of all ____________ and keep ____________ at all times in order to prevent patients falls, injury, and possible litigation.
2. When transporting the patient, the physical therapy aide must always use ____________, ____________, or ____________ to protect the patient.
3. The physical therapy aide should always be prepared in case of fire. To do this, you should know where the ____________ ____________ are located and the hospital ____________ ____________ including ____________ ____________.

◆ ◆ LEARNING ACTIVITY 9-2

Safety

Read the narrative, then write answers to the numbered questions. You should try to find answers at the health care facility, from classroom information, or from independent research.

Narrative

Martha and Ben are spending their first day at Riverside Community Hospital. Their first days are pretty scary, and they aren't entirely comfortable, even though everyone has been very nice to them and the hospital director even welcomed them with a little speech. Ms. Green, the physical therapist to whom they are assigned, says, "The first thing we need to mention is fire safety. Let's look at the fire extinguisher in this hall and see what kind it is." Martha and Ben know that there are four common types of fire extinguishers. Ms. Green says,

(1) "What are the common classes of fire extinguishers, and what type of fire is each used for?" Between them, Martha and Ben manage to answer the questions and make a good first impression.

There is much more to discuss about fire safety, but Martha and Ben now move along with Ms. Green to the lobby of the hospital. Here she stops and says, "Safety is such a big subject that we must learn about it in every part of the hospital. But there are a few general safety rules that apply wherever you are. One of them is, never run in the halls, and never rush around corners and through doors.

(2) Why is this an important rule?

Another general rule is, if something is spilled, clean it up at once because someone might slip and fall. A third general rule is, do not engage in horseplay or practical jokes in the health care facility.

(3) What is horseplay?

Ms. Green then takes the students by the Physical Therapy area and introduces them to Ms. Jones, another physical therapist. Ms. Jones is placing a patient in a wheelchair. She makes it look very simple, but Martha remembers the correct procedure and notes that Ms. Jones is careful to use good body mechanics as she guides the patient into the chair.

(4) Define "bodymechanics."

As they continue on their walk through the hospital, Ben notes information about OSHA posted in the employees' lounges. He knows that the OSHA is a federal program to ensure that employees work in safe and healthful conditions.

(5) Name three areas of the hospital that an OSHA inspector might check.

As Martha and Ben leave the hospital to return to school, Ben says, "I guess I just hadn't thought that much about safety until now, but I'm glad Ms. Green made us aware of it right away. I feel much better about observing now, and surely we'll be able to keep from causing any serious accidents."

◆ ◆ LEARNING ACTIVITY 9-3

Infection Control

Read the narrative, then write answers to the numbered questions. You should try to find answers at a health care facility, from classroom information, or from independent research.

Narrative

Claire and Bob are assigned to Infection Control for the rest of the week. Although they will be on this service for only three days, Mr. Kennedy, the nurse epidemiologist, is waiting to take them with him as he makes his rounds. They know that he is responsible for monitoring all patient infections, but he has mentioned that he is trying to cut down on the number of nosocomial infections at Riverside Community.
(1) Why might a patient be more likely to be infected in a hospital than at home?

Nosocomial infections are not Mr. Kennedy's only problem. There are two patients with classic signs and symptoms of infection that are not yet diagnosed. These are a serious problem because he doesn't know whether they will require isolation and, if so, what type of isolation will be needed.
(2) What steps must be taken in strict isolation?

Mr. Kennedy tells Claire and Bob about a series of infections they had on Unit 4 last year. Two patients developed a communicable disease, called typhoid fever. It took real detective work to figure out how the bacteria were spread. Finally, it was found that one of the employees was an asymptomatic carrier of typhoid.
(3) What is a "carrier" of a disease?

Mr. Kennedy says to Bob, "You know that one means of preventing the spread of pathogens is sterilization. Since it is impossible to sterilize living tissue,
(4) How can we achieve surgical asepsis?

REVIEW QUESTIONS

1. Briefly explain what the term *environment* means.
2. List the 10 environmental factors of concern to the members of the physical therapy team.

a. ________	f. ________
b. ________	g. ________
c. ________	h. ________
d. ________	i. ________
e. ________	j. ________

3. A range of between ____ and ____ degrees F is generally maintained in most air-conditioned health care facilities.
4. ________ is defined as the amount of moisture in the air.
5. ________ refers to the movement of air.
6. ________ is a negative environmental factor that can affect one's health.
7. Whose responsibility is it to provide a safe environment?
8. List at least three types of patients who are more at risk of having an accident than others:
   a. ______________________________
   b. ______________________________
   c. ______________________________
9. List at least three ways the physical therapy aide can assist in preventing fires in the office:
   a. ______________________________
   b. ______________________________
   c. ______________________________
10. The practice of good _____ ________ and using good _____ ________ to perform one's work is part of providing a safe environment.
11. ________ is defined as the proper relationship of the body segments to one another.
12. ________ is one of the simplest methods for preventing the spread of diseases and germs.
13. ________ ________ includes the techniques and skills used to render any medical setting free of disease-causing microorganisms.
14. List the five environmental conditions necessary for a microorganism to live and grow:

a. ______________	d. ______________
b. ______________	e. ______________
c. ______________	

15. To be effective, how long should a medical handwash take?

10

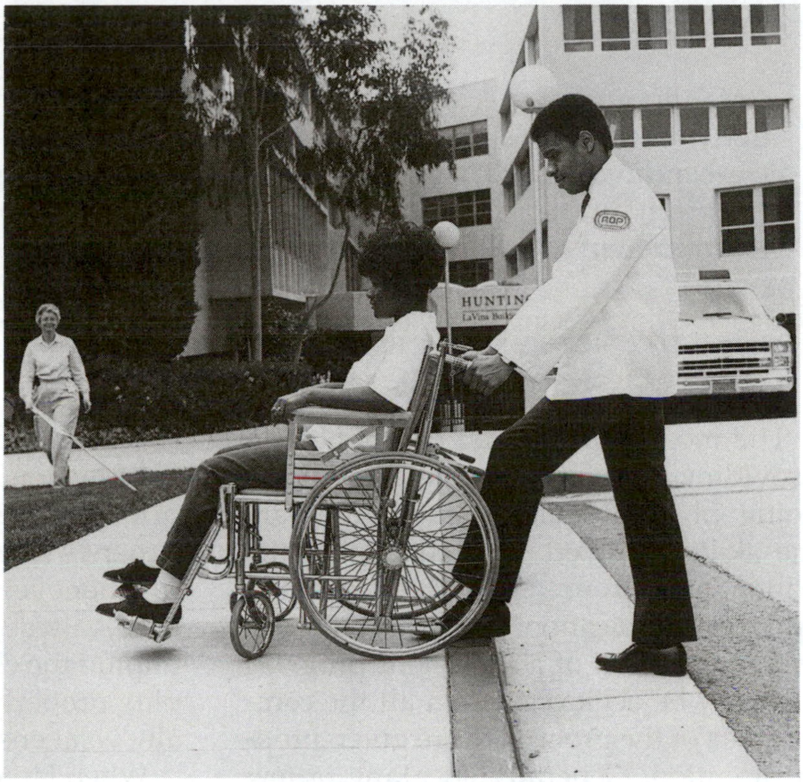

Preparation for Patient Care

OBJECTIVES

Upon completion of this chapter, you should be able to:

1. List and explain the three fundamental components to providing care to patients undergoing physical therapy modalities.
2. Describe the role body mechanics play in physical therapy.
3. Explain the purpose of patient preparation and identify the physical therapy aide's role in preparing the patient for physical therapy treatments.
4. Describe patient preparation for transporting patients via a cart and a wheelchair.

KEY TERMS

Ascending
Body mechanics
Descending
Draping
Environment
Gurney
Lifting
Squatting
Transferring
Transporting
Verbal command

The most fundamental component in providing proper care to patients undergoing physical therapy modalities are the skills involved with managing the patient's **environment,** body mechanics, and communication. Safe and correct implementation of a treatment program can only be achieved when all the components of the procedure are given proper attention. Generally speaking, a few minutes taken at the start of a procedure to plan the steps involved and to prepare for the actual procedure increases the likelihood of a safe, efficient, and effective implementation.

MANAGEMENT OF THE ENVIRONMENT

Managing and maintaining the organization of the work area provides the greatest protection of the patient and staff, and creates an environment for efficiency. Achieving these goals is the responsibility of all staff members. However, you should always remember that the person using the area or the equipment is the individual most responsible for making sure that all equipment is returned to its proper storage place in proper functioning condition and that the area is left clean and ready for the next patient.

All equipment should be periodically checked and inspected for wear and malfunction. It should also be inspected prior to patient use to ensure the patient's safety.

Whenever electrical equipment is used, always make sure to plug and unplug the electrical cord by holding the plug properly. Pulling on the cord generally weakens its attachment to the plug.

When large pieces of equipment, such as the diathermy machine, is used in the treatment of a patient, always remember to position the equipment and patient to allow easy accessibility. Should the patient need assistance quickly, improperly placed equipment may tend to hamper the ability to provide assistance quickly and efficiently. The floor should also remain uncluttered in order to avoid any tripping by the patient or the staff.

Preparing the Area

Prior to initiating any patient care, transfer, or treatment, the bed or **gurney** and surrounding areas must be readied. Enough room should be provided for unimpeded movement. Staff and patients should be able to move around and maneuver within the area without bumping into or tripping over any equipment or other supplies. Equipment and furniture not needed as part of the transfer or treatment, such as any diathermy machines or mobile foot stools, should be moved far enough out of the area to not present a danger to either the patient or yourself.

After the area has been properly arranged, you should prepare the specific equipment necessary for the treatment. This will avoid the possibility of leaving a patient alone or unguarded or interrupting the treatment once it has begun. Any supplies necessary in a treatment area, such as linens or pillows, should also be prepared before the patient arrives in the treatment area.

BODY MECHANICS

The use of proper posture and body mechanics is necessary in order to limit stress and strain on the musculoskeletal structures. Whenever you are required to lift, push, or pull a patient, the stresses and strains upon the musculoskeletal system tend to increase. Proper posture and the use of **body mechanics** are based upon the alignment and functioning of the musculoskeletal system. They include the understanding of four very important principles, including (1) using larger and stronger muscles to perform heavy work; 2) maintaining the center of gravity of the body close to the center of the base of support; (3) keeping the combined center of gravity of the aide and patient centered within the base of support; and (4) having a base of support that is of the appropriate size and shape.

Lifting

All **lifting** should be initiated from a **squatting** position. The aide's feet are generally placed in a stride position, slightly apart, in order to widen the base of support in the anterior and posterior and lateral directions. The trunk must be erect so that the muscles have only to maintain the erect position and not have to work extra hard in order to extend the trunk during the lifting motion. Beginning from a squatting position allows you to reach the object or person to be lifted. Do not squat so deeply that the leg muscles are put at a disadvantage in regaining the upright position.

You should always be as close as possible to the object or person to be lifted since this allows the center of gravity to be maintained within the base of support. Bending the hips and knees in a squat allows the aide to get close enough to the object or person to permit lifting using the strong leg muscles. Always remember that when you carry patients or objects, keeping them close to the midline of your body, also helps to maintain the combined center of gravity within the base of support.

Transferring

The act of **transferring** a patient requires special movements that move the center of gravity away from the center of the base of support, possibly causing a loss of balance. By increasing the size of the base of support and setting your feet in stride and slightly apart, you are provided with a larger base of support. Your feet should also be free to move as the situation requires, allowing the base of support to be reestablished under the moving center of gravity. Crossing the legs during movement should be avoided since it tends to decrease the size of the base of support and may also lead to tripping. Whenever possible, always use quick shuffling movements when required to move your feet.

Moving Large Pieces of Equipment or Furniture

If you are required to move a large piece of equipment or furniture or to guard a patient during ambulation, always remember to position yourself facing the direction of the movement in order to determine if the path is free from obstruction. In addition, being behind an object to be moved allows for more freedom in the lifting or pushing motion and uses larger muscles and body weight more efficiently.

If you are required to guard the patient during gait training, make sure you position yourself at an approximate 45-degree angle, slightly to the side and rear of the patient. If the patient happens to fall forward or backward, your position is close enough to the plane of the fall to support the patient before she falls directly to the floor. If the patient falls from side to side, your position will again allow proper support and break the fall. Again, the base of support must be wide enough to support shifts in the center of gravity if the patient should start to fall. Your feet should not be crossed during ambulation nor should they interfere with the patient's feet or ambulatory devices.

In all cases, movements should be properly planned and the area prepared for use prior to starting. Utilizing proper body mechanics and safety precautions will enhance the safety and effectiveness of the patient's treatment as well as assist you in providing that treatment.

◆ VERBAL COMMANDS

Patients must know what they are expected to do and when they are to do it during transfers and treatment. This understanding is paramount to the patient's effective participation in his treatment. **Verbal commands** on the part of the aide focus the patient's attention on specifically desired actions. Instructions to the patient should be simple and in language he can understand in order to avoid confusion. If the patient understands medical terminology, medical terms may be used. In most cases, however, lay language will be required. In some cases, the need for foreign language instructions may also be necessary.

Whenever you are asked to provide commands, you must make sure they are specific. Counting to five does not tell a patient to do anything specific. If the patient is to look up at the count of five, count to five and then say, "Look up." "Look up" is a specific command; it tells the patient what to do without requiring him to translate the word "five" into the specific command "look up."

As a physical therapy aide, you should describe to the patient the general sequence of events that will occur. In addition, the patient should also be instructed in his expected responses. This helps the patient to learn the skill for future independent use and thereby to increase the safety of the immediate task performance. Therefore, always make sure you determine that the patient understands your instructions. Asking the patient "Do you understand the instructions?" does not always ensure understanding. Having the patient repeat the instructions in the proper order provides an opportunity for mental rehearsal of the task in addition to indicating an appropriate level of understanding.

Always remember to speak clearly and vary your tone of voice as the situation requires. Sharp commands will generally receive quicker responses, while a soft command will elicit a slower response. Make sure that the patient can hear the commands. If she cannot hear or does not understand the spoken word, you may use gestures and demonstrations to convey the necessary meaning.

◆ PATIENT PREPARATION

For the most efficient use of treatment time, it is important that patient preparation be completed prior to transport and treatment. To do so, you should notify the nursing staff or your department's transport person of the preparation requirements well in advance of the scheduled treatment time. You must convey to the appropriate personnel that the patient should be properly dressed for transfer and treatment; this is necessary for the patient's right to modesty, for enhanced and beneficial treatment, and for safety.

All hospital gowns have been designed for ease in dressing and accessibility during nursing care. They may not provide the most effective **draping** during the movements required for transfers and treatment, but proper securing of the ties may assist in providing some additional coverage. A robe, housecoat, or two hospital gowns, one opening in the front and the other opening in the back, may also be used. If necessary, a sheet or towel may also be used for draping.

Patient preparation also involves dressing the patient in the appropriate attire such as slacks or shorts if the lower extremities must be observed or examined. If a female patient's upper trunk must be observed, a halter top is considered appropriate. Shoes and socks that offer support are also required if the patient is to ambulate or practice standing transfers. When a patient is dependent and working on a mat program only, slippers may be used as they are easier to take off and put on as necessary. In all cases, the decision about proper attire must be dictated according to the patient's needs, his ability to manipulate the clothing, and the requirements of the treatment.

Preparing the patient for her treatment also involves taking into consideration the variety of settings in which he or she may be receiving treatment. In some cases, either intravenous tubes, chest tubes, catheters, or combinations of any one of these should be present. Therefore, whenever you are required to position, transfer, or treat the patient, care must be taken not to disrupt the setup of vital medical equipment.

During and after patient transport, transfers, or repositioning, attention should always be paid to appropriate draping. In some cases, even shorts or a halter top may limit observation. Draping by sheet may be necessary. The aim is to never expose any part of the body, except for the part that is receiving treatment. The purposes of draping are to protect a patient's modesty, provide warmth, and protect wounds, scars, and stumps. Edges should be tucked under the patient to avoid inadvertent exposure. When repositioning a patient, advance planning is required in order to maintain appropriate draping during the movement.

◆ TRANSPORTING

Transporting, or taking the patient from one area to another, is frequently necessary. A cart, gurney, or wheelchair may be necessary for safety or because of hospital regulations. The patient should be transferred to an appropriate manner with proper draping during the transfer and transport. Always remember to lock the brakes on the cart or wheelchair before beginning the transfer and to adjust the patient's clothing, draping, and medical accessories so that they will not become tangled in the wheels or drag on the floor during the transport. A mattress pad on the cart and a wheelchair cushion may also be used for the patient's comfort and protection. Additional pillows and padding can be used for comfort and protection as necessary.

Safety belts should also be used to secure the patient whenever it becomes necessary to transport or transfer him. There may be circumstances that require the use of restraints that the patient cannot release. If a cart has side rails, they should also be used. Arms and legs should be kept within the cart or wheelchair so that they do not get injured during the transport.

Transporting Via a Cart

Carts or gurneys may be moved so that the patient is moving feet first, with the aide or therapist pushing from the head of the cart. The pace should be slow and steady; quick, jerky movements should be avoided so as not to upset a patient or make him nauseated. Always remember to maintain control of the cart at all times. This means turning corners cautiously and avoiding bumping into walls or other objects.

Transporting Via a Wheelchair

Using a wheelchair properly requires that the patient be seated well back on the seat and that the lower limbs be placed on the footrests or leg rests. Wheelchairs should also be pushed at a slow and steady pace, avoiding any quick or jerky movements. Control of the wheelchair, especially when turning corners, should always be maintained in the same manner as a cart or gurney. Refer to Procedures 6, 7, 8 and 9 for instructions on **ascending** and **decending** a wheelchair..

◆ SUMMARY

In this chapter, we discussed the importance of preparing for patient care. We explained the three fundamental components to providing care to patients undergoing physical therapy modalities, including management and maintenance of the environment and care of the equipment. We also talked about how to prepare the patient area, including both the treatment room and the equipment. Finally, we talked about body mechanics as it relates to patient preparation, including the proper steps to take when lifting and transferring patients.

PROCEDURE #6: Descending a Wheelchair from a Curb

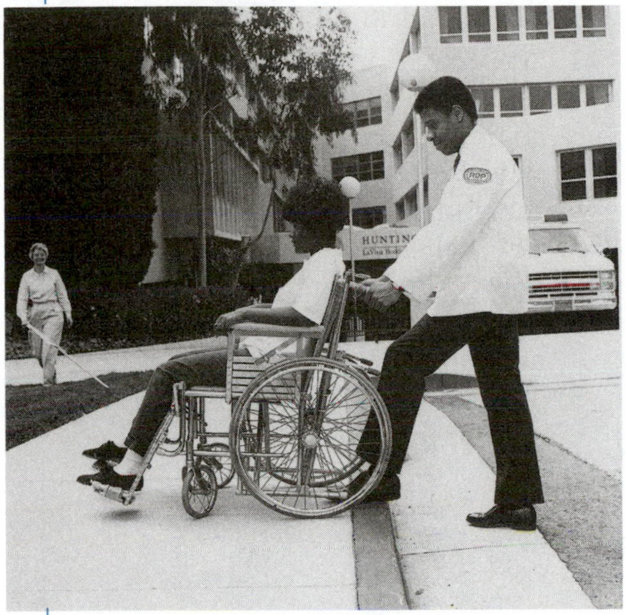

Figure 10-1 Starting position to descend curb backwards.

1. Position the wheelchair so that the patient is facing away from the curb, Figure 10-1.
2. While facing the wheelchair, carefully step off the curb backwards.
3. Holding onto the handles of the wheelchair, slowly lower the rear wheels to the street by rolling them smoothly off the edge of the curb, Figure 10-2.
4. Continue to slowly roll the wheelchair backward without allowing the front wheels to fall until the front wheels are clear of the curb.
5. Slowly lower the front wheels until all four wheels are securely on the lower level, Figure 10-3.

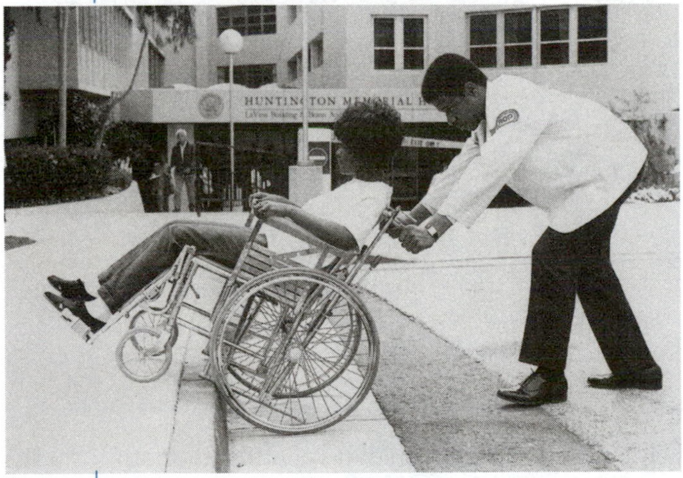

Figure 10-2 Rear wheels lowered to the street.

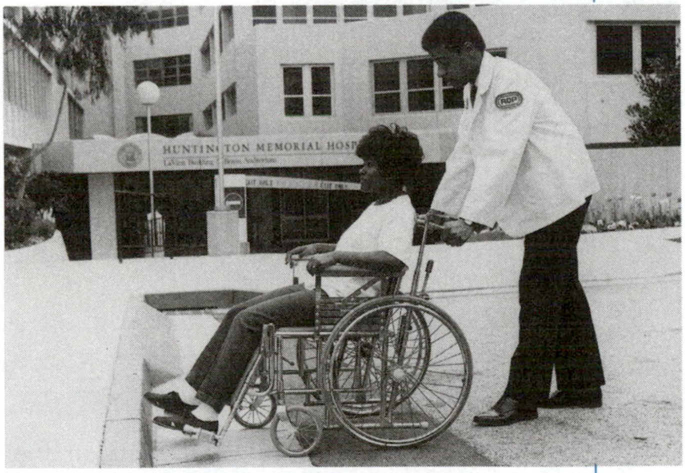

Figure 10-3 Completion of descending wheelchair from the curb in a backward manner.

PROCEDURE #7: Alternate Method for Descending a Wheelchair from a Curb

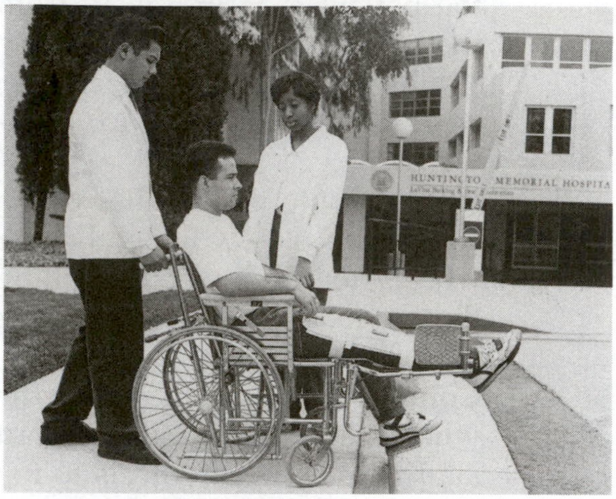

Figure 10-4 Tilting the wheelchair to descend the curb in a forward manner.

1. Approach the curb forwards, Figure 10-4, then tilt the wheelchair backward so that the front wheels are about eight inches off the ground.
2. The wheelchair is then rolled slowly and smoothly off the curb into the lower level, Figures 10-5 and 10-6.
3. The front wheels are then lowered to the ground.

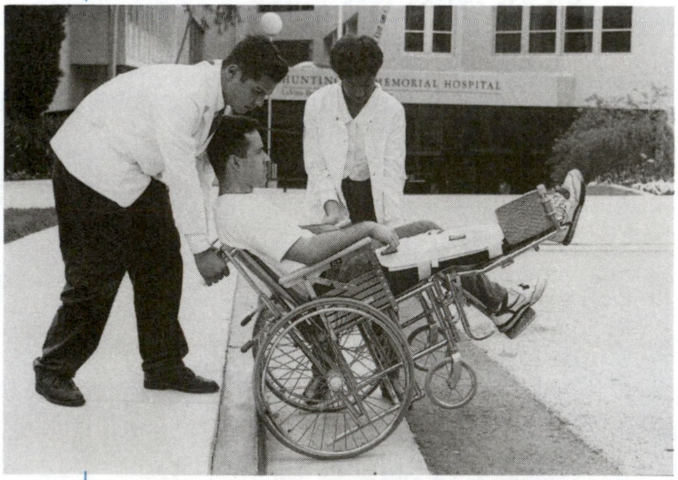

Figure 10-5 Rolling the wheelchair off the curb.

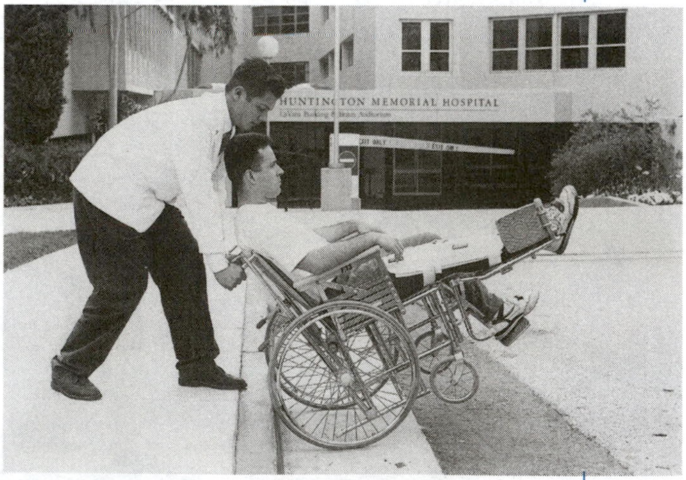

Figure 10-6 Completion of descending the curb in a forward manner.

PROCEDURE #8: Ascending a Wheelchair up a Curb

1. Tilt the wheelchair backward onto the rear wheels, Figure 10-7.
2. Standing on the curb, carefully lift and roll the wheelchair backward up the curb, Figure 10-8.
3. When all four wheels are clearly over the curb, the front wheels can be lowered, Figure 10-9.

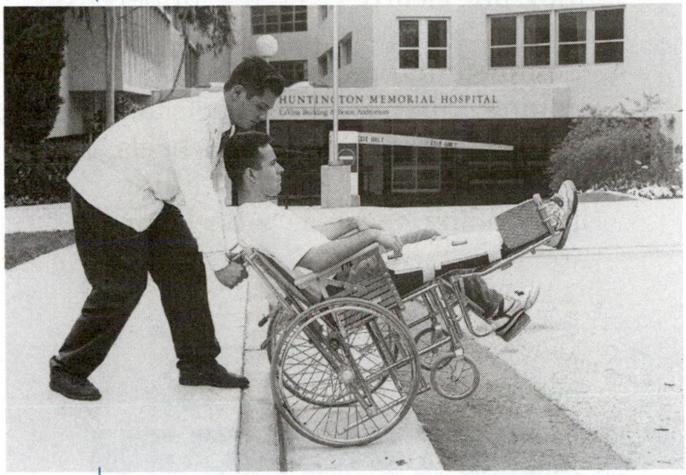

Figure 10-7 Tilting the wheelchair to begin ascending the curb in a backward manner.

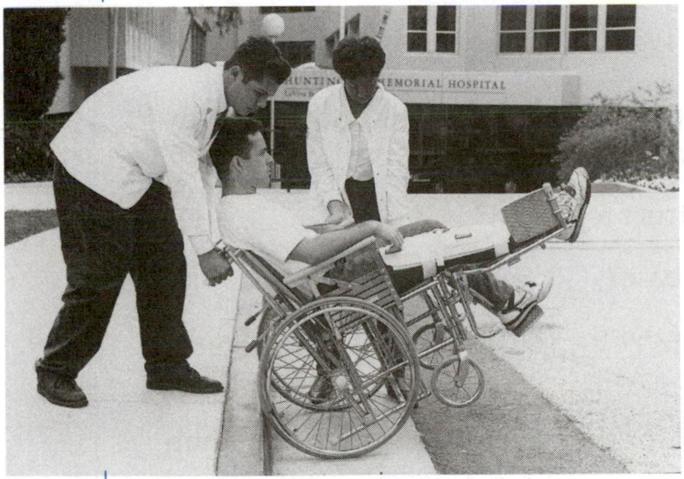

Figure 10-8 Rolling the wheelchair up the curb.

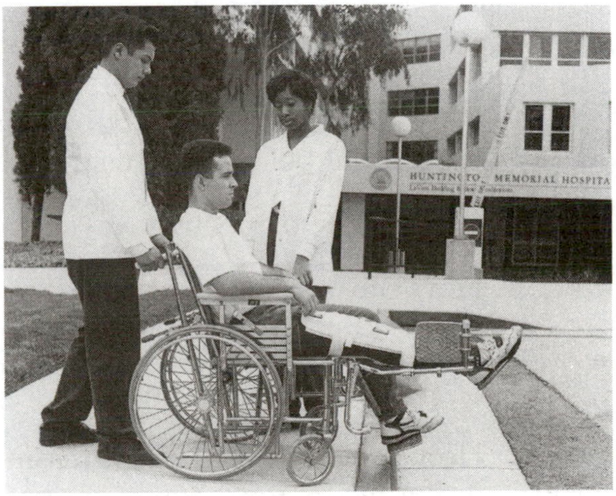

Figure 10-9 Completion of ascending the curb backward.

PROCEDURE #9: Alternate Method for Ascending a Wheelchair Up a Curb

1. Approach the curb forwards.
2. While facing the curb, carefully tilt the wheelchair backward onto its rear wheels, so that the front wheels can clear the curb.
3. The wheelchair is then wheeled forward, placing the front wheels on the upper level as soon as they are clearly over the upper level.
4. Complete the procedure by continuing to wheel the wheelchair forward until the rear wheels contact the curb, and then lifting and rolling the rear wheels up and over the curb.

◆ ◆ LEARNING ACTIVITY 10-1

Questions to Answer

Answer the following questions as briefly as possible.

1. Why should an activity be explained and the instructions understood by the patient before treatment begins?
2. What are two effective ways to instruct a patient?
3. How can you help put a patient at ease?
4. Why is to so important for you to know the purpose and desired results of an activity or treatment?
5. How can you avoid embarrassment for the patient when preparing him or her for treatment or examination?
6. How can the physical therapy aide assist the therapist before the patient is treated?
7. When you are assisting the patient to dress, which limb should be placed into the clothing first?
8. How are patient errors in procedure dealt with?

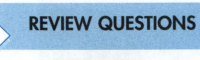

REVIEW QUESTIONS

1. The three components of preparation for the patient undergoing physical therapy treatments include __________, __________, and __________.

2. Preparing the patient's area for treatment always involves creating a __________ environment.

3. __________ __________ is necessary in order to limit stress and strain on the body's musculoskeletal structures.

4. The proper practice of __________ __________ involves the implementation of __________ important principles.

5. All lifting should be initiated from a __________ position.

6. The physical therapy aide should always be as __________ as possible to the object or person being lifted.

7. Whenever transferring is required, the center of gravity should be __________ from the center of the base of support.

8. When guarding a patient during gait training or ambulation, the physical therapist aide should always position herself at an approximate _____ -degree angle to the side and rear of the patient.

9. __________ __________ are always used to focus the patient's attention on specifically desired actions.

10. The physical therapy aide should always describe the general __________ __________ __________ that the patient is expected to follow.

11. Patient preparation should always be completed __________ to transport or treatment.

12. Three modes of transporting a patient include a __________, __________, and a __________.

13. The physical therapy aide should always remember to __________ the brake whenever transferring a patient is required.

11

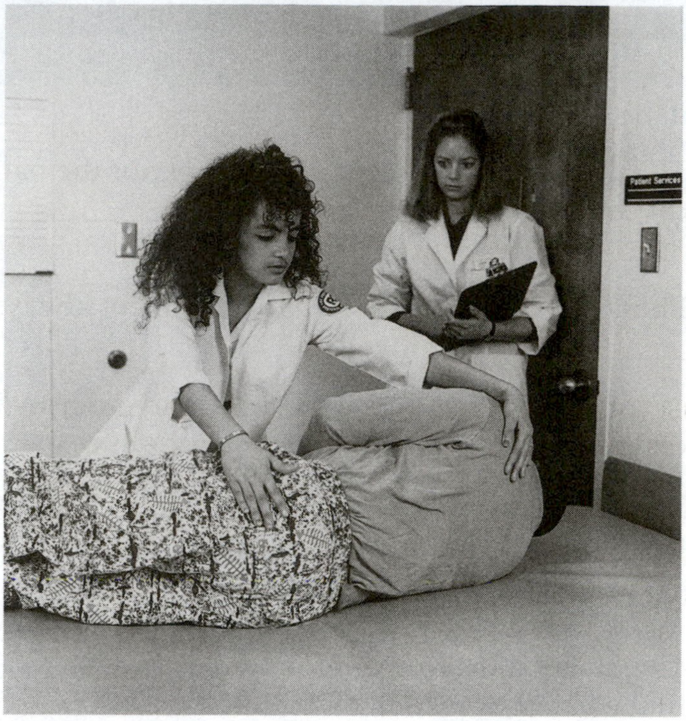

Turning and Positioning the Patient

OBJECTIVES

Upon completion of this chapter, you should be able to:

1. Describe the purpose of turning and repositioning the debilitated patient and explain the physical therapy aide's role in its function.
2. Describe how to turn a patient in the supine position.
3. Describe how to turn a patient from a supine position to a prone position.
4. Describe how to turn a patient from a prone position to a supine position.
5. Explain how a patient is turned using a floor mat.
6. Explain how to turn a patient from a supine position to a side-lying position.
7. Describe a side-lying position.
8. Explain how to return a patient from a sitting position to a supine position.

KEY TERMS

Circulation
Debilitation
Floor mat
Pivoting
Prone
Side-lying position
Supine

Because of the nature and **debilitation** of some illnesses and injuries, patients frequently are unable to turn in bed or position themselves properly. Frequent turning or repositioning of the dependent patient prevents the development of pressure sores and skin breakdown. A patient who is confined to the bed for any period of time should be turned or repositioned at least every two hours. If a patient has problems such as poor **circulation,** fragile skin, or decreased sensation, more frequent repositioning may be required. And whenever repositioning or turning is undertaken, time should also be allocated to proper observation and inspection of the skin over the area in which the patient may have been lying. By taking a few extra moments to examine the area for color and integrity, you may prevent the possibility of skin breakdown later on.

When sitting, a patient must be able to relieve pressure on the buttocks and sacrum at least every ten minutes. Push-ups using the armrests, leaning first to one side and then to the other, and leaning forward are ways in which to relieve pressure in the sitting position.

Proper positioning involves making the patient as comfortable as possible, thus preventing the development of any deformities and pressure sores as well as providing the patient access to her environment. In order to achieve these goals, the patient and environment must be properly handled. This means that when turning and repositioning is required, the patient must be lifted rather than dragged across the sheets to prevent any skin irritation. Wrinkles in the sheets, blankets, and clothes, should be avoided since they can increase the potential for pressure on a small area causing skin irritation. Pillows and rolled blankets or towels may also be used to support body parts to avoid possible strain on ligaments, nerves, and muscles, Figure 11-1.

When using pillows as a means of support or to provide relief to bony areas or areas of potential skin breakdown, it is important to place them proximally and distally to the involved area. Refer to Procedures 10 and 11.

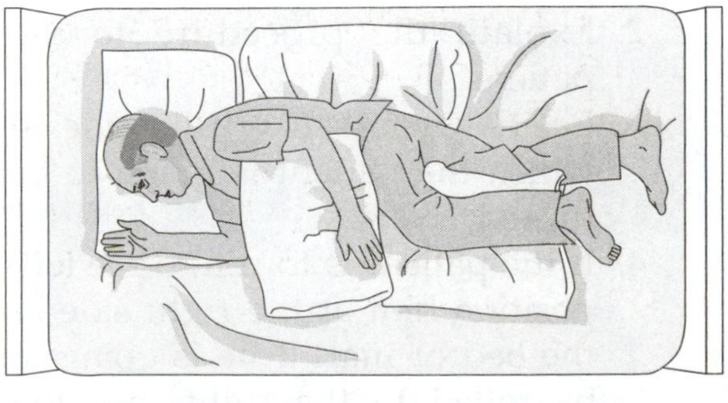

Figure 11-1 Lateral/side-lying position.

PROCEDURE #10: Positioning the Patient in the Supine Position

1. Wash your hands, identify the patient, and provide for privacy.
2. Place the patient's shoulders so that they are parallel to the hips, with the spine straight.
3. Place a pillow under the patient's knees in order to relieve strain on the lower back, Figure 11-2.

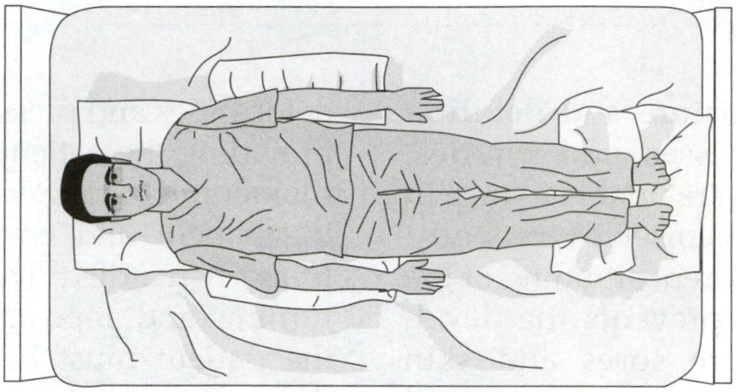

Figure 11-2 A client in **supine** position. The head and arms may be elevated slightly with a pillow, and the arms may also be supported with pillows. A trocanter roll may be placed along the side of the patient's thighs to keep legs in good alignment.

PROCEDURE #11: Turning the Patient From a Supine Position to a Prone Position

1. Wash your hands, identify the patient, and provide for privacy.
2. Explain the procedure to the patient.
3. Position yourself on the side to which the patient is going to be turned.
4. If the patient is to roll to the left, position him at the right side of the bed or mat. If he is going to be rolled to the right, position him at the left side of the bed or mat.

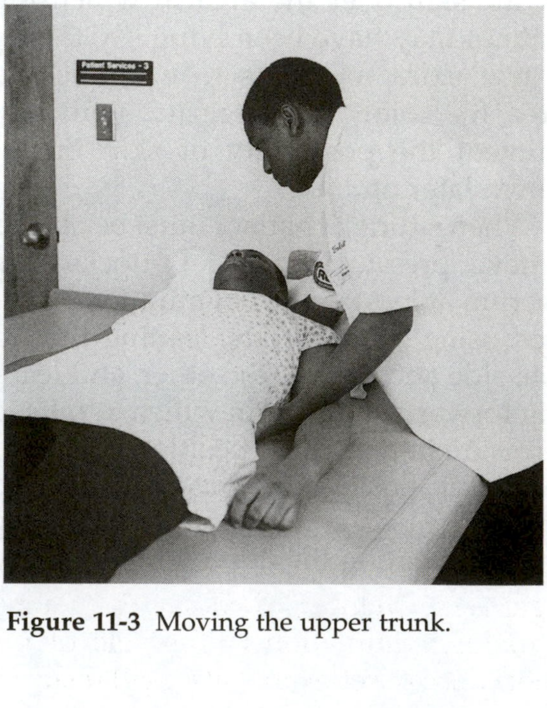

Figure 11-3 Moving the upper trunk.

5. Move the patient to the edge of the bed in three separate stages; first move the upper trunk (Figure 11-3), then move the lower trunk (Figure 11-4), and finally, move the legs (Figure 11-5).
6. Adduct the left upper arm so that the hand can be placed under the left hip with the palm against the hip.
7. The right lower leg is then crossed over the left lower leg so that the right ankle is resting on top of the left ankle.
8. The right arm is then adducted so that the hand is at the hip with the palm against it.

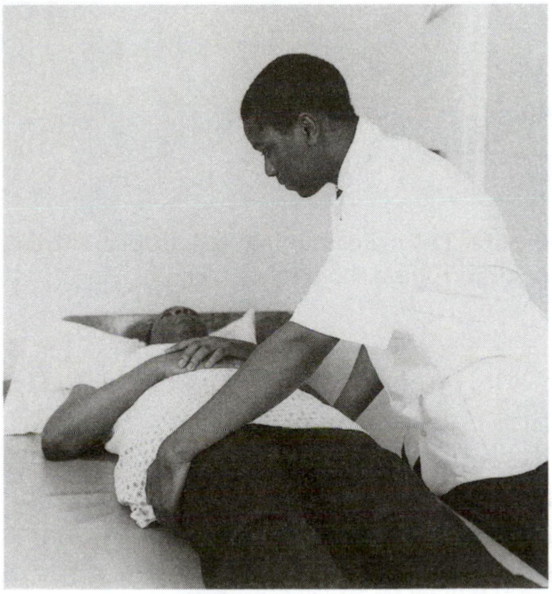

Figure 11-4 Moving the lower trunk.

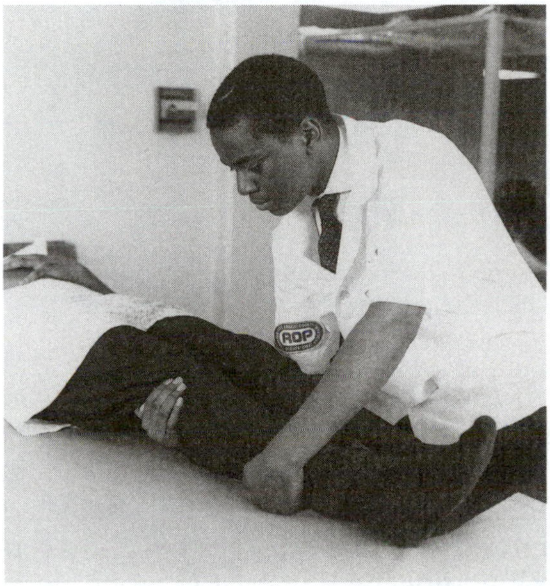

Figure 11-5 Moving the legs.

TURNING AND THE SUPINE POSITION

When sheets or blankets are used, they should not be tightly tucked in at the foot of the bed, as this may contribute to a decreased ankle dorsiflexion motion. Footboards are occasionally used to maintain the foot in its neutral or anatomical position. These are usually ineffective since the patient tends to push against the board and the ankle is again in plantar flexion. For some patients, stimulation to the sole of the foot causes a reflex that also will result in ankle plantar flexion.

It is important that you position yourself on the side to which the patient is going to be turned, Figure 11-6. If the bed is narrow or does not have a guardrail, someone should stand next to the patient in order to prevent him from falling while you are moving to the other side of the bed. The second person can assist with the positioning of the pillows and turning the patient. If a pillow is to be placed under the patient for the final positioning, make sure it is positioned so that it will be in the proper position as the patient is rolled.

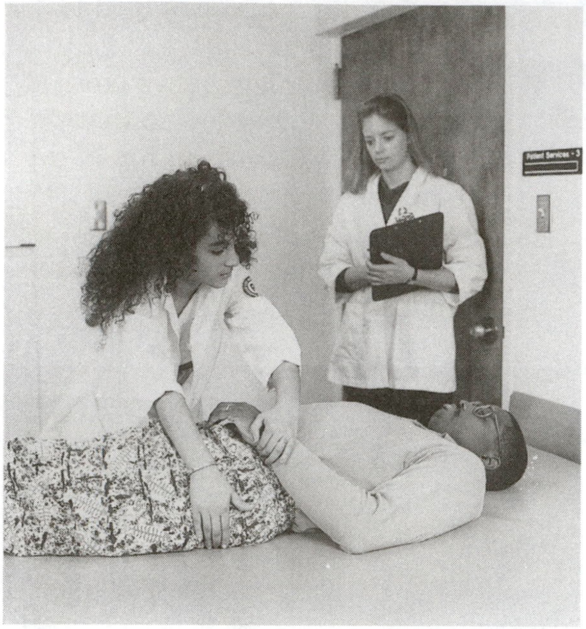

Figure 11-6 Positioning yourself on the side to which the patient is being turned.

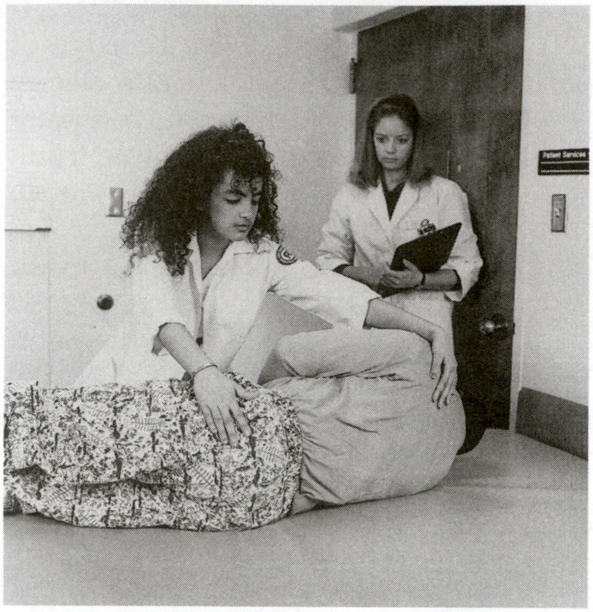

Figure 11-7 Positioning the upper extremity prior to rolling the patient.

If the patient has control of his head, chances are that he will be able to assist in turning both his head and neck in the direction of the roll as it is initiated, Figure 11-7. If he does not have this control, you or the therapist must be aware that the face will be subject to some rubbing on the mattress or mat during the roll. When you are ready to initiate the movement, make sure you let the patient know; give a preparatory count and then a specific verbal command. The verbal command should be one which is a direct clue to the task.

If you are working with a therapist, she will be the one to initiate the actual roll by placing her hands on the patient's back. Once the patient reaches the halfway point, he may finish the roll uncontrolled as a result of the pull of gravity. Therefore, the therapist will begin to rotate her hands as the patient reaches the side-lying position so that they are on the anterior surface of the patient, controlling the second half of the roll (see Figures 11-8 and 11-9).

Once the roll has been completed, the first body segment to be repositioned is the head. It must be placed in a comfortable position, facing to one side. There should be no pressure on the eyes, nose, or mouth. After this has been done the hands should be removed from under the hips and placed in a position of slight abduction, approximately 20 to 30 degrees. Finally, the feet should be uncrossed if they remain crossed after the roll is finished and placed approximately six to eight inches apart.

◆ TURNING IN THE PRONE POSITION

Patients that are positioned in the **prone** position lie with their shoulders parallel to their hips and the spine straight. The head may be turned to either the right or left side, or may be maintained in the midline with a small pillow or towel placed under the forehead in order to increase comfort. Refer to Procedure 12.

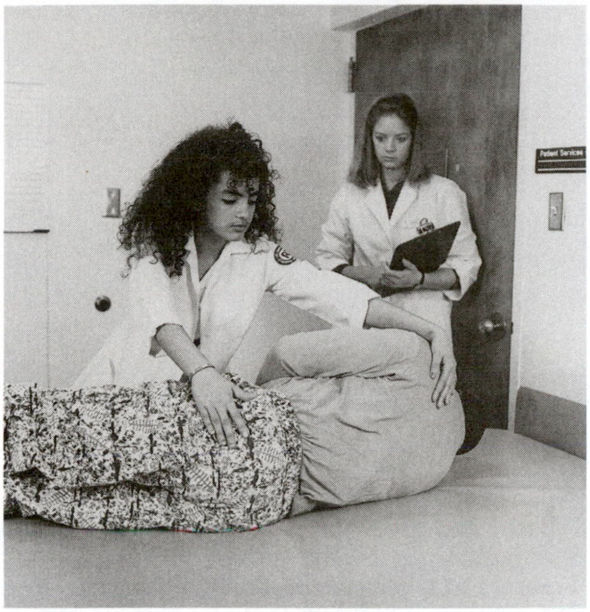

Figure 11-8 Physical therapy aide's hand position for first part of roll.

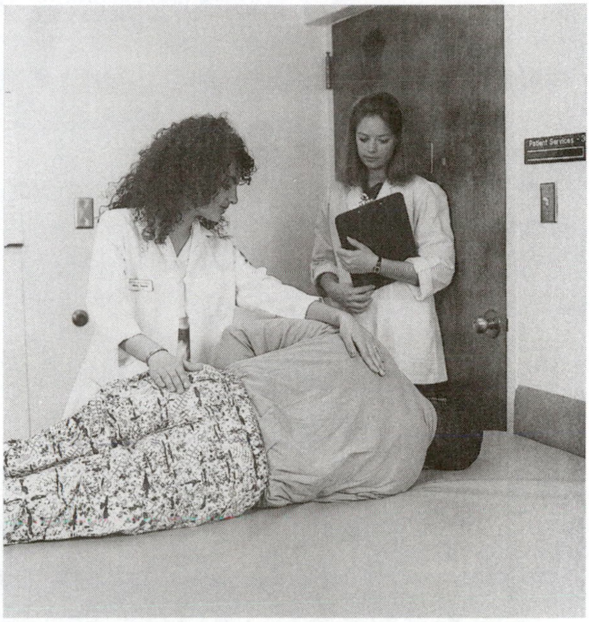

Figure 11-9 Physical therapy aide's hand position for second part of roll.

PROCEDURE #12: Positioning the Patient in the Prone Position

1. Wash your hands, identify the patient, and provide for privacy.
2. Place the patient's arms alongside his trunk or above his head.
3. Place a pillow under the patient's trunk, either lengthwise or crosswise. Lengthwise may be more comfortable if the patient has limited neck mobility. Crosswise positioning, using a pillow, may be more comfortable for a patient suffering from low back pain.
4. Position the patient's feet over the end of the table, Figure 11-10. A pillow may be placed under the lower legs to avoid the possibility of plantar flexion of the ankle, Figure 11-11.

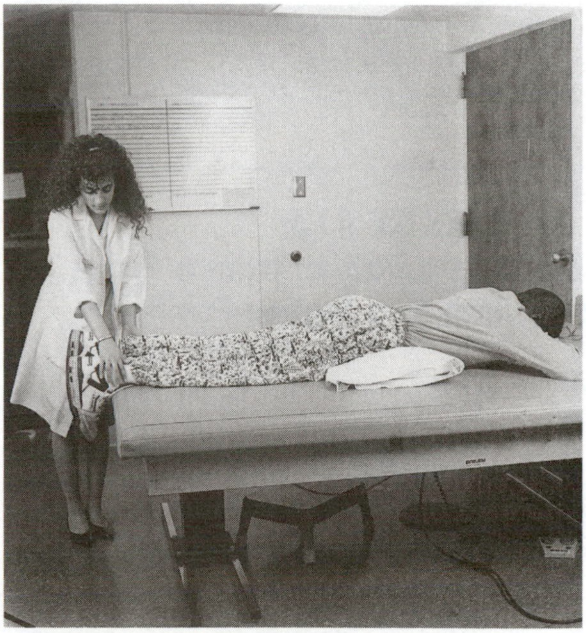

Figure 11-10 Prone position with arms overhead, pillow under hips, and feet off end of table.

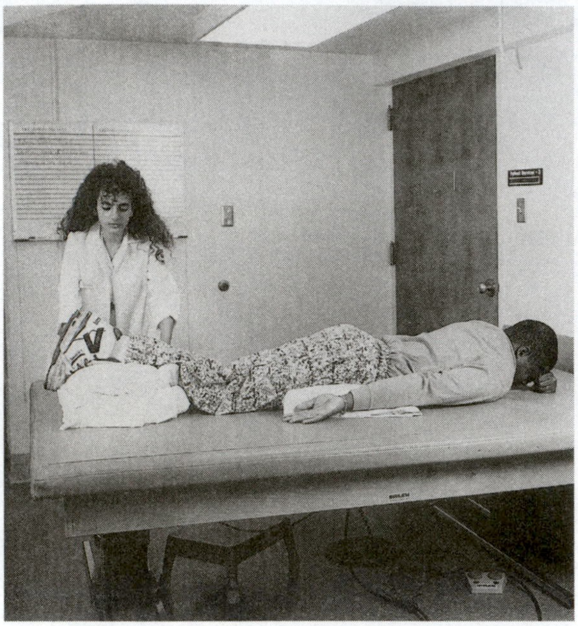

Figure 11-11 Prone position with arm alongside the pillow under legs.

Turning from the Prone Position to the Supine Position

In many ways, rolling the patient from the prone position to the supine position is simply the reverse of rolling from the supine to the prone position. The patient's initial position is prone. The beginning steps of moving to one side of the bed and of placement of the patient's hands remain the same. The crossing of the lower extremities is usually unnecessary. Refer to Procedure 13.

PROCEDURE #13: Turning a Patient from a Prone Position to a Supine Position

1. Wash your hands, identify the patient, and provide for privacy.
2. If you are working with a therapist, she should stand on the side to which the patient will roll.
3. Position the patient's head so that he is looking up and over his shoulder as he is being turned toward the therapist (Figure 11-12).
4. Guard the patient on the appropriate side of the bed while the therapist moves to the other side

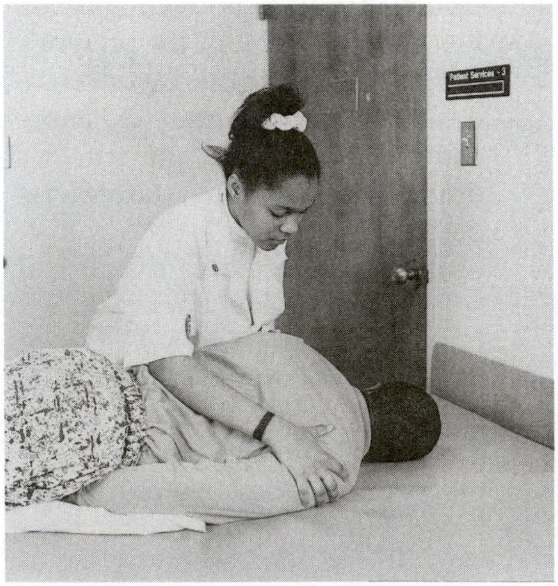

Figure 11-12 Positioning head and upper trunk for rolling patient to supine position.

of the bed.

5. The therapist then reaches over the patient and places her hands on the patient's anterior surface. As the patient reaches the side lying position, Figure 11-13, the therapist rotates her hands so that they are on the posterior surface of the patient and she can then control the second half of the roll. From another angle, the complete procedure can be seen in Figures 11-14, 11-15, and 11-16.

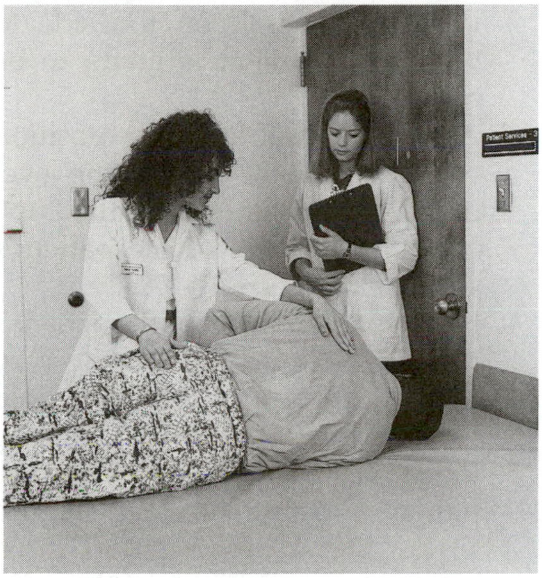

Figure 11-13 Positioning lower trunk for rolling patient to supine position.

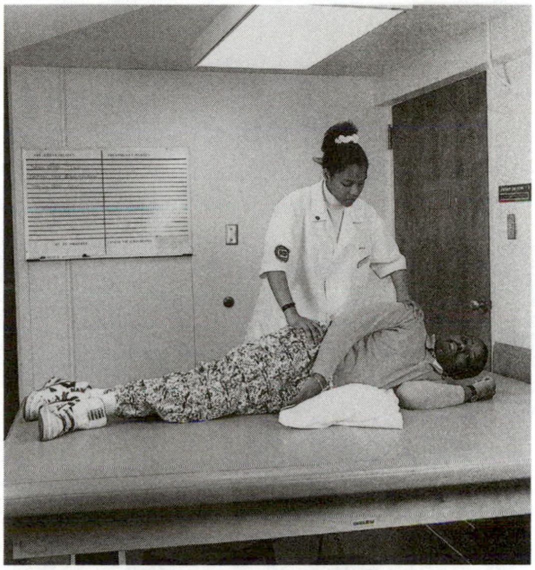

Figure 11-15 Physical therapy aide's hand position to initiate rolling patient to supine position.

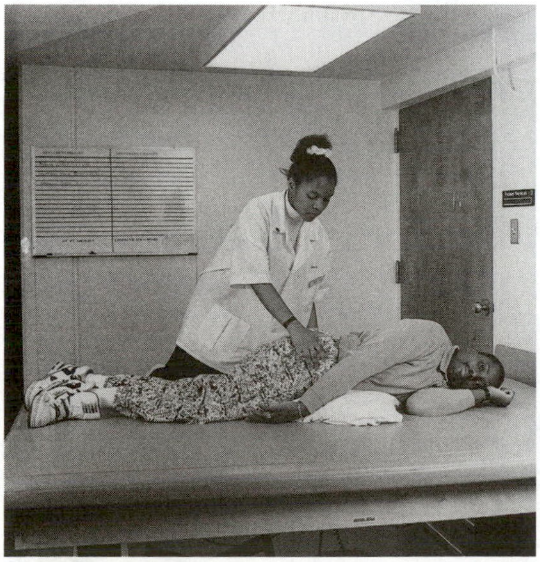

Figure 11-14 Starting position to roll patient from prone to supine position.

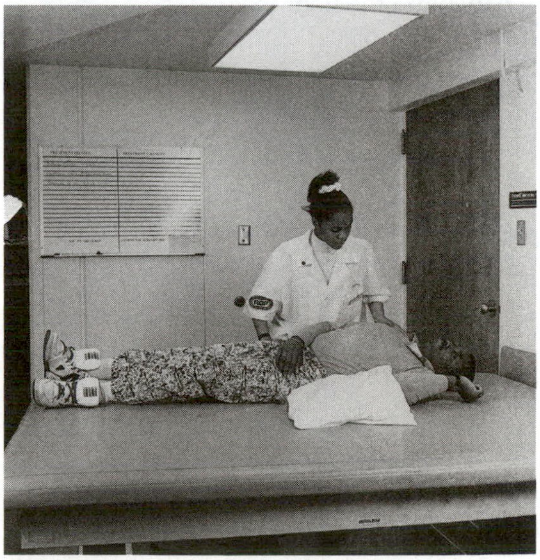

Figure 11-16 Physical therapy aide's hand position to complete rolling patient to supine position.

TURNING ON THE FLOOR MAT

When you are required to turn a patient on the **floor mat,** the same steps are followed as when turning a patient on a bed. Refer to Procedure 14.

PROCEDURE #14: Turning the Patient on the Floor Mat

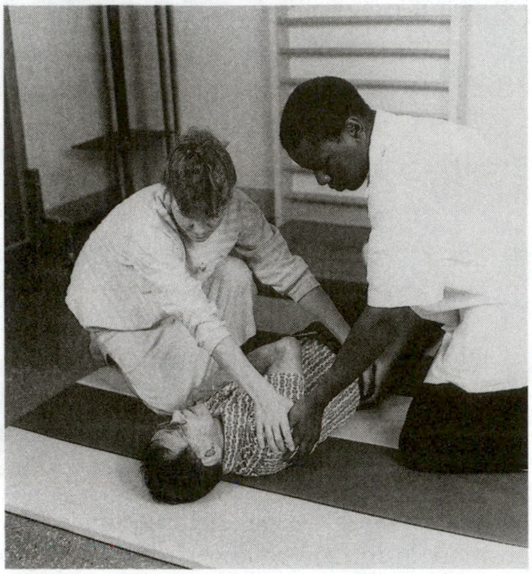

Figure 11-17 Starting position for turning patient on the floor mat.

1. Wash your hands, identify the patient, and provide for privacy.
2. Position yourself on the side to which the patient is going to be turned.
3. Assume a half-kneeling position with the "down" knee at the level of the patient's hips and the "up" knee at the level of the patient's shoulders, Figure 11-17.
4. Place your left hand on the patient's right hip, Figure 11-18, being very careful to hold the patient's right hand on top of the hip.
5. Place your right hand on the patient's right shoulder, Figure 11-19. The hand position must rotate at the midpoint of the roll.
6. Move out of the patient's way as he is turned in order to allow him to complete the roll without rolling onto you.

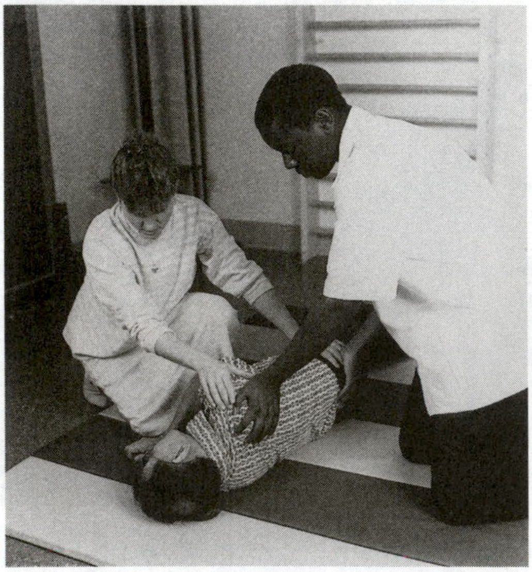

Figure 11-18 Turning patient from a supine position to a prone position on the floor mat.

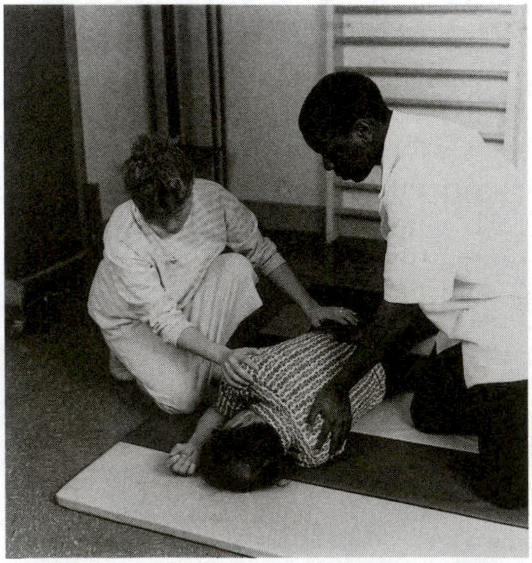

Figure 11-19 Completing the turn from the supine to the prone position on the floor mat.

TURNING FROM A SUPINE POSITION TO A SIDE-LYING POSITION

In the **side-lying position,** the patient remains resting on his side for some time. Therefore, adjustments involving rolling may have to be made during the procedure. Side-lying can be accomplished from either the supine or the prone position; however, it may be more comfortable for the patient and easier for yourself if the patient rolls to side-lying from the supine position.

When the patient is to be positioned on his left side, his initial position is supine and to the right side of the mattress. The left arm is abducted to a 45-degree angle. The right lower leg is crossed over the left lower leg at the ankle, and the right hand is placed against the right hip with the palm against it. Refer to Procedures 15 and 16.

RETURNING FROM A SITTING POSITION TO A SUPINE POSITION

There are several methods that can be used to bring a patient back to a sitting position from a supine position. The method generally depends upon the patient's functional abilities and his medical problem. In all cases, however, a patient should never be left unguarded in the sitting position if he cannot maintain the position safely.

If a patient has enough strength, he can come to the sitting position by doing a sit-up in bed. If slight assistance is necessary, such as for a medical problem involving general weakness, a trapeze bar can be used. In some cases, a patient can do a sit-up or use a trapeze bar while you provide assistance at the same time. Refer to Procedure 17.

Another method of assisting the

PROCEDURE #15: Turning the Patient from a Supine Position to a Side-lying Position

1. Wash your hands, identify the patient, and provide for privacy.
2. Assume a position on the side to which the patient is turning.
3. With your left hand, grasp the patient's right hip, being careful to hold his right hand between your hand and his hips.
4. With your right hand, grasp the patient's right shoulder.
5. Roll the patient until he reaches the side-lying position, Figure 11-20.

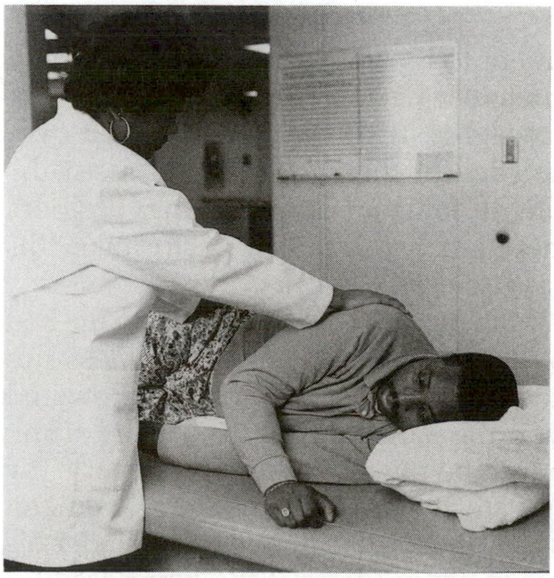

Figure 11-20 Turning the patient to the side-lying position.

PROCEDURE #16: Positioning the Patient in the Side-lying Position

1. Wash your hands, identify the patient, and provide for privacy.
2. Place a pillow under the patient's head. If the patient is being placed in side-lying forward, place the pillow in front of him and bring the uppermost arm forward to rest on the pillow, Figure 11-21. If the patient is being placed in a side-lying inclined backward, place the pillow behind him, with the uppermost arm extended and supported by the pillow.
3. If necessary, rotate the uppermost trunk by bringing the lowermost shoulder forward.
4. Flex the uppermost leg and rest it on the pillow.

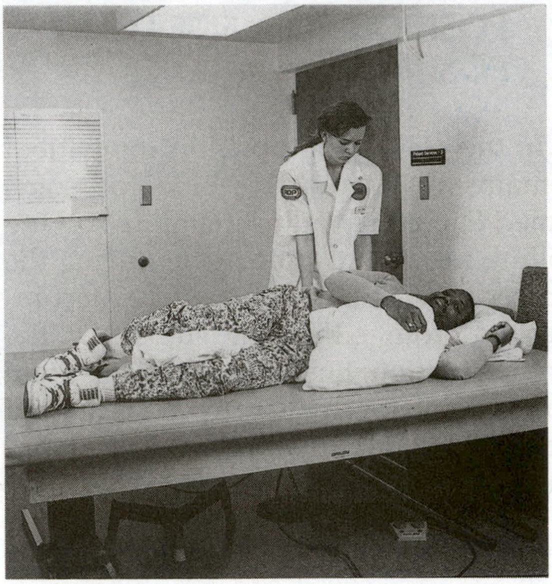

Figure 11-21 The side-lying position, inclined forward.

5. To avoid excessive pressure on the bottom leg, do not allow the uppermost leg to lie directly on top of the bottom leg.

patient to the sitting position is teaching him to use his lower extremities as counterweights. If the legs are lowered over the edge of the bed, this will assist the patient to come to a sitting position. There are two ways of performing this maneuver.

If the patient is able to **pivot** in the bed so that he is lying across it, his legs can then be put into a position to be lowered over the edge of the bed. The trunk should be raised at the same time as the legs are lowered. If necessary, you can assist him by putting your arm under his legs in order to assist the lower leg and by placing your other arm behind his back and head in order to assist the trunk raising, or both. Any of these movements will reduce the strain on the patient's abdominal and hip flexor muscles. For some patients who are too weak to pivot in the bed, assistance may be necessary throughout the entire maneuver. Refer to Procedure 18.

SUMMARY

In this chapter, we described the purpose, preparation, and skills involved in properly turning and positioning the patient. This included how to turn and reposition the patient, how to turn a patient in the supine and prone positions, how to turn and position the patient in the side-lying position, and how to reposition the patient from a sitting position to a supine position.

PROCEDURE #17: Returning the Patient from a Sitting Position to a Supine Position

1. Wash your hands, identify the patient, and provide for privacy.
2. Put your arm behind the patient's back and push or pull to assist him up, Figure 11-22.
3. If a trapeze bar is not available, you can stabilize your arm in front of the patient and allow him to pull himself up using your arm.
4. Do not do the patient's work by pulling your arm back as he holds onto your arm; rather, allow the patient to achieve the full sitting position, Figure 11-23.

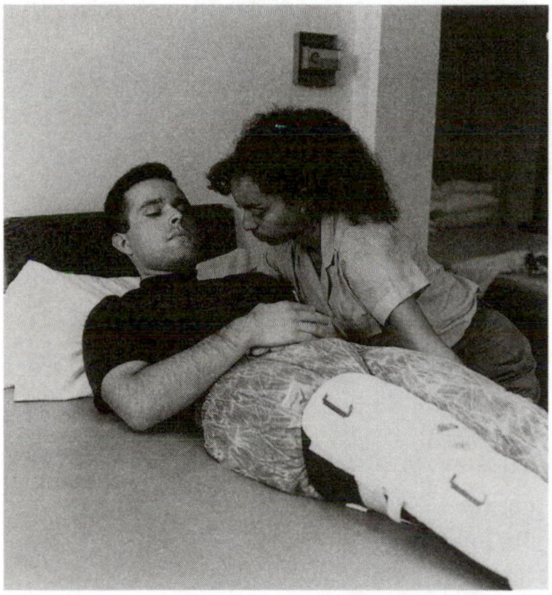

Figure 11-22 Starting position to come to a sitting position.

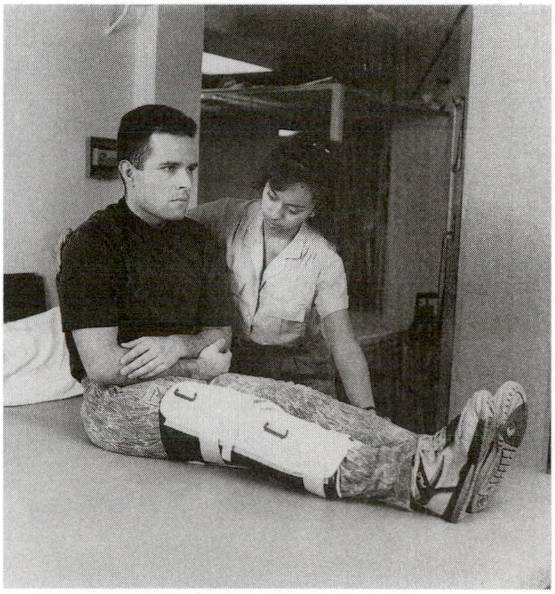

Figure 11-23 Completion of coming to a sitting position.

PROCEDURE #18: Alternate Method for Returning the Patient from a Sitting Position to a Supine Position

1. Wash your hands, identify the patient, and provide for privacy.
2. Have the patient assume a side-lying position, Figure 11-24.
3. Assist the patient to flex the hips and knees to a 90-degree angle. This places the lower legs over the edge of the bed.
4. The patient then pushes or pulls himself to a sitting position, Figures 11-25, 11-26, and 11-27.

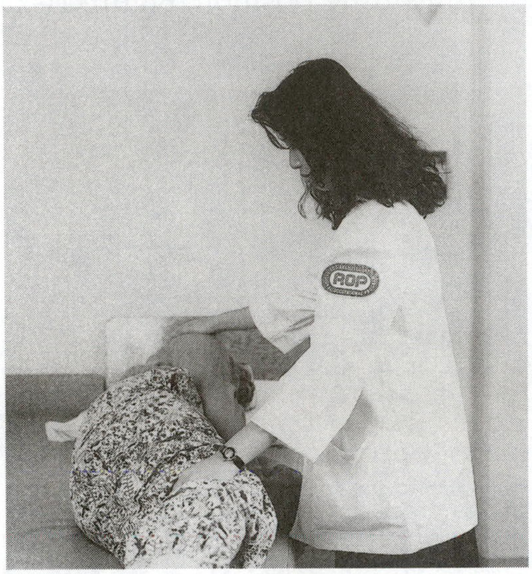

Figure 11-24 Pivoting on bed to lower the legs.

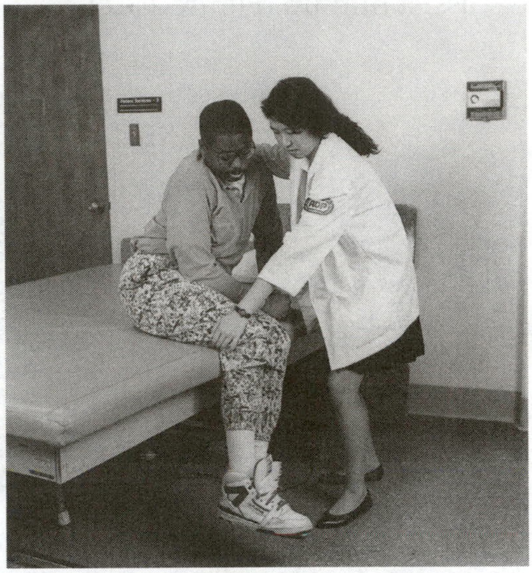

Figure 11-26 Physical therapy aide assisting patient to adjust position.

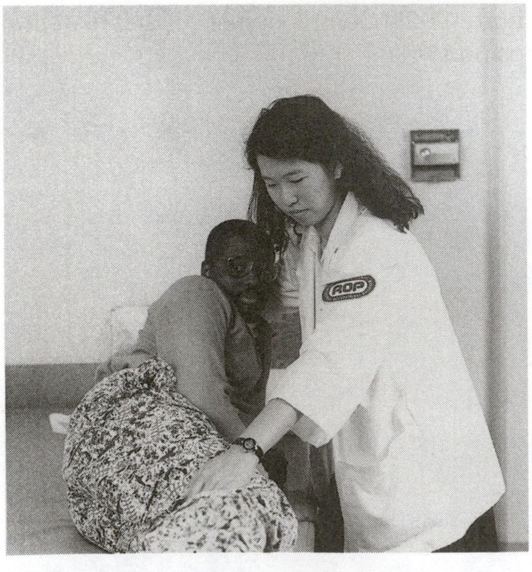

Figure 11-25 Physical therapy aide assisting the patient to raise trunk.

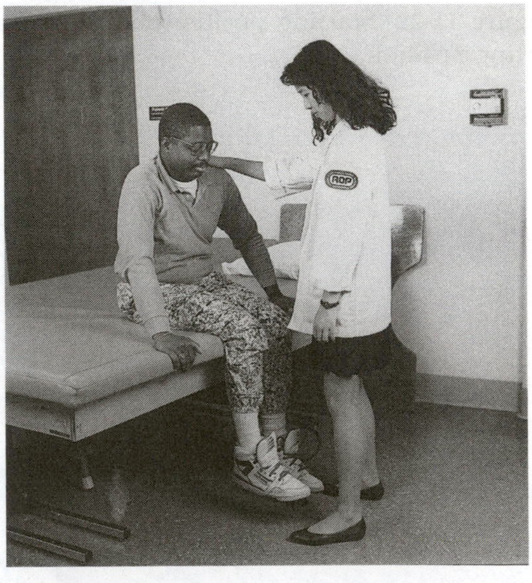

Figure 11-27 Achieving a full upright sitting position.

◆ ◆ LEARNING ACTIVITY 11-1

Terms to Define

Match the term with its definition.

a. ADL
b. disability
c. dangling
d. ambulate
e. decubitus ulcer
f. contracture
g. prong
h. personality
I. Fowler's position
j. supine
k. foot drop
l. psychological exam

_______ 1. assessment of individual's behavior in a given situation
_______ 2. lying on the back looking upward
_______ 3. patient in a sitting position in bed
_______ 4. failure to maintain foot in the normal flexed position
_______ 5. sum total of activities, attitudes, and interests that distinguish one individual from others
_______ 6. walking
_______ 7. bedsore
_______ 8. lying on the face looking downward
_______ 9. shortening of muscles
_______ 10. inability to perform physical or mental activities normally done
_______ 11. activities of daily living
_______ 12. sitting on the edge of the bed with legs hanging down

◆ ◆ LEARNING ACTIVITY 11-2

Positioning

Describe how you would use pillows, towel rolls, and sheets to position the following:

1. A patient with low back pain—in prone for comfort only.
2. A patient with a head injury and in a coma—side-lying position.
3. A patient with an ankle sprain—in supine for comfort only.

◆ ◆ LEARNING ACTIVITY 11-3

Transfers

Make a list of steps for each of the transfers listed below. Try not to leave out any steps.

1. From the bed to the wheelchair.
2. From the wheelchair to a treatment table.
3. From the parallel bars to a wheelchair.

REVIEW QUESTIONS

1. Frequently turning and repositioning a dependent patient prevents __________ and __________.
2. When sitting, a patient should be able to relieve pressure on the buttocks and sacrum at least every __________ minutes.
3. Placing a patient in a __________ position means that the shoulders are parallel with the hips.
4. If a patient is to be rolled to the left, she should begin the roll on the __________ side of the bed.
5. Placing a patient in a __________ position means that the shoulders are parallel to the hips with the spine straight.
6. Whenever the physical therapy aide turns the patient from a supine position to a prone position, the lower extremities should be __________ in order to prevent them from dragging.
7. When turning a patient, the physical therapy aide should always remember to position herself to the __________ in which the patient is going to be turned.
8. In turning the patient from a supine position to a side-lying position, the patient's left arm should be __________ to a __________-degree angle.
9. The side-lying position requires the use of __________ for proper placement of the patient's head, trunk, and extremities.
10. If a patient is able, the physical therapy aide should allow him to __________ in turning and repositioning.

12

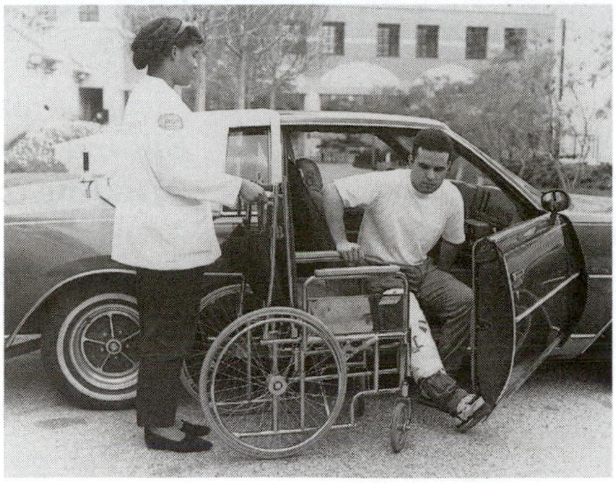

Transferring the Patient

OBJECTIVES

Upon completion of this chapter, you should be able to:

1. Discuss the importance of properly transferring a patient.
2. Describe the role body mechanics play during the transfer procedure.
3. Identify different types of transfers.
4. Briefly discuss the difference between an unassisted and an assisted bed to wheelchair transfer.
5. Explain an assisted wheelchair to parallel bar transfer.
6. Describe an assisted wheelchair to treatment table transfer.
7. Describe a modified standing transfer.
8. Briefly discuss the following transfers: standing toilet, standing car, and bathtub transfer.
9. Explain the difference between an assisted and an unassisted sitting transfer from the bed to the wheelchair.
10. State the purpose and use of a drawsheet transfer.
11. Define a pneumatic lift transfer and briefly discuss its purpose, operation, and usage.
12. Briefly discuss the physical therapy aide's role in a one-person transfer from the floor to the wheelchair.

KEY TERMS

Body mechanics
Drawsheet transfer
Efficiency
One-person transfer
Parallel bars
Pneumatic lift transfer
Sitting transfer
Sliding board
Sliding transfer
Standing transfer
Transfer
Transfer belt
Treatment table

Transferring a patient in and out of a wheelchair, bed, or any other immobile object requires an understanding of two basic theories: first, you should have a thorough grasp of the importance of safety and efficiency, and, second, you will need to have a complete understanding of the importance of body mechanics and the role it plays in the correct and safe transferring of your physically challenged or disabled patients.

The purpose of **body mechanics** is to provide you with the knowledge and understanding of how to correctly position and move your own body, that is, your trunk, legs, and arms, in order for you to achieve the best possible leverage with the least stress and fatigue. Both you and the patient should be able to move in ways that take advantage of gravity and momentum.

Most transfers that require little, if any, active participation by the patient are called "dependent" transfers. These would include any transfer that required the use of the aid of one or more individuals, such as yourself, to complete the transfer. Transfers falling into this category include a **sliding transfer** from a cart or gurney or a bed, a three-man carry, a dependent standing pivot transfer, and the pneumatic lift transfer. Transfers that require some patient participation include the two-man lift, the sliding board transfer, and the assisted standing pivot transfer.

It should be noted that the goal of any assisted transfer is to gradually reduce the assistance necessary until such time as the patient can perform the transfer independently. Assistance may be provided through the use of physical assistance with a maneuver, or verbal reminders of the steps involved. It is also important to always keep the patient informed about the transfer and what he can expect to do. Explanations should be understandable, and commands and counts used to synchronize the actions of all participants should be clear, firm, and concise.

TYPES OF TRANSFERS

There are two basic types of **transfers:** standing and sitting. In a **standing transfer,** the patient takes his or her weight on one or both legs and comes to an upright position prior to sitting down again in the new place. In a **sitting transfer,** the patient does not rise, but moves her hips sideways from one surface to another, generally by taking the weight through the arms. Normally, sitting transfers are used by patients who cannot stand such as those patients suffering from paralysis or having an amputation of the lower extremity(ies).

◆ PREPARATION FOR BEGINNING TRANSFERS

Prior to beginning any transfer, there are certain preparations that will need to be made. First, you should always check the equipment and its position. Make sure it is stable and firm. If you are using a bed during the transfer, you will want to make sure that if it is on casters, they are locked. If not, make sure the bed is pushed against a wall. If you are using a wheelchair, you must make sure that its brakes have been locked.

Always make sure that the transfer surfaces you are using are of the same height. A hospital bed, for example, can be lowered to the height of a wheelchair; also, by placing a raised seat on a toilet seat, you can bring it up to the height of a wheelchair seat. Also remember to keep the transfer surfaces as close together as possible. Removable armrests and swing-away detachable footrests on the wheelchair allow it to be positioned close to the bed or toilet. A **sliding board,** or a thin board that is placed across the two surfaces over which a patient may slide, can also be used to close the gap between them completely.

When positioning your equipment, always remember that it must be placed according to the patient's physical limitations or disability. The patient with one side stronger than the other, such as a hemiplegic, will generally prefer to move toward her stronger side during the transfer. If the wheelchair faces the foot of the bed when this patient transfers out of the bed to her wheelchair, then the wheelchair will need to face the head of the bed when the patient wants to return to bed (Figure 12-1).

Footwear, both for your patient, and yourself, is extremely important during the transfer. Always make sure that both of you are wearing shoes that fit snugly and have a low, wide heel. Also, in case the patient has been prescribed a brace or other prosthesis, make sure that it has been applied prior to the transfer.

Since the patient should know what she is expected to do during the transfer, it is important that you carefully explain and teach the process one step at a time. Instructions should be simple and repeated whenever necessary. They should also be consistent from one time to another. Never try to hurry the patient; allow him time enough to complete each step in a systematic and

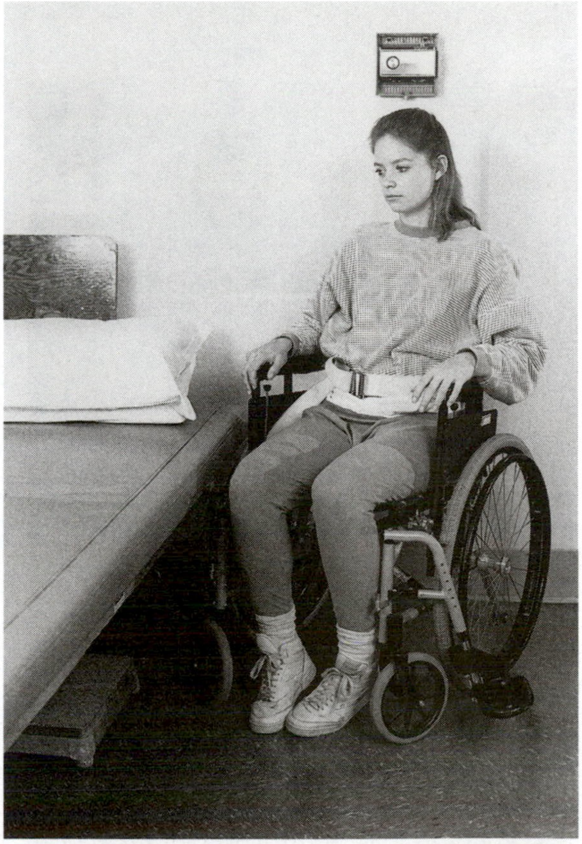

Figure 12-1 Position of wheelchair relative to bed.

methodical manner.

Since safety and **efficiency** is of the utmost importance during the transfer procedure, you should always make sure that you place yourself in the right position for assistance to the patient and for safety for both of you during the procedure. This is accomplished by standing close to the patient. If you allow yourself to stand apart from him, the strain on your back is much greater. Therefore, stand with a broad base of support, keeping your feet slightly apart with one foot ahead of the other. This position allows you to maintain your balance and affords you the ability to quickly and easily shift your weight whenever necessary.

Whenever you are required to transfer the patient from the bed to a wheelchair, you should always remember to assist her at the waist, and never hold onto her at the shoulder. If a **transfer belt** is available, you may use it to assist in the transfer. Make sure it is securely fastened around the patient's waist since this will give you a better grip on the patient without restricting the use of her arms (Figure 12-2A, B, and C).

As we have previously discussed, the use of proper body mechanics is of the utmost importance when transfer techniques are employed. Therefore, when you are required to implement these techniques, always make sure that you keep your back straight, with your hips and knees slightly bent. Straightening your legs as you help the patient into the standing position will prevent you from injuring or straining your back as you complete the transfer. Lifting with your legs is also much less strenuous than lifting with your back muscles. Let the patient see the surface to which he is

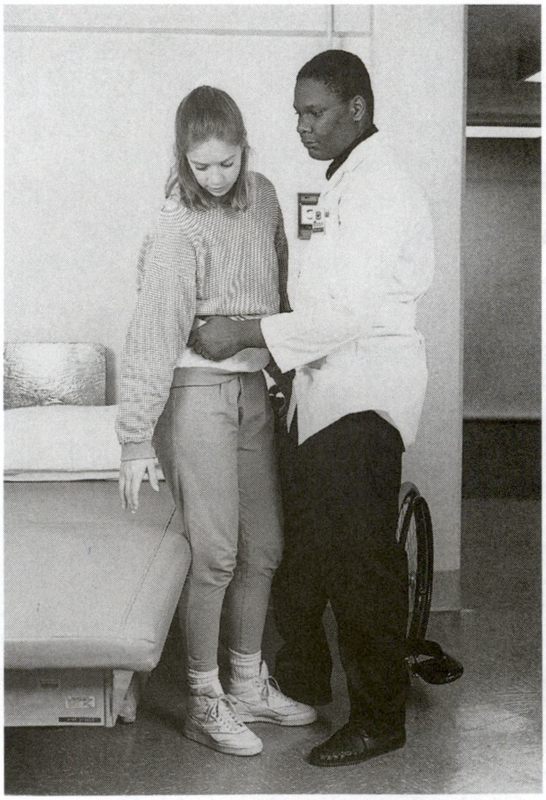

Figure 12-2A Lifting with a transfer belt.

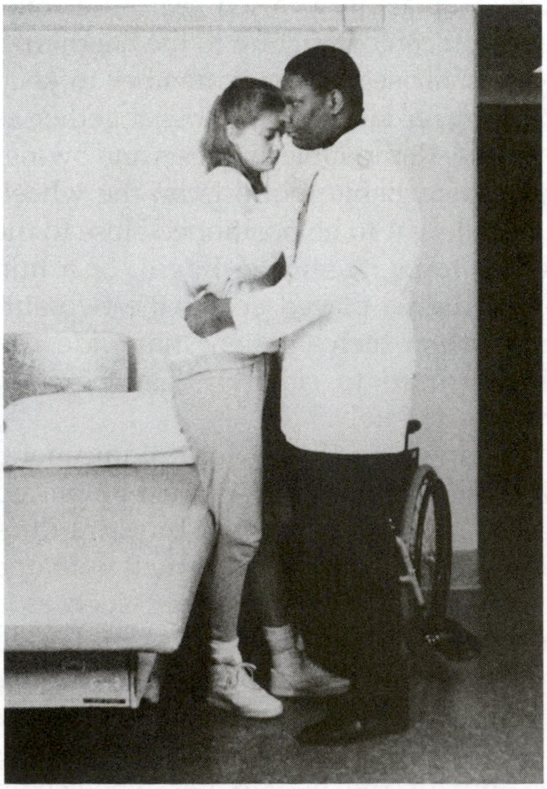

Figure 12-2B Pivoting.

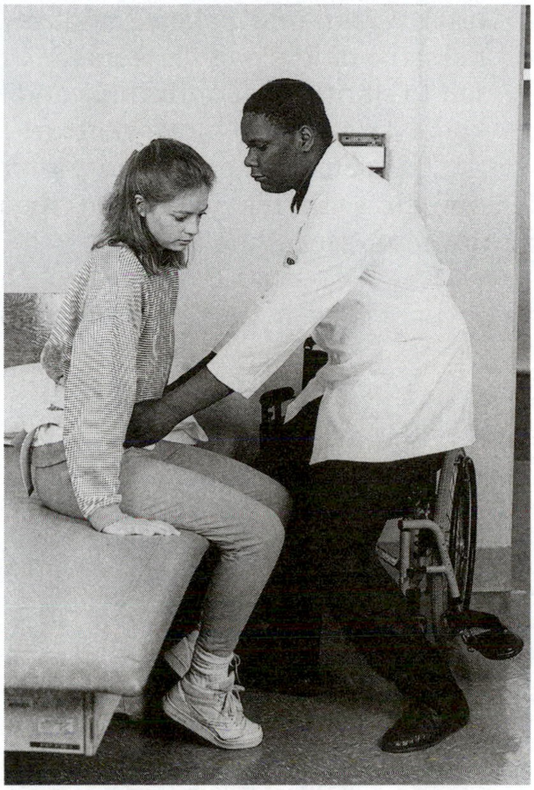

Figure 12-2C Transferring from the wheelchair to the bed using the transfer belt.

being transferred, and never obscure his vision since not being able to see the place in which he is going can sometimes frighten him.

Finally, you should always remember that the exact manner in which the patient is to be transferred will always depend upon his abilities, the environment, and any other circumstances unique to that particular patient. Following simple and proper transferring techniques will assist both you and the patient to complete the procedure in a safe and efficient manner.

STANDING TRANSFERS

Bed to Wheelchair: Unassisted

Some patients will have the ability to transfer themselves unassisted from the bed to the wheelchair. If this is the case, the rule of thumb is if the transfer is being completed for the first time, you will want to stay close and supervise the patient during the procedure. Once you have properly instructed him on the technique and have seen him complete the tasks, you should allow him to finish the transfer on his own. Refer to Procedure 19.

PROCEDURE #19: Unassisted Bed to Wheelchair Transfer

1. Have the patient slide forward to sit on the edge of the bed and put his feet on the floor with the stronger leg slightly behind and apart from the weaker one. Then have him lean forward, see Figure 12-3A.
2. The patient then stands by pushing down with his arms and, at the same time, straightening his legs.

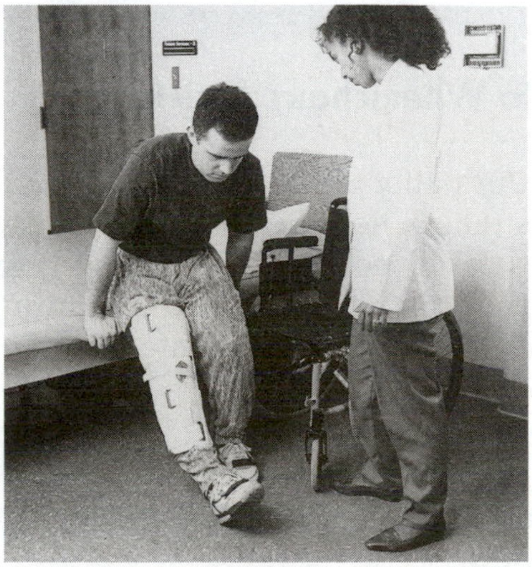

A

Figure 12-3 Unassisted standing transfer from bed to wheelchair.

3. After the patient stands, have him reach for support to the far side armrest of the wheelchair. Then have him step or pivot his back to the wheelchair, see Figure 12-3B.
4. To complete the transfer, the patient bends forward to improve his leverage and balance and, at the same time, slowly lowers himself to sit by bending his hips and knees and easing himself down. At the same time, he supports himself with his hands on the armrests, see Figure 13-3C.

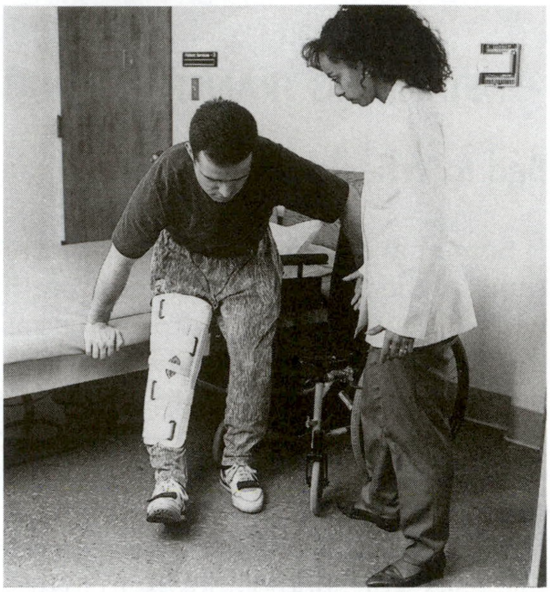

B

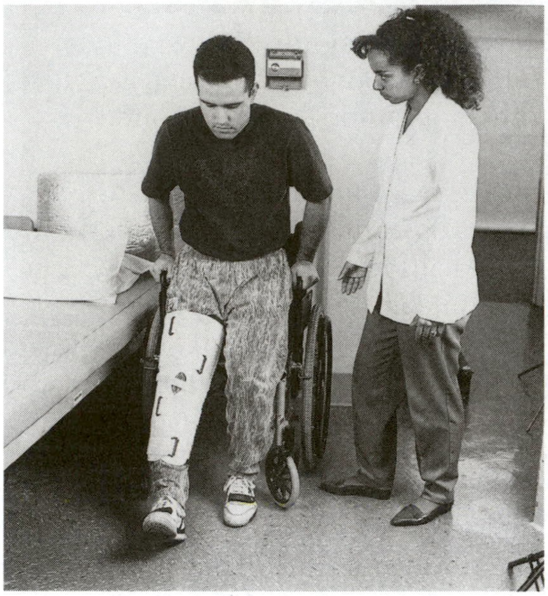

C

Figure 12-3 Unassisted standing transfer from bed to wheelchair (continued).

Bed to Wheelchair: Assisted

If your patient does not have the sufficient strength necessary to bring himself from a lying position to a sitting position, you will need to assist him during the bed to wheelchair transfer. Refer to Procedure 20.

Wheelchair to Treatment Table: Assisted

Whenever your patient is required to use a **treatment table,** you should always make sure that there is a stool with four rubber-tipped legs available for his use. Before beginning the procedure, make sure that the wheelchair is placed sideways next to the treatment table, with the patient's stronger side nearest the table.

To dismount from the table, assist the patient to move to the edge, slide down onto her feet, and proceed with the basic transfer. Refer to Procedure 21.

PROCEDURE #20: Assisted Bed to Wheelchair Transfer

1. Keeping your back straight and your feet slightly apart, bend your hips and knees in order to become more level with the patient.
2. Using your transfer belt or gripping the patient around the waist with one hand and under the thighs with the other, assist the patient to come into a sitting position at the edge of the bed.
3. While bending your hips and knees, place your feet so that you have a good broad base of support and your knees are blocking the patient's knees. Lift the patient by the waist or by the belt as you straighten your hips and knees and carefully rise with the patient into the standing position. Remember to keep slightly to the side in order to give the patient room enough to move and thus enable him to see the area to which he is being transferred.
4. Position yourself so that you are standing close to the patient, making sure that you still have a broad base of support and, if necessary, are still using your knees to support the patient's knees. Together, allow both yourself and the patient to pivot or turn, slightly shifting the weight from one side to the other and taking tiny steps.
5. As the patient bends forward to sit, slowly bend your hips and knees, gently easing the patient to the seat and helping him in sliding back into the wheelchair.

PROCEDURE #21: Assisting Patient from the Wheelchair to the Treatment Table

1. Wash your hands, identify the patient, and provide for privacy.
2. Place a step stool alongside the treatment table.
3. If the patient has one weak leg, use your knees to block hers, while she steps onto the stool with her strong leg.
4. If a transfer or gait belt is available, use it to assist in the transfer.
5. Complete the transfer by assisting the patient to turn her back toward the treatment table and helping her into a sitting position.

Wheelchair to Parallel Bars: Assisted

Refer to Procedure 22.

Modified Standing Transfer

Refer to Procedure 23.

PROCEDURE #22: Assisting the Patient from a Wheelchair to the Parallel Bars

1. Wash your hands, identify the patient, and provide for privacy.
2. Make sure the wheelchair brakes are applied and that the footrests are swung out to the side.
3. Assist the patient to the front edge of the wheelchair.
4. With his feet flat on the ground and under his hips, ask the patient to place his hands on the bars.
5. Assist the patient to complete the maneuver by bending your hips and knees in order to bring yourself to the patient's level, Figure 12-4.
6. Block the patient's knees in order to prevent him from falling.

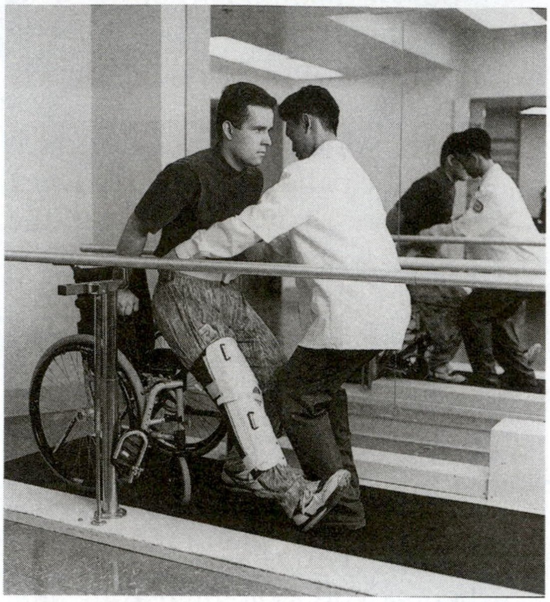

Figure 12-4 Standing from a wheelchair to the parallel bars.

7. Using the patient's belt or his waist, assist him to rise with you from his wheelchair to the bars.

PROCEDURE #23: Modified Standing Transfer

Depending upon the patient's specific disability or injury, some variations of the standing transfer technique may be necessary. A patient suffering from hemiplegia, for example, may have total or partial paralysis in one arm and one leg. If indeed, this is the case, the following procedure may be followed (assume the nonfunctional side is the right side):

1. To sit up in bed, the patient moves toward his left side.
2. The patient then grips his weak right arm with his strong left hand and places it across his abdomen.
3. The patient then moves his left foot under the knee of the weak right leg. He then slides his good foot down under the calf to the ankle. Crossing the ankles so that the involved leg can be supported by the noninvolved one, he lifts or slides both legs over the edge of the bed.
4. Holding onto the edge of the mattress with his left hand and bending his head forward, the patient should lean with his weight against the left forearm and left elbow as he brings the left leg to the floor.
5. The patient completes the transfer by pushing on his left forearm and coming into a sitting position while straightening his left elbow.

Standing Toilet Transfer

The same minimum locomotion potentials that are necessary for a patient's standing transfer from a bed to a wheelchair are required for a standing transfer from the wheelchair to a toilet. The patient should have the use of one good leg, one good arm with a hand able to grip firmly, and a good sitting balance.

Bathrooms may vary in size and the arrangement of fixtures. While the patient may have to practice the transfer technique in the hospital bathroom, the method which he ultimately learns should be suitable for his bathroom at home.

Preferably, the toilet seat should be approximately 50 centimeters above the floor. If it is lower, a raised toilet seat may be used without any difficulty (see Figures 12-5A, 12-5B, and 12-5C).

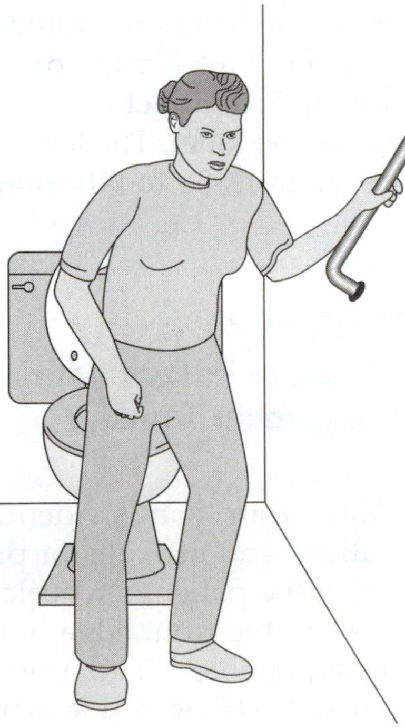

A

Figure 12-5 Unassisted standing transfer from the toilet to the wheelchair.

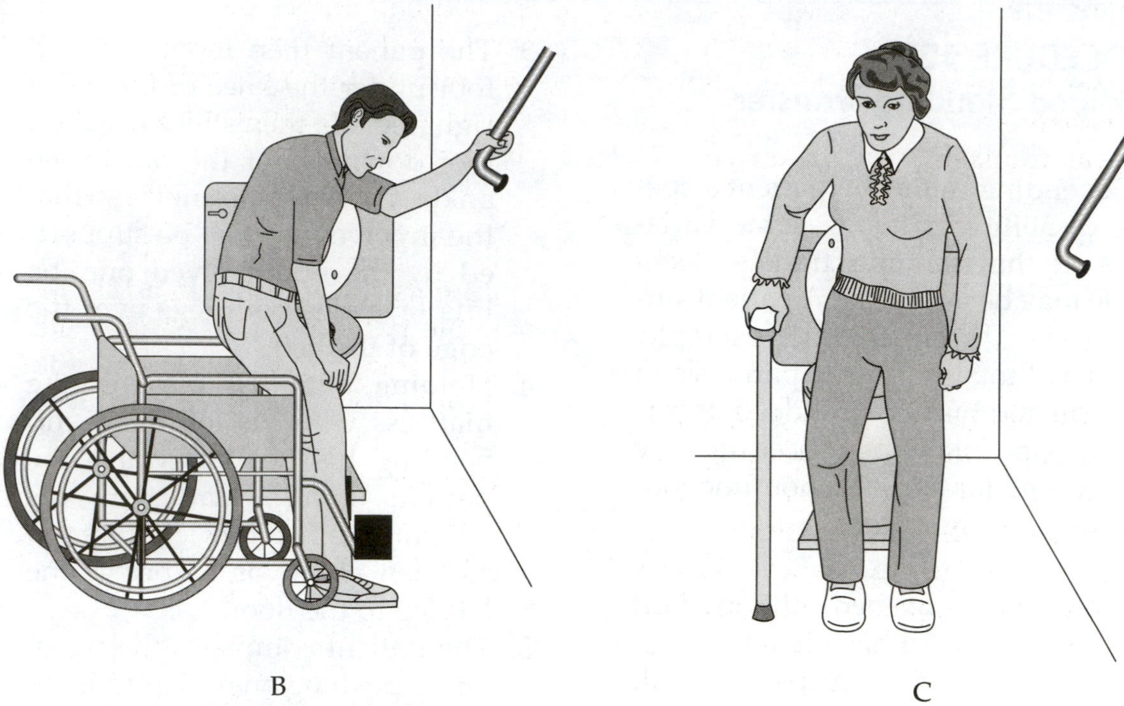

Figure 12-5 Unassisted standing transfer from the toilet to the wheelchair (continued).

A 45-degree angle wall handrail or a right-angle handrail should be placed on the wall that is closest to the side of the toilet bowl. The rail is mounted on the wall with the lower part of the bar placed about 5 centimeters behind the front edge of the toilet. The length of the bar can vary from 50 to 90 centimeters. Refer to Procedure 24.

Standing Car Transfer

Patients who have disabilities involving paralysis of the lower extremities may still be able to drive a car with an

PROCEDURE #24: Assisting the Patient with a Standing Toilet Transfer

1. Wash your hands, identify the patient, and provide for privacy.
2. Bring the patient's wheelchair as close to the front edge of the toilet as possible. Make sure that the patient's stronger side is brought nearest to the toilet.
3. Lock the wheelchair brakes and swing the footrests to the outside.
4. Have the patient grasp the handrail firmly and assist him to pull himself up to a standing position.
5. Assist the patient so that his body weight is borne entirely or as much as possible on his stronger leg, and his trunk is bent slightly downward. This will establish the patient's center of gravity closer to the grip on the wall bar.

automatic transmission. With the aid of special hand controls, the patient can apply the brakes and accelerate the car with his hands.

The car transfer is an advanced and more difficult mode of transfer and is generally only accomplished unassisted by patients with strong upper extremities and good body control. Refer to Procedure 25.

PROCEDURE #25: Standing Car Transfer

1. Whether or not the patient is the driver or the passenger, he should always enter the car through the right front door, since the steering wheel on the left side frequently hampers or inhibits the transfer. In addition, if the patient is a passenger, the rear doors may not open wide enough to allow proper positioning of the wheelchair for the transfer.
2. The door should be opened as wide as possible, Figure 12-6A. If he wishes the patient may use the edge of the door after the window has been rolled down, the back of the car seat, the door frames of the car, or the seat of the wheelchair for support, Figure 12-6B.
3. The patient turns his back to the car seat and sits down, Figure 12-6C. He then swivels on the seat in order to bring both feet inside, lifting up his involved leg with his hands, if necessary.
4. To leave the car, the patient reverses the process.

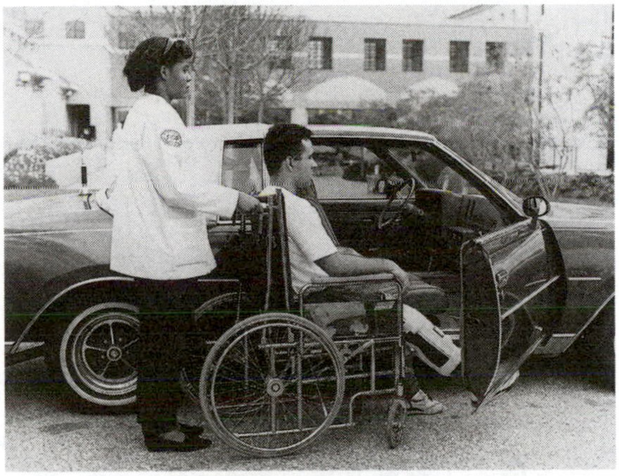

A

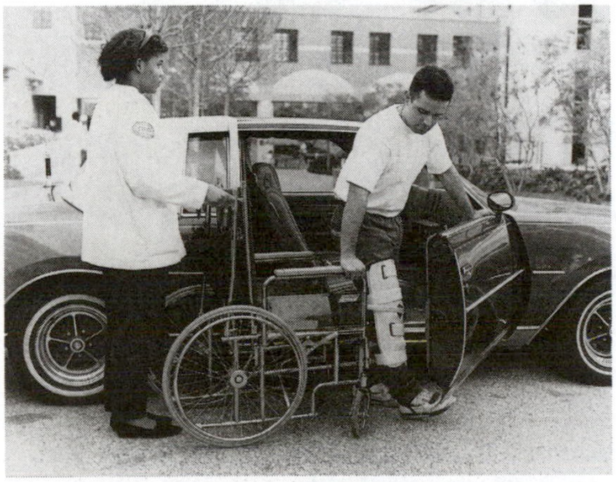

B

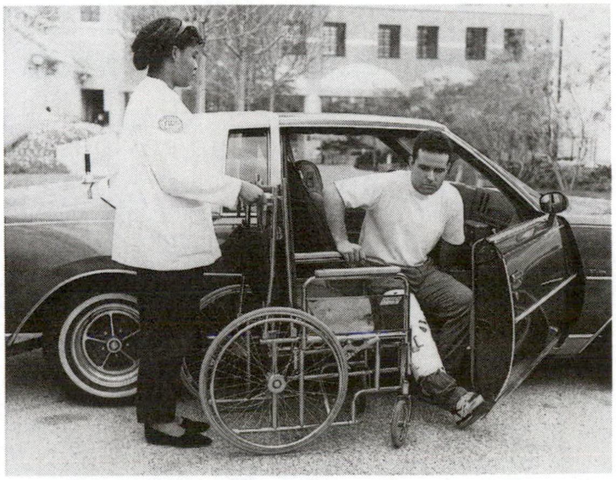

C

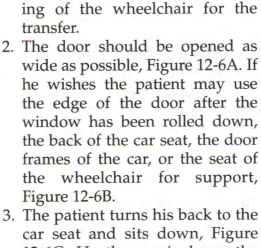

Figure 12-6 Standing transfer from a wheelchair to a car.

BATHTUB TRANSFERS

For patients who may be spending either a prolonged period of time in the hospital or whose disability may be chronic, or long lasting, certain daily tasks, such as bathing, must be addressed. For the patient who is confined to a wheelchair, the standing transfer from a wheelchair to a bathtub may be a bit more difficult than some of the other standing transfers already discussed. This patient will need good balance and sure footing; therefore, the person who may be able to perform a standing transfer from a wheelchair to a bed may not be able to use this type of transfer. If the patient is unable to perform this transfer, the use of a sliding board may help to diminish the risk of falling.

The major difference with this type of transfer is that, unlike other transfers, it is generally made toward the weaker side. The reason for this is that it seems to be much easier for the patient to get into the bathtub than to get out of it. Therefore, when the patient returns from the bathtub to the wheelchair, he can move with his better side first. Refer to Procedures 26 and 27.

Often, it may be difficult to place the proper chair beside the bathtub in the bathroom. The patient may also experience difficulty in sliding across the chair and the edge of the bathtub onto the chair in the tub. If this is the case, it may be easier to teach the patient a sliding-board transfer.

PROCEDURE #26: Assisting the Patient with a Bathtub Transfer

1. Wash your hands, identify the patient, and provide for privacy.
2. Place a sturdy chair of the same height as the bathtub edge inside the tub, on a bath mat, Figure 12-7, and another one beside the tub. Make sure both chairs have rubber tips on the legs, in order to avoid any possibility of slipping.
3. Place a tread tape under the bath mat in the tub to avoid any slipping of the mat.
4. If necessary, have the patient hold onto the bars on the walls for greater security.
5. Assist the patient to assume a sitting position on the chair in the tub.

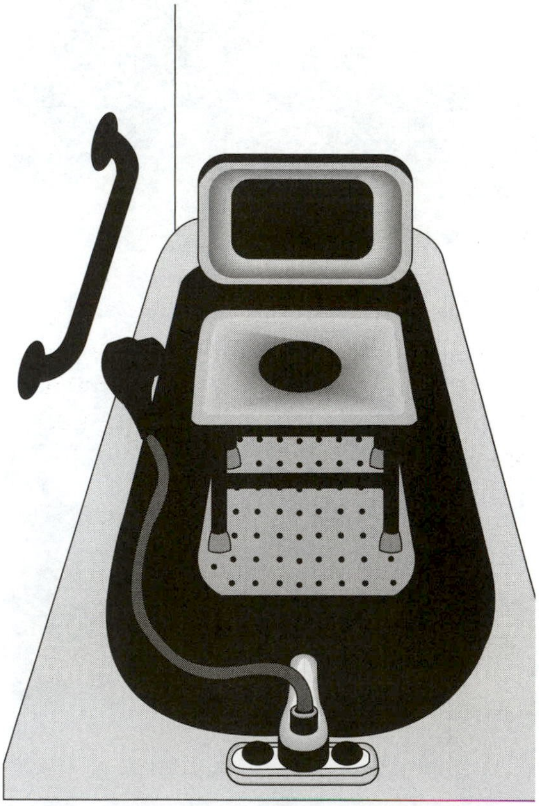

Figure 12-7 Bathtub with chair and bath mat in it.

PROCEDURE #27: Assisting the Patient with a Bathtub Transfer Using a Sliding Board

1. Wash your hands, identify the patient, and provide for privacy.
2. Obtain a sliding board. It is usually made out of lightweight pine, approximately two centimeters in thickness in the middle and beveled lengthwise approximately one centimeter at both ends.
3. If the patient is sitting in a wheelchair, bring it as close to the edge of the tub as possible.
4. Apply the wheelchair brakes and remove or swing the footrests out to the side.
5. Place one end of the board securely under the patient's buttocks on the wheelchair seat and the other end on the chair in the bathtub.
6. Pushing down on the board with one hand, place the other hand on the wheelchair seat, and assist the patient to slide over to the edge of the bathtub, and to place the leg closest to the bathtub in it.
7. The patient then grips the handrail on the edge of the tub and slides his buttocks onto the chair in the tub.
8. The transfer is completed by the patient bringing his second leg over the edge of the bathtub.

◆ SITTING TRANSFERS

Patients experiencing weakness or paralysis in both lower extremities are generally unable to support their body weight with their legs, even for only a few moments. Therefore, it may be necessary to complete a transfer from a sitting position.

Bed to Wheelchair: Unassisted

Whenever the patient is to be moved unassisted from the bed to the wheelchair, the wheelchair should be placed against the bed sideways. The armrest and the footrest of the wheelchair that are located nearest the bed should be removed and the brakes locked. Refer to Procedure 28.

PROCEDURE #28: Unassisted Transfer from Bed to Wheelchair

1. The patient leans forward and pushes down with his fists onto the mattress, carefully shifting his hips until they are angled toward the wheelchair. With the arm closest to the wheelchair, he supports himself on the wheelchair seat.
2. Still leaning forward, the patient pushes down forcefully with one arm on the bed and the other on the wheelchair seat and slides his buttocks from one surface to the other. As the patient shifts his position, he adjusts his legs. He should avoid pushing on the backrest of the wheelchair for support during the transfer.
3. To complete the transfer, the patient then replaces the armrest, and, pushing down on it with his hands, slides back into the chair and adjusts his legs with his arms, if necessary, Figures 12-8A through E.

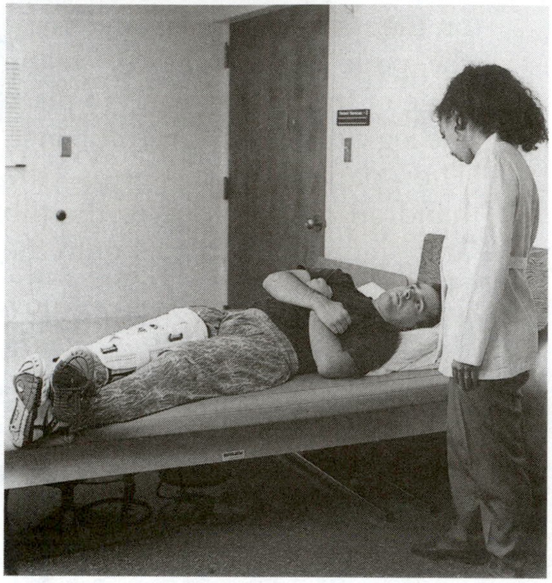

A

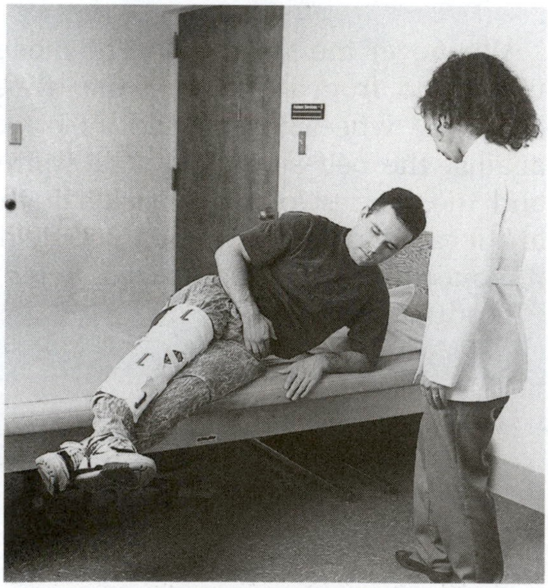

B

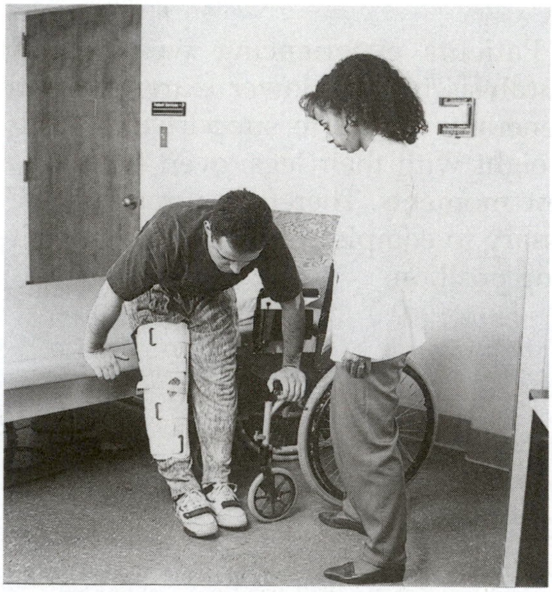

C

Figure 12-8 Unassisted sitting transfer from the bed to the wheelchair.

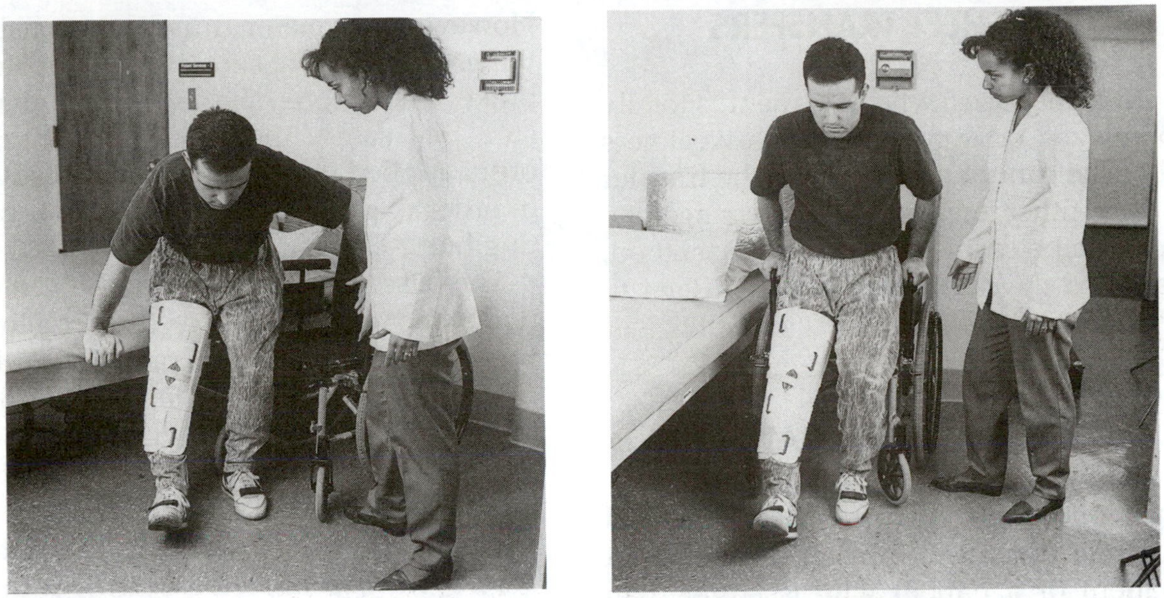

D E

Figure 12-8 Unassisted sitting transfer from the bed to the wheelchair (continued).

Bed to Wheelchair: Assisted

If the patient's arms are not strong enough to lift his body, he may have to be assisted in moving from the bed to the wheelchair.

Finally, you should always remember that the same principles of good body mechanics that are applied for a sitting transfer from the bed to the wheelchair, whether assisted or unassisted, also apply to sitting transfers from the wheelchair to the toilet or from the wheelchair to a car. Refer to Procedure 29.

PROCEDURE #29: Assisted Transfer from Bed to Wheelchair

1. To assist the patient in this transfer, you will first have to bring yourself to the level of the patient. To perform this task, you should bend at your hips and knees to lower yourself. Then grip the transfer belt or grasp the patient around her waist and assist her in angling her hips toward the wheelchair. You should also be supporting the patient's knees with your knees in order to prevent her from sliding forward.
2. Again, using the transfer belt or gripping the patient at her waist, assist her in sliding her buttocks to the wheelchair. At the same time, allow her to see the surface toward which she is being transferred. Throughout this procedure, always make sure that you are assisting the patient to lean forward, so that she can maintain her trunk balance.
3. To complete the transfer and assist the patient to move back into the chair, you should push your knees against hers, continually making sure that she keeps leaning forward and pushes down on the armrests with her hands.

DRAWSHEET TRANSFERS

In some cases, when a patient is totally paralyzed or experiences such weakness that she cannot participate in the transfer at all, other means of transferring may have to be employed. One such method, is called the **drawsheet transfer.** Refer to Procedure 30.

PNEUMATIC LIFT TRANSFER

A **pneumatic lift** provides a method for one person to transfer a dependent patient or a patient who is larger than herself. This mechanical system has caster wheels, which make it easier for positioning and moving the patient. However, one major drawback to using the pneumatic lift is that it does not have brakes. Therefore, she aide must make sure that safety measures are continuously applied throughout this procedure in order to prevent the patient from getting hurt.

The base of the pneumatic lift can be widened to fit around the patient's wheelchair or any other piece of equipment. It is generally in the narrow position when the patient is being moved, in order to make the maneuvering easier. The long lever attached to the base is turned and moved from one side to the other to increase or decrease the width of the base (Figures 12-9A through D). Refer to Procedure 31.

PROCEDURE #30: Assisting the Patient with a Drawsheet Transfer

1. Wash your hands, identify the patient, and provide for privacy.
2. Roll the patient to one side.
3. Place a folded sheet under the patient's back.
4. Gently roll the patient to the other side of the bed and unfold the drawsheet.
5. Two persons must perform the transfer, one on each side of the patient's bed. They hold either side of the drawsheet and carefully slide the patient from the bed to the gurney or treatment table.

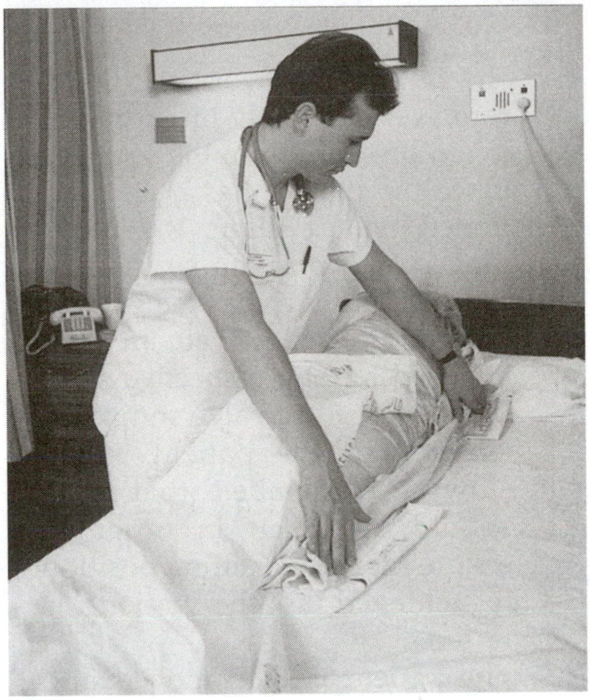

Figure 12-9A Roll patient toward you and place sling smoothly under patient's body.

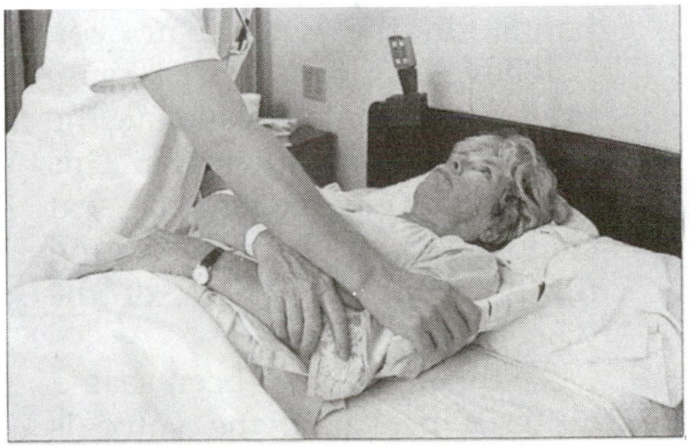

Figure 12-9B Position sling smoothly under hips.

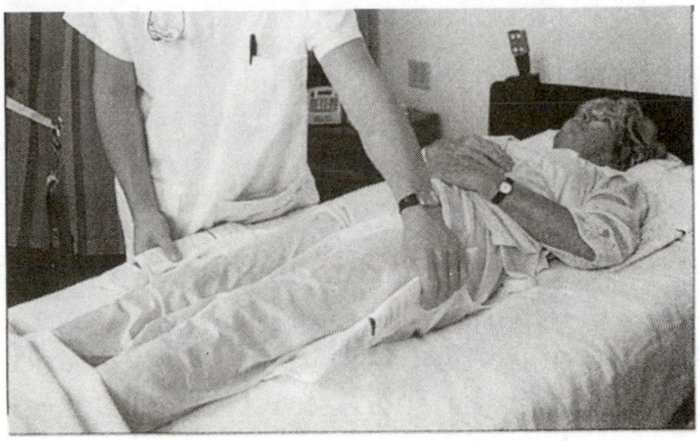

Figure 12-9C Make sure top of sling is positioned under shoulders so it extends above them.

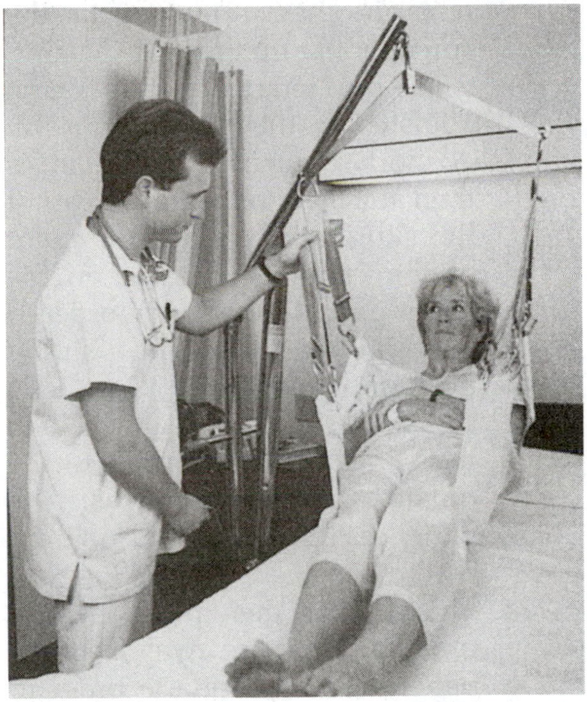

Figure 12-9D Lift patient free of bed. (Second physical therapy aide is out of camera range.)

PROCEDURE #31: Transferring the Patient Using the Pneumatic Lift

1. The valve on the front of the upright is closed in order to allow the lift to be raised and then opened slowly in order to lower the patient. After checking that the valve is closed, the aide "pumps" the handle to raise the lift.
2. The sling on which the patient rests is then attached to the spreader bar on the lift by chains, with the length of the chain adjusted to the patient's height. A short segment of the chain is then attached to the upper part of the sling, and a longer segment of the chain is attached to the lower part of the sling in order to suspend the patient in a sitting position.
3. The hooks are then attached to the sling from the inside to the outside. By doing this, the patient is less likely to be injured by the hook.
4. The sling is then positioned so that the seams are away from the patient. This is done in order to avoid pressure areas. Slings are made of a variety of fabrics and may either be one piece or two piece. When the patient is in bed, the sling is placed under her by rolling her to one side, positioning the sling, and then rolling her to the other side. The sling may be left under the patient when she is in the wheelchair; therefore, it is extremely important to avoid pressure from the seams.
5. Once the patient has been positioned on the sling, the lift is moved into position so that the spreader bar is across the patient. Both ends of each chain are then attached to their respective sides of the sling. The valve should be closed and the patient raised slowly. Remember that care should be taken in order to ensure that a safe sitting position is achieved as the patient is raised.
6. The patient is then moved into position over the seat of a locked wheelchair.
7. The valve is opened slowly in order to lower the patient into the wheelchair.
8. In order to properly seat the patient in the wheelchair, you will have to apply slight pressure in the horizontal plane at the patient's knees and thighs. This pushes the patient into the seat completely, with her back resting firmly against the back of the wheelchair.
9. Once the patient has been seated in the wheelchair, the valve is closed in order to avoid striking the patient should the lift arm continue to lower. The chains are then removed from the sling. The transfer is completed by moving the lift away from the wheelchair and placing the patient's feet properly onto the footrests.

ONE-PERSON TRANSFER FROM FLOOR TO WHEELCHAIR

Occasionally a patient may fall out of or tip over the wheelchair. If the patient is unable to transfer from the floor to the wheelchair, you may have to perform a **one-person transfer.** Refer to Procedure 32.

SUMMARY

In this chapter, we described the purpose, preparation, and skills involved in properly transferring the patient. First we discussed the role body mechanics play during the transfer procedure. Then we identified several different types of wheelchair transfers, including the unassisted and assisted bed to wheelchair transfer, an assisted wheelchair to parallel bar transfer, and an assisted wheelchair to treatment transfer. We also talked about a modified standing transfer, a standing toilet transfer, a standing car transfer, and a bathtub transfer. We also talked about how to perform a drawsheet transfer, a pneumatic lift transfer, and finally the physical therapy aide's role in a one-person transfer from the floor to the wheelchair.

PROCEDURE #32: One Man Transfer from Floor to Wheelchair

1. When using this transfer, the wheelchair should be positioned on its back, at the patient's buttocks. The patient's ankles are then placed over the front edge of the wheelchair seat. You will then have to perform a series of short lift and scooting maneuvers in order to move the patient into the wheelchair. This is accomplished by placing one arm under the patient's knees and the other under her upper trunk and neck.
2. After you have placed yourself into a half-kneeling position to help provide a stronger lifting posture, lift the handles of the wheelchair, bringing it to an upright position. As you are bringing the wheelchair up, begin to move out of the half-kneeling position to a standing position.
3. As the wheelchair begins to approach the upright position, shift one arm to guard the patient's upper trunk. This will prevent you from falling forward.

REVIEW QUESTIONS

1. Transferring patients requires an understanding of __________, __________, and __________.
2. __________ __________ require little, if any, active participation by the patient.
3. The goal of any assisted transfer is to __________ the assistance and __________ independence.
4. The two basic types of transfers are __________ and __________.
5. It is important to always check the __________ of the wheelchair before starting any transfer to or from it.
6. A __________ __________ may be used to assist the patient transferring from the bed to the wheelchair.
7. When transferring from the bed to the wheelchair unassisted, the patient should slide __________ to the edge of the bed.
8. When assisting the patient to transfer from the bed to the wheelchair, the physical therapy aide should always keep his back __________ and hips and knees __________.
9. When using the parallel bars, the patient always starts from a __________ position.
10. A standing toilet transfer requires the use of a __________-degree angle wall handrail.
11. When making a standing car transfer, the patient always enters the car through the __________ front door.
12. A bathtub transfer is generally made toward the patient's __________ side.

SECTION V

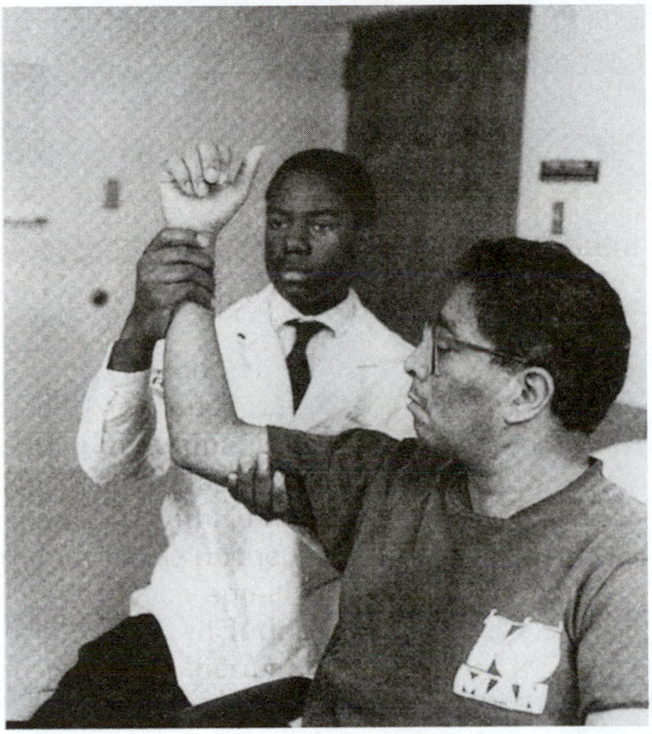

PHYSICAL THERAPY MODALITIES

13

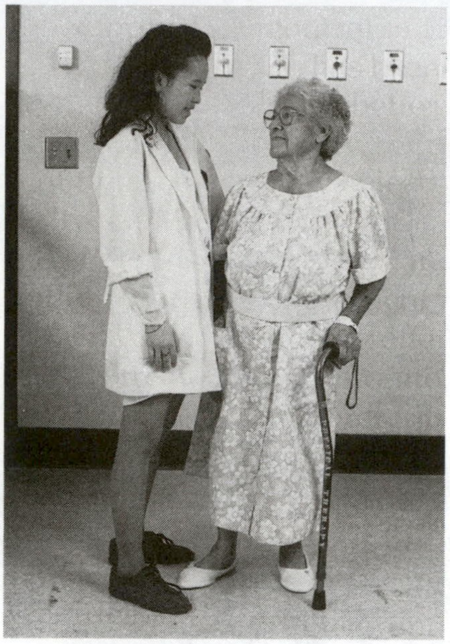

Assisting with Ambulation and Gait Training

OBJECTIVES

Upon completion of this chapter, you should be able to:

1. Define the term ambulation and discuss the physical therapy aide's role in assisting the patient with it.
2. Briefly explain how to choose the appropriate ambulatory device for a patient's use.
3. Identify four basic ambulatory devices and briefly discuss the physical therapy aide's role in assisting the patient to use them.
4. Delineate the difference between a two-point, three-point, and four-point gait as each relates to crutch walking.
5. Describe the difference between a swing-to and a swing-through gait, and briefly explain how each relates to crutch walking.
6. Briefly explain the physical therapy aide's role in assisting the patient to walk up and down stairs using crutches.
7. Define what it meant by the term *gait*.
8. Briefly explain what a normal gait is and discuss the differences between a normal gait and the following abnormal gaits: coxalgic gait, painful-knee gait, sacroiliac gait, and a flexed-hip gait.
9. Describe the gait of a patient with hemiplegia.
10. Describe the gait of a patient with Parkinson's disease.

KEY TERMS

- Ambulation
- Ambulatory device
- Axillary crutches
- Cane
- Crutch
- Crutch walking
- Four-point gait
- Gait pattern
- Hemiwalker
- Lofstrand crutch
- Parallel bars
- Swing-through gait
- Swing-to gait
- Three-point gait
- Two-point gait
- Walker

Ambulation is a term that means *to walk.* It is a functional activity that some patients may be able to accomplish, but for others, because of physical limitations or disabilities affecting the lower extremities, may be completely impossible or only possible with the aid of an assistive device. The ambulatory aid or device a patient needs depends on the type of disability she may have. Ambulation aids can be prescribed by a physician only after a careful evaluation of the patient's general condition and the specific gait disability.

Generally speaking, assistive devices are used to make safe ambulation possible. The three main indications for such devices include a decreased ability to bear weight on the lower extremities, resulting from structural damage of the skeletal system; muscle weakness or paralysis of the trunk or lower extremities; and poor balance in the upright posture. These devices may also be used to increase the patient's base of support, allowing a redistribution of weight within the base of support and a larger area within which the center of gravity can shift without the patient's losing balance.

Whenever an **ambulatory device** is used, the amount of energy the patient puts out is generally very high. This, coupled with the necessity of having to learn a new sequence of walking, can cause the patient to tire quite rapidly. Therefore, in early training sessions, the patient usually requires greater concentration in order to learn the proper gait.

Under the supervision and guidance of a physical therapist, you may be allowed to introduce the patient to the proper use of ambulatory aids. You should remember, however, that some of these patients may be so weakened by disease or prolonged bed rest that a preambulatory therapy program may be necessary before ambulation training begins. Such a program may consist of range of motion and strengthening exercises for the upper extremities, especially for the muscles extending to the elbow and the muscles depressing the shoulder.

TIPS ON PREAMBULATION TEACHING

Part of the preambulation may consist of teaching the patient newly acquired **gait patterns.** To provide maximum stability, this often begins with bringing the patient to the parallel bars since they require the least amount of coordination by the patient. By practicing on the parallel bars, the patient can become accustomed to the upright posture and learn the sequence for gait or walking in relative safety. Also, assistive devices or aids may be fitted while the patient stands between the parallel bars.

Whatever device may be prescribed for the patient's use, it is the task of the physical therapy team member to describe and demonstrate its proper use to him, as well as the appropriate gait sequence, before ambulation begins. Usually, a demonstration is the primary method of instruction, but a verbal description reinforces the demonstration. Verbal descriptions should always be kept to a minimum. Observing other patients who may be using the same or similar devices can also be a useful method of instruction.

Once a patient has become proficient on level surfaces, instruction or teaching in the use of stairs, curbs, ramps, and doors can be given. The patient should be taught to climb and descend stairs on the right-hand side since this is the usual method used throughout the United States. Teaching the patient to sit down and stand up when using armless chairs, low or soft sofas and chairs, toilets, and car seats may also be necessary. In addition, the patient should also be instructed on how to protect herself during a fall and how to get up after the fall has occurred.

Finally, it is important to teach the patient how to check his ambulatory aid for its safe operation and use. Wing nuts used on crutches, for example, often loosen with prolonged use. The rubber tips of assistive devices will not grip the floor properly if they become too worn or dirt fills their grooves. The patient should also be warned to avoid small throw rugs that may slip or become entangled when the ambulatory aid is placed on them.

◆ CHOOSING THE APPROPRIATE DEVICE

As we have previously discussed, the type of ambulatory device or aid the patient uses, is generally dependent upon the type or disability she has. Some devices provide more stability and support than others; some require more coordination. As the patient's limitations decrease, she may also progress from a device that provides more stability and support to one that provides less. Other patients may continue to use the same aid throughout the entire time an assistive device is required. Some of the more frequently used devices include parallel bars, walkers, crutches, and canes.

Parallel Bars

Parallel bars, as we have already stated, are generally used as the first step in teaching the patient to ambulate (see Figures 13-1A and B). Because of their stability, they tend to give the patient a sense of security, as well as assisting the patient in initial standing and walking.

The use of parallel bars actually helps the patient to propel himself forward more with his hands than with his legs. To induce him gradually to place more body weight on his lower extremities, encourage him to put the palm of his hands on the bars without gripping them.

The height and width of the bars are extremely important. They should be adjusted to fit the individual patient, with the height being such that the elbows are bent 25 to 30 degrees when the patient is standing and holding on to the bars with his hands.

Walker

After the patient has been able to

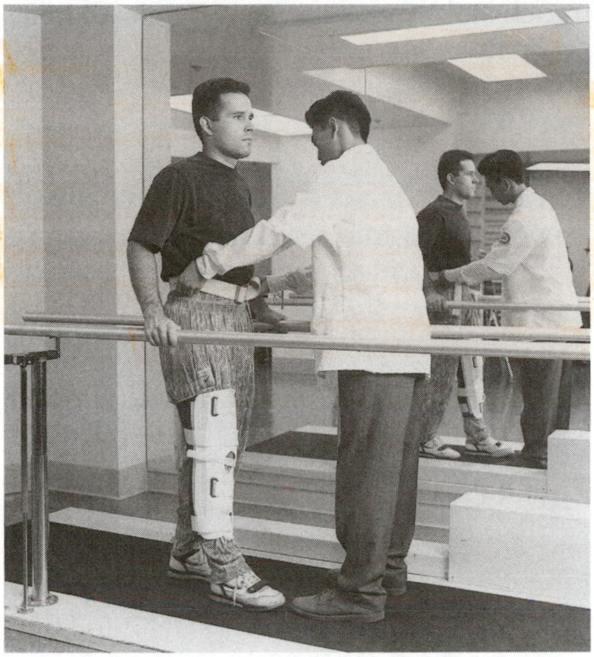

Figure 13-1A Physical Therapy (PT)—the department where the patient learns how to use his body again and becomes strong after an accident or surgery.

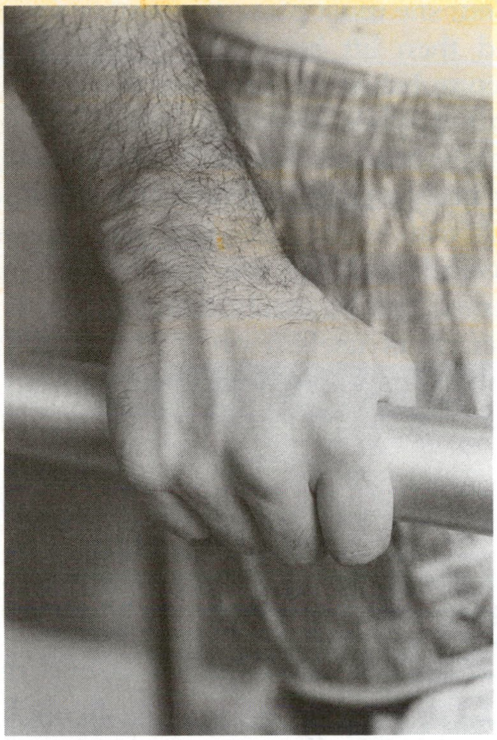

Figure 13-1B Patient standing with a standard walker.

master the parallel bars, the next step is to instruct her in the use of a **walker.** Generally made of aluminum, this device consists of a frame with four adjustable legs (Figure 13-2). Each of the legs has a rubber tip in order to prevent sliding.

The walker serves the same function as the parallel bars but is not as stable. It can be used at home and in the hospital and can be easily transported. The height of the walker should be adjusted to the individual patient, so that the elbow can be flexed 25 to 30 degrees when the patient is standing with her hands on it.

When ambulating with a walker, the walker is first lifted with both hands and then placed forward 25 to 30 centimeters. Then it is stepped into, first with the stronger leg and then with the weaker leg.

If the patient can only bear weight on one lower extremity or has one leg ampu-

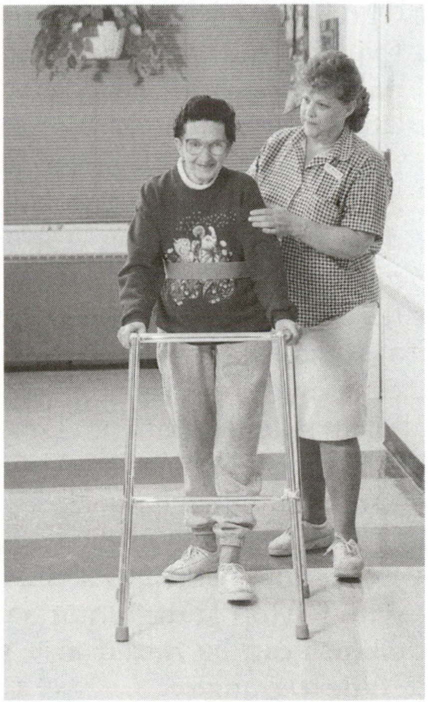

Figure 13-2 Older patients may need help to remain physically active. The walker provides support and stability, giving the patient more confidence in walking.

tated, she must place the walker forward and then lift her body weight. This is accomplished by pressing down on the walker while stepping into it with the weight-bearing extremity. The lifting of the body weight is done by the shoulders.

A walker may be used only on level ground and, as we previously mentioned, can be easily transported, however, it is useless on stairs. A hinged walker may be occasionally used for stair walking, but it does not provide as much stability as the standard walker.

Walkers are moist helpful in the early stages of training for patients who will eventually be able to use lesser ambulatory aids such as crutches or a cane. However, it is used frequently as a permanent walking aid for elderly people who are confined to a specific area of the home or hospital or who have difficulty with balance and coordination. Refer to Procedure 33.

PROCEDURE #33: Assisting the Patient to Ambulate with a Walker

1. Wash your hands, identify the patient, and provide for privacy. Obtain the necessary equipment.
2. Explain the procedure to the patient.
3. Check the walker. Make sure the rubber suction tips are secure on all the legs. Check for rough or damaged edges on the hand rests.
4. If possible, position the patient in a standing position, a wall or chair may be used for support. Make sure the patient is wearing walking shoes with a one to one-and-one-half inch heel.
5. Check the height of the walker to see if the hand rests are level with the top of the femur and the elbows can be flexed at a 25- to 30-degree angle.
6. Start with the walker in position; the patient should be standing inside the walker.
7. Tell the patient to lift the walker and place it forward so the back legs are even with the patient's toes.
8. Instruct the patient to transfer her weight forward slightly to the walker.
9. Instruct the patient to use the walker for support and to walk into the walker.
10. Repeat steps 7 through 9. While the patient is using the walker, you should walk to the side of and slightly behind her. Be alert at all times and be ready to catch the patient if she starts to fall.
11. Check the patient constantly to see that she is lifting the walker to move it forward. Also make sure the patient is placing the walker just up to the toes and is not attempting too large a step.
12. Note the patient's progress and report any problems to the therapist.
13. Replace the equipment.

◆ CRUTCHES

Once the patient is secure with the walker, he is ready to begin ambulating with **crutches.**

There are two basic types of crutches. The first, called **axillary crutches,** can be made of wood or aluminum, and are generally used for patients who will need crutches for a relatively short period of time. They are easier to use than forearm crutches, but are also more restrictive. The second type of crutch, called a **Lofstrand crutch,** are recommended for patients who will need crutches permanently or for long periods of time, and who have the stability, strength, and coordination to use them. These crutches, commonly referred to as "forearm" crutches, allow the patient greater maneuverability and are less wearing on the patient's clothing.

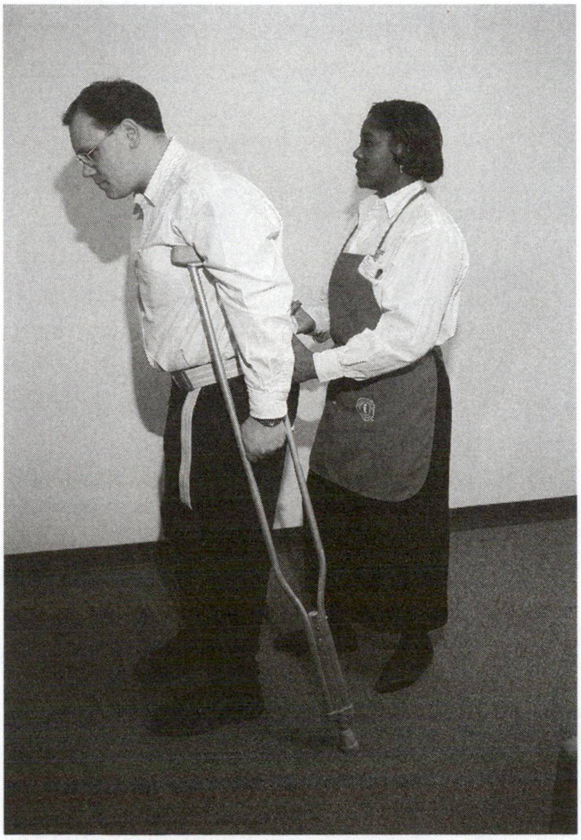

Figure 13-3A Crutch walking.

Crutch Walking

The standard axillary crutch is composed of two uprights and an adjustable bottom, which are secured to the uprights with two screws, an axillary crossbar joining the uprights at the upper end, and a handgrip that can be adjusted (Figures 13-3A and B). They must be rubber-tipped at the bottom in order to not slip on the floor. In crutch walking, the patient shifts about 50 percent of the weight-bearing load from his legs to his arms and crutches. Therefore, the crutches must be fitted to the individual patient.

In the standard position, the tips of the crutches should be approximately 15 to 20 centimeters in front and 15 to 20 centimeters to the side of the toes. A "tripod" base is formed with the patient's feet and the crutches. To place the body center of gravity more toward the base of the tripod, you must ask the patient to bring his hips forward. You should also instruct him to look straight ahead in the direction he will walk, not down at the tip of the crutches and his feet as he may have a tendency to do.

You must instruct the patient not to bear weight on the axillary crossbar

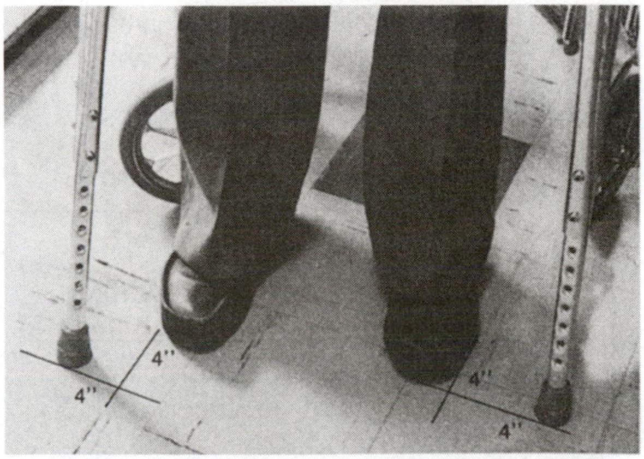

Figure 13-3B Patient standing with axillary crutches.

since this can cause undue impairment of the nerves or arteries that supply the arm and hand, causing the patient to complain of numbness in his arms or hands.

Different types of gaits may be used with crutches, depending upon the patient's disability or limitations. If one leg is not affected and the patient can tolerate full weight bearing, the crutches are moved forward with the affected limb. This is called a **three-point gait** (Figure 13-4). This type of gait is generally used for patients who have had hip or knee surgery.

Another gait, called the **four-point gait,** is usually indicated for a patient who is able to move her legs alternately, but may not be able to bear the full weight on either leg without the support of crutches (Figure 13-5). With this gait, the legs and crutches move in the sequence of left crutch-right foot, right crutch-left foot. Hence, when the patient is using the crutches in this manner, you can assume that she is actually ambulating with four legs. In the four-point gait, only one leg or crutch is off the floor at one time, leaving three points for support, and thereby creating a very stable and safe gate.

The **two-point gait** is a modification of the four-point gait and is closest to the natural rhythm of walking. In this gait, the right crutch and left leg move together and the left crutch and the right leg move together (Figure 13-6).

For patients who may suffer from

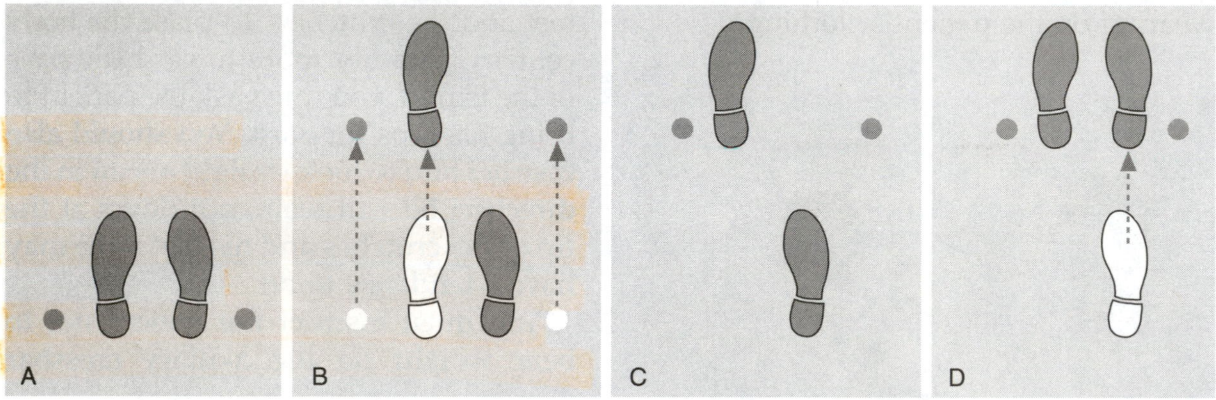

Figure 13-4 Three-point gait.

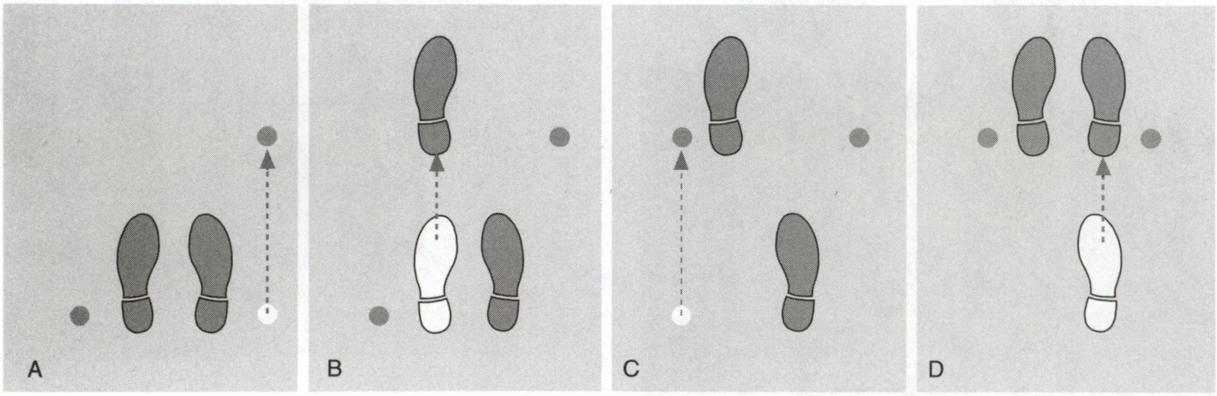

Figure 13-5 Four-point gait.

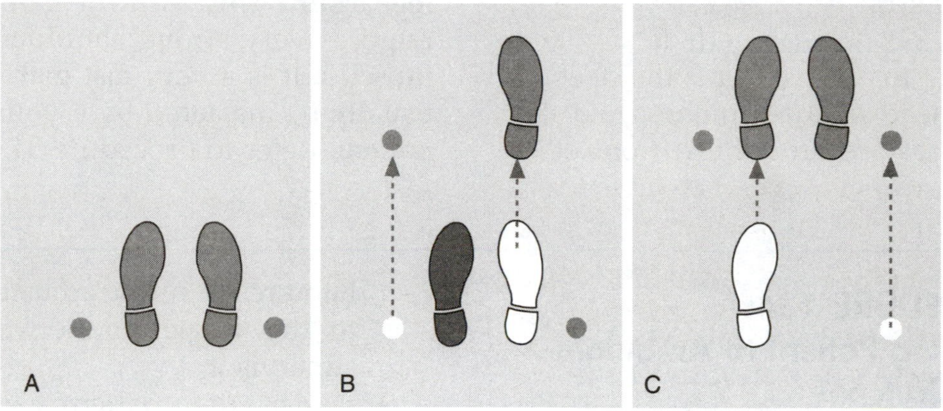

Figure 13-6 Two-point gait.

paralysis of both lower extremities or who are unable to move the legs alternately, the swing-to or swing-through gaits may be used.

In the **swing-to gait,** the patient assumes a standing position and places her full body weight down on the handgrip of the crutches by extending her elbows (Figure 13-7A). While standing, she thrusts the pelvis forward in order to place the center of gravity behind her hip joints. With the feet placed firmly in line with the crutches, the patient lifts her body and swings forward (Figure 13-7B). At that point, both crutches are moved forward again to end directly

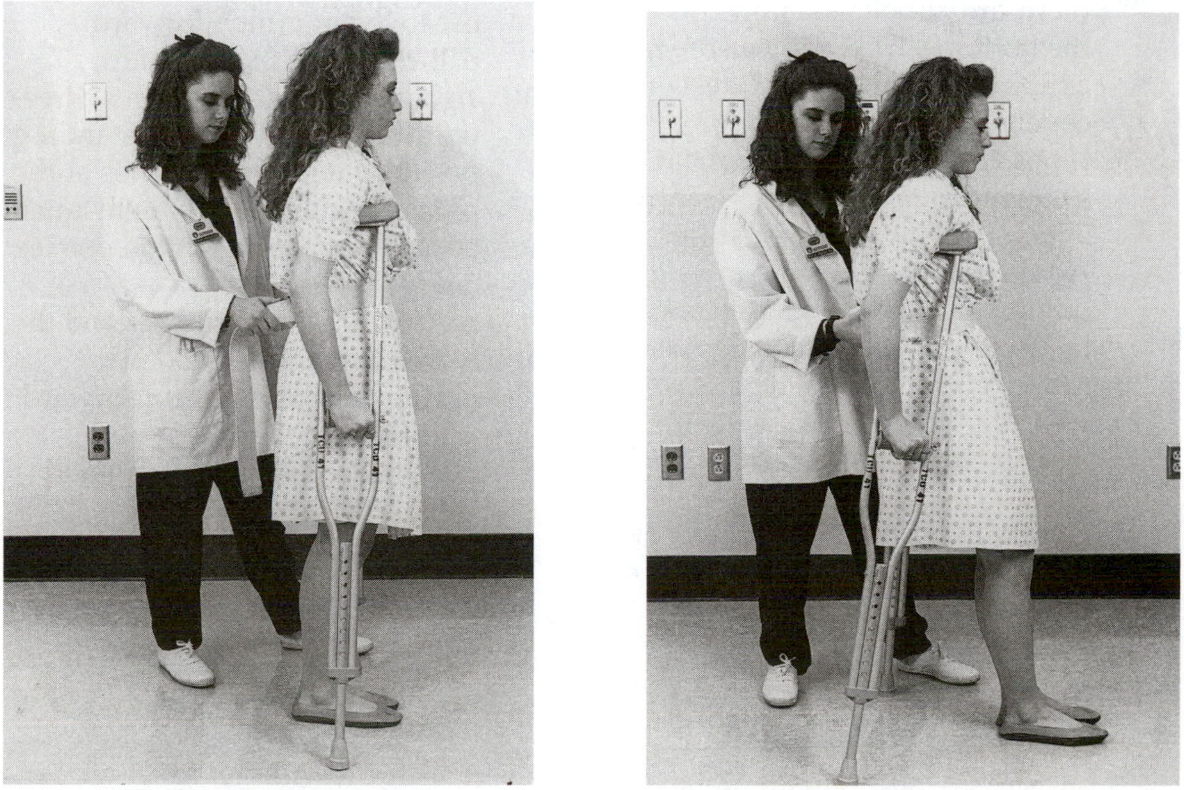

A B

Figure 13-7 The swing-to gait.

under the arm.

The **swing-through gait** is similar to the swing-to gait except the feet are placed ahead of the crutches, and then the crutches are brought in front of the feet again. This form of gait generally requires very strong shoulder and arm muscles. It is a very fast gait, but it can usually be mastered by a young, strong patient. Refer to Procedure 34.

PROCEDURE #34: Assisting Patient to Ambulate with Crutches

1. Wash your hands, identify the patient, and provide for privacy. Obtain the necessary equipment.
2. Explain the procedure to the patient.
3. Check the patient's order or obtain authorization from your supervisor to ascertain which gait the therapist taught the patient.
4. Check the crutches. Make sure there are rubber suction tips on the bottoms. Check to be sure the axillary bar and hand rest are covered with padding.
5. If possible, position the patient in a standing position leaning against a wall for support. Advise the patient to bear weight on the unaffected leg. A chair can be used for additional support.
6. Make sure that the patient is wearing walking shoes with a one to one-and-one-half inch heel.
7. Check the measurement of the crutches: position crutches four inches to the side of the feet; make sure there is a two-inch gap between the axilla and the axillary bar or rest. If the length must be adjusted, check with your supervisor; the elbow must be flexed at a 30-degree angle. If the hand rest must be adjusted to get to this angle, check with your supervisor.
8. Assist the patient with the required gait. The gait used depends on the patient's injury and condition and is determined by the therapist or physician.
9. To assist the patient with a four-point gait, start in a standing position with the crutches at the patient's sides. The patient must be able to bear weight on both legs.
   a. Move right crutch forward.
   b. Move left foot forward.
   c. Move left crutch forward.
   d. Move right foot forward.
10. To assist the patient with a three-point gait, start in a standing position, with the crutches at the patient's side. The patient must be able to bear weight on one leg only.
    a. Advance both crutches and the weak or affected foot.
    b. Transfer body weight forward to the crutches.
    c. Advance unaffected or good foot forward.
11. To assist the patient with a two point gait, start in a standing position with the crutches at the patient's side. The patient must be able to bear weight on both legs.
    a. Move the right foot and left crutch forward at the same time.

b. Move the left foot and right crutch forward at the same time.

12. To assist the patient with a swing-to gait, start in a standing position with the crutches at the patient's side.
    a. Balance weight on one foot or both feet. Move both crutches forward.
    b. Transfer the weight forward.
    c. Use shoulder and arm strength to swing the feet up to the crutches.
13. To assist the patient with a swing-through gait, start in a standing position with the crutches at the patient's side.
    a. Balance the weight on one foot or both feet.
    b. Advance both crutches forward at the same time.
    c. Transfer the weight forward.
    d. Use shoulder and arm strength to swing up to and through the crutches, stopping slightly in front of the crutches.
14. While using the crutches, do not allow the patient to rest her body weight on the axillary rest. The shoulder and arm strength should provide the movement on the crutches.
15. Check to be sure that the patient is not moving too far at one time. Distances should be limited. If the patient attempts to move the crutches too far forward, it is very easy for her to lose balance and fall forward.
16. Check the patient's progress and report it to therapist.
17. When the patient is finished using crutches, replace all equipment.

Crutch Walking and Chairs

Another problem a patient experiences with crutch walking is the use of a chair. In addition to learning how to walk with the crutches, the patient must also be instructed in how to sit down and stand up from chairs of varying heights. Such techniques are taught at the beginning of the crutch ambulation program so the patient can practice them when she stops to rest during an ambulatory session.

It is important to remember that the mode of getting in and out of a chair with crutches will depend greatly on the type of chair and the patient's limitations. Generally speaking, the method safest for the patient is usually the preferred one. The chair should be well supported and should not be allowed to slide. The crutches should be removed from under the arms and held in one hand, freeing the other hand for support when the patient sits down. With her free hand, the patient should push down on the chair seat or armrest in order to support her weight. Finally, she lowers herself into the chair by gradually flexing the elbow. To stand up from the chair, the patient follows the reverse order of sitting down.

If the patient is required to use the Lofstrand type of crutch, she will find greater support than that of the standard axillary type. Instead of one point of support, like the handgrip of a crane, these forearm crutches have two points, the handgrip and the forearm cuff (Figure 13-8). As with the standard axillary

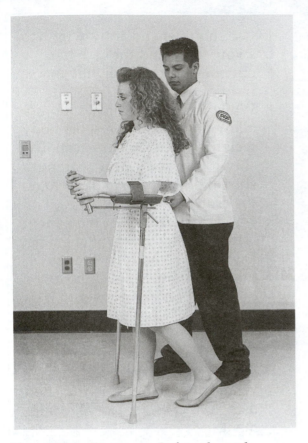

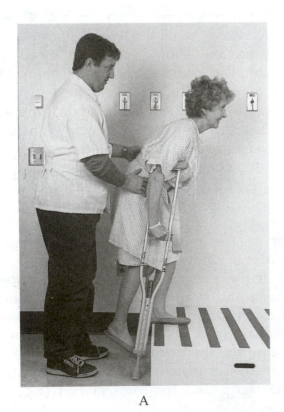

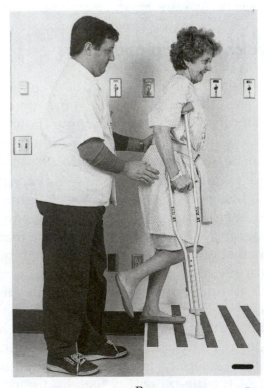

Figure 13-8 Forearm or Lofstand crutches.

crutches, rubber tips prevent slipping on the floor, and the forms of gait are the same as with the axillary crutches.

Stair Walking and Crutches

If the patient finds herself in a position where stair walking is required, you will have to remind her that the stress is always on the leg that does the lifting of the body weight by extension in the hip and knee. When walking upstairs, the good leg must be placed on the next higher step first (Figure 13-9A) while the ambulatory aid supports the impaired leg on the step below. The walking aid and the impaired leg must be brought up together (Figure 13-9B). When walking downstairs, the impaired leg comes first with the ambulatory aid while the good leg has to bear the body weight when flexed with the hip and knee (Figure 13-10). Refer to Procedure 35.

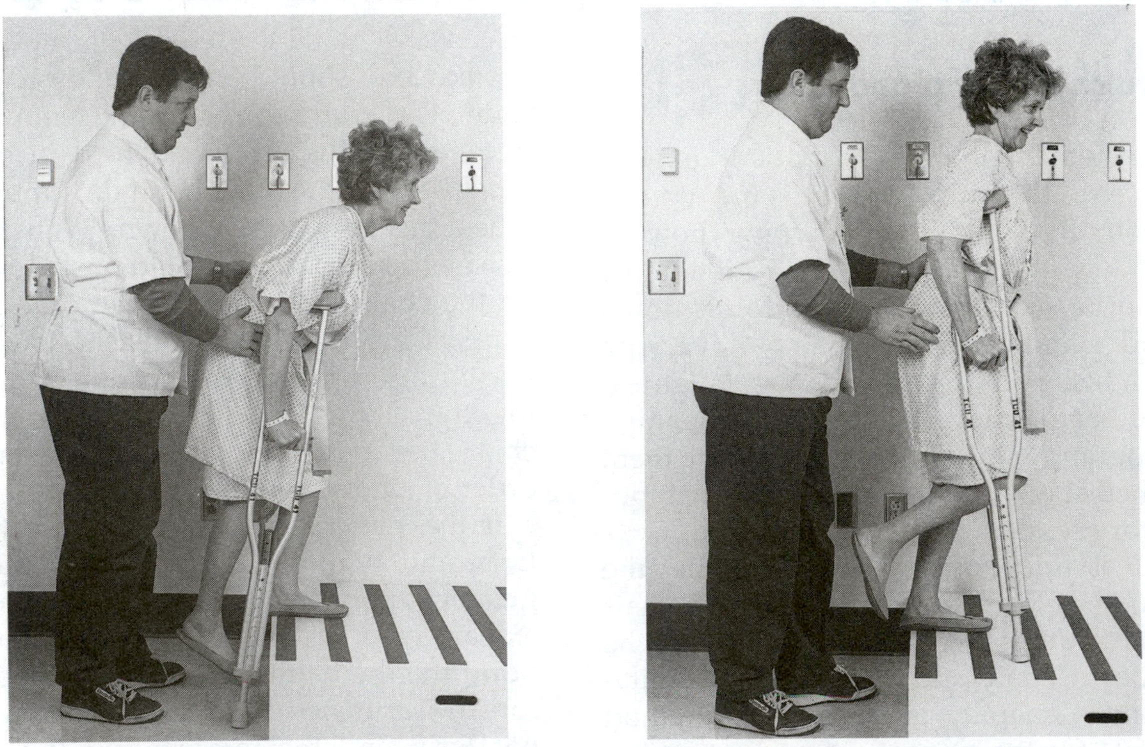

A B

Figure 13-9 Going upstairs with crutches.

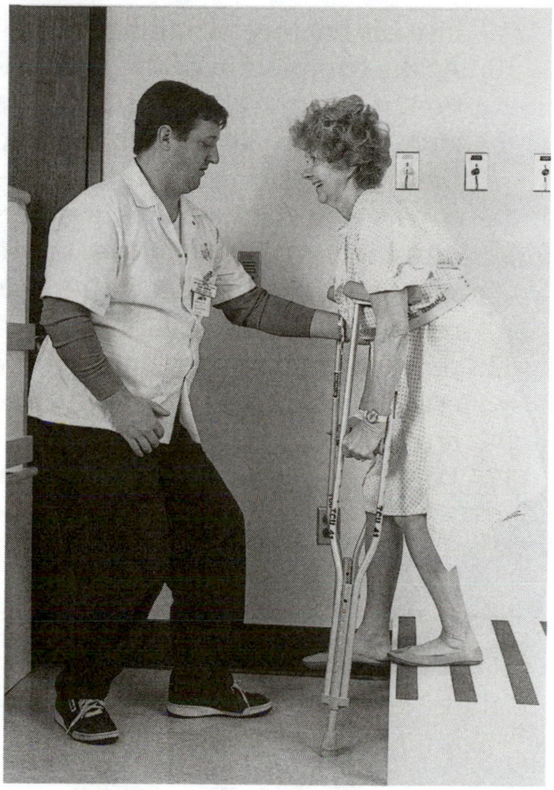

Figure 13-10 Going downstairs with crutches.

PROCEDURE #35: Ambulating a Patient Using Crutches

1. Check the doctor's orders in order to ensure proper authorization for the use of crutches and to determine what type of gait should be taught.
2. Obtain the proper crutches. You will need to make sure that they are the proper size and both bottom ends have rubber suction tips. Also make sure that the axillary bar and handrests are covered with padding.
3. Wash your hands.
4. If at all possible, have the patient stand leaning against a wall for ample support. Advise him to bear weight on the unaffected leg. If necessary, you may use a chair for additional support.
5. Make sure that the patient is wearing sturdy walking shoes, with a heel that is no more than one-and-one-half inches high.
6. Check the measurement of the crutches. This is accomplished by positioning the crutches four inches in front of the patient's feet and moving them four inches to the side of the foot. There should be no more than a two-inch gap between the axilla (armpit) and the axillary bar. The elbow is then flexed to a 30-degree angle. Any adjustment to the handrest should be cleared by your immediate supervisor.
7. Assist the patient with the appropriate gait, that is, four-point, three-point, two-point, swing-to, or swing-through.

8. While ambulating with the crutches, remind the patient that he must never rest his body weight on the axillary rest of the crutches, and his shoulder and arm strength should provide the movement of the crutches.
9. During the ambulation process, be sure to check to see that the patient is not moving too far at one time. If he does attempt to move too far too quickly, slow him down so that he does not lose his balance or fall forward.
10. At the completion of the ambulation, report the patient's progress and tolerance to the activity to the therapist or your immediate supervisor. At that time, a determination will be made as to whether or not the patient is ready for a more advanced gait.
11. After the patient has finished the crutch walking, replace the crutches to their proper location.
12. Wash your hands.

◆ CANES

The use of a **cane** as an ambulatory aid is a convenient device for relieving one extremity of some weight-bearing load. Constructed of either wood or aluminum, this device is also able to provide the patient with continuous stability.

The length of a cane should always be adjusted so that the elbow is bent approximately 25 to 30 degrees when standing with the cane (Figure 13-11). In most physical therapy departments, adjustable aluminum canes are also available for patient training and measurements.

The cane should always be used in the hand opposite the impaired leg. There are several reasons for this. First, the leg and opposite arm move together in normal walking. Second, a wider base is provided in order to increase stability. Finally, the shift of the center of gravity from one side to the other is eliminated. Refer to Procedure 36.

When we speak of a cane, we are generally referring to a unilateral walking aid. Therefore, an axillary or forearm crutch can be used like a cane. When these are used properly, approximately 20 to 30 pounds of stress is placed on the cane and about 40 pounds of stress is placed onto the forearm crutch.

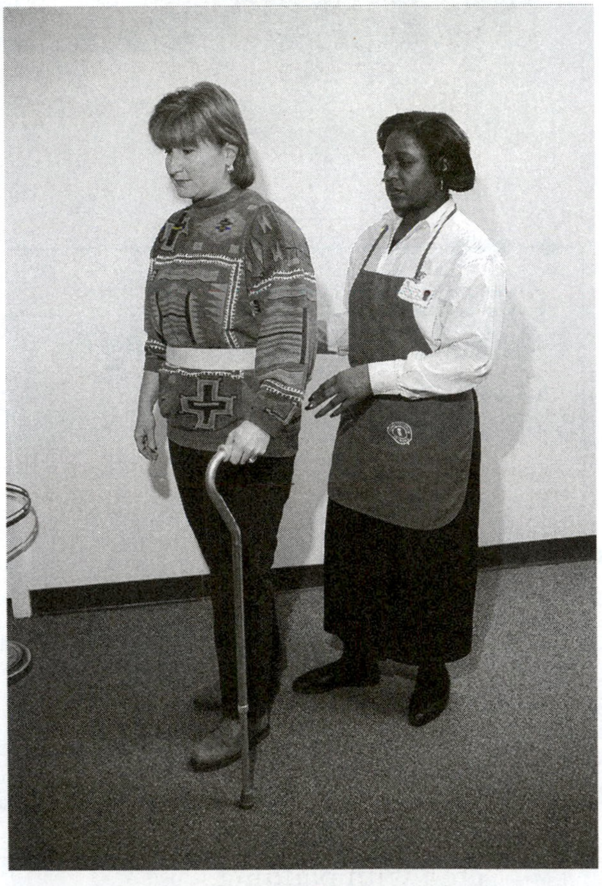

Figure 13-11 Using various types of canes.

In order to assure more stability in

PROCEDURE #36: Ambulating a Patient Using a Cane

1. Check the doctor's orders to make sure the patient should be ambulated with a cane and determine what type of gait should be taught.
2. Obtain the appropriate cane. Check its size and make sure that it has a rubber suction tip. If the patient needs additional stability, use a tripod or quad cane.
3. Wash your hands.
4. If at all possible, try to position the patient in a standing position, using the wall of a chair for additional support. Make sure the patient is wearing shoes with a heel no more than one to one-and-one-half inches high.
5. Check the height of the cane to make sure that the top of it reaches the femur and that the patient's elbow is flexed at a 25 to 30 degree angle.
6. Instruct the patient to use the cane on the unaffected side.
7. Assist the patient with her gait, as necessary.
8. While ambulating with the cane, try to make sure that the patient does not try to take too large a step since this may cause her to lose her balance or fall.
9. Note the patient's progress and report it to the therapist or your supervisor.
10. Replace the cane, as necessary, to its proper location.
11. Wash your hands.

elderly people, a three- or four-legged cane may be used. This type of ambulatory aid is most useful on level ground, but its greatest limitation is that it only allows for a slow gait. Hence, if the patient were to try to walk faster, a rocking action from the two rear legs to the front legs or leg might develop. This rocking action defeats the goal of the increased stability, or the very purpose of the use of the cane.

The three- or four-legged cane is extremely useful for most elderly people since their gait tends to be slower anyway. Also, people who suffer from hemiparesis after a stroke may derive greater benefit from this type of cane since it can also be used on stairs with a very wide or low step (Figure 13-12).

Another type of ambulatory walking aid that may be used as a cane is the

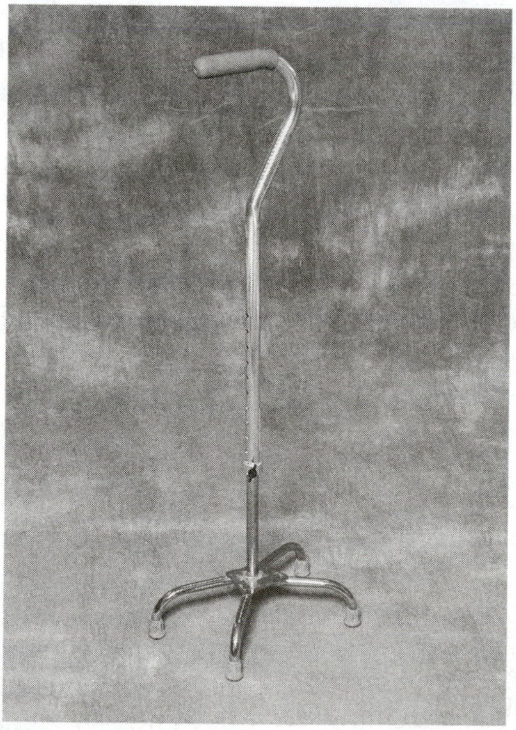

Figure 13-12 Four-point (quad) cane.

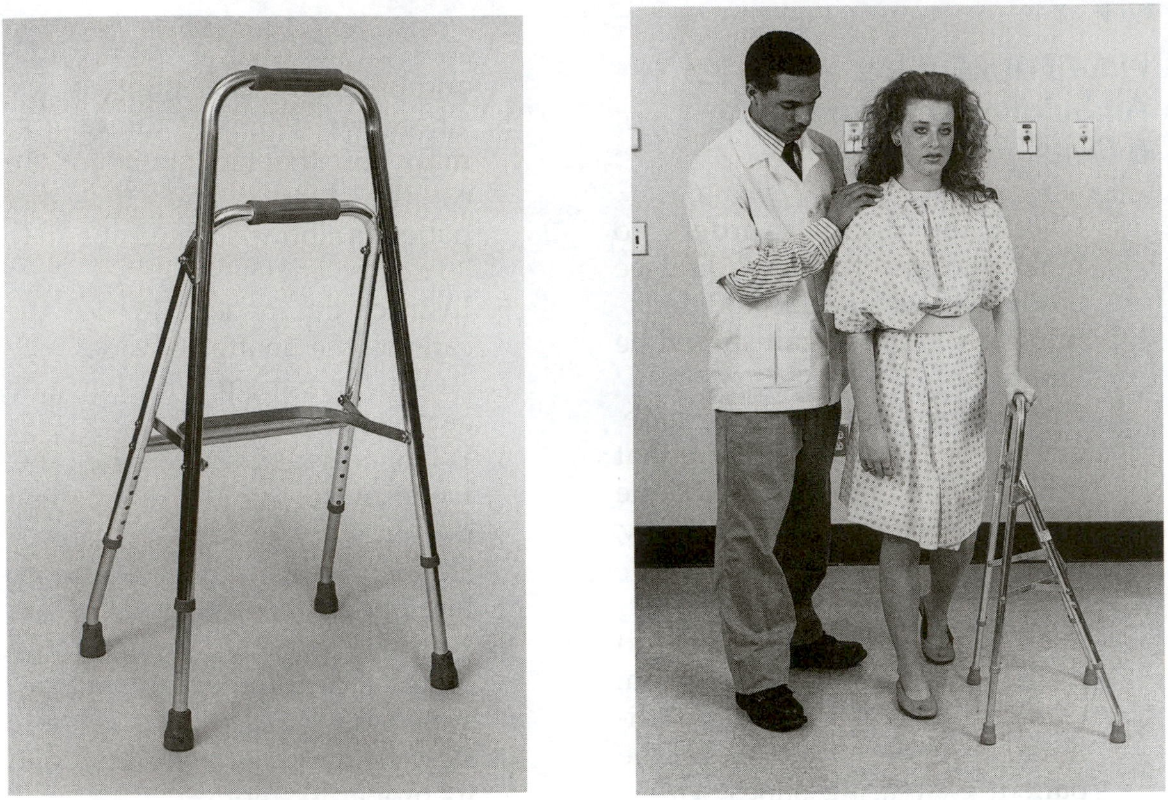

A B

Figure 13-13 (A) The hemiwalker; (B) in use.

hemiwalker (Figure 13-13A). With this device, the patient holds the walker like a cane (Figure 13-13B), on the opposite side with one hand. Increased stability is gained, but the patient can only ambulate slowly. The walker has four points of contact with the floor, but, again, a faster gait could result in a rocking motion that would eliminate the stabilizing effect. Refer to Procedure 37.

◆ GAIT TRAINING AND GAIT DEVIATIONS

Having an understanding of the normal human gait provides the physical therapy aide with a basis for the treatment and management of gait deviations that may occur in patients with impairment of the function of the lower extremities.

The human gait is the result of a series of rhythmic alternating movements of the arms and legs and the trunk. These various movements create a forward motion of the body. They mainly occur between the legs, pelvis, and spine, as well as between the arms, shoulders, and spine. A person walking at a speed to which she is accustomed swings the arm and shoulder forward as the leg of the opposite side is brought forward. The same phase relationship between the arms and legs is present in running although the extent of the movement is greater.

Each human being has a slightly different walking pattern than that of other human beings. Differences in the walking pattern are relatively small, yet the

PROCEDURE #37: Ambulating a Patient Using a Walker

1. Check the doctor's orders to obtain proper authorization for the walker.
2. Bring the walker to the patient.
3. Wash your hands.
4. Check the walker to ensure that it is in proper working condition. Make sure that the rubber suction tips are secured on all of the legs.
5. If possible, have the patient stand, using the wall or a chair to lean against. Make sure the patient is wearing sturdy shoes with heels no higher than one to one-and-one-half inches.
6. Check the height of the walker to make sure that the hand rests are level to the top of the patient's femur and that the patient's elbows are flexed at a 25- to 30-degree angle.
7. Start moving with the walker with the patient standing inside of it.
8. Instruct the patient to lift the walker and place it forward so that the back legs are even with his toes. Follow that command with instruction to transfer his weight forward slightly to the walker.
9. Tell the patient to use the walker for support and to walk into it.
10. Remain with the patient while he continues to practice using the walker. Since use of this ambulatory device may seem difficult at first, you should remain alert at all times and be ready to catch the patient if he starts to fall.
11. Determine the patient's progress and tolerance to the activity and report it to the therapist or your supervisor.
12. Replace the walker to its proper location.
13. Wash your hands.

principal pattern is the same for all of us. Generally speaking, individual particularities of the walking pattern do not mature until about the age of seven. Prior to that time, the youngster's body undergoes experimentation in order to find the best pattern for his own body build.

◆ THE NORMAL GAIT

The normal gait cycle consists of two major phases: the *stance phase* and the *swing phase*. The *gait cycle* is the time interval between successive heel strikes of the same foot. The stance phase begins when the heel of the shoe of one extremity strikes the floor and ends when the toes of the same foot leave the ground. The swing phase begins with lifting the toes off the floor and ends when the heel again strikes the ground after the leg has been brought forward.

The stance phase (Figure 13-14), consists of the following components: the *heel strike*, when the heel contacts the floor; the *midstance*, when the sole of the foot is flat on the ground and the body weight is directly over the stance-phase leg; and the *toe push-off*, when the heel of the stance-phase leg rises from the floor

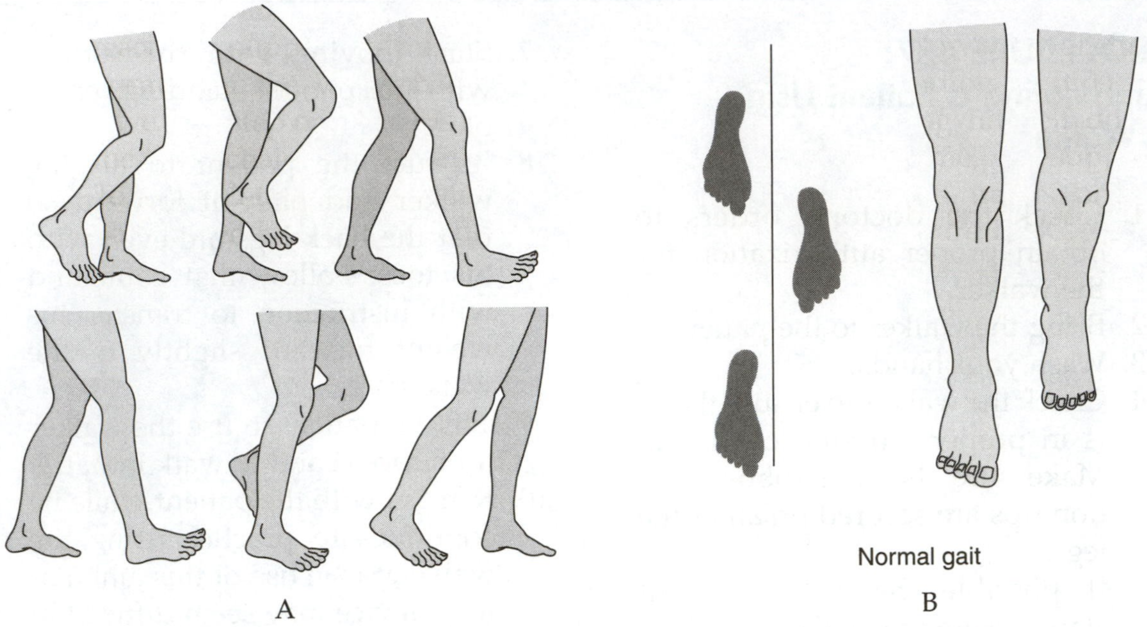

Figure 13-14 Normal gait.

and the body is pushed forward by the ball of the foot that is still in contact with the ground. At this exact moment, the body is propelled forward by the forceful action of the calf muscles and hyperextension of the hip.

The stance phase terminates and the swing phase begins when the entire foot rises from the ground. During the swing phase, the leg must be accelerated in order to get in front of the body, ready for the next heel strike. To clear the ground in the swing phase, the leg has to be shortened by the hip and knee flexion. The leg is then brought in front of the body and in front of the leg of the other side. The swing phase ends at the exact moment of the heel strike.

There is also a rotation of the pelvis around the spine in the horizontal plane (Figure 13-15). This rotation is generally six to eight degrees. The rotation comes to a complete stop at the exact time of the heel strike. As full weight is placed on the leg in the midstance phase, the rotation of the pelvis in the horizontal plane is reversed. As the leg of the other side goes into the swing phase, the pelvis on the side starts to rotate forward.

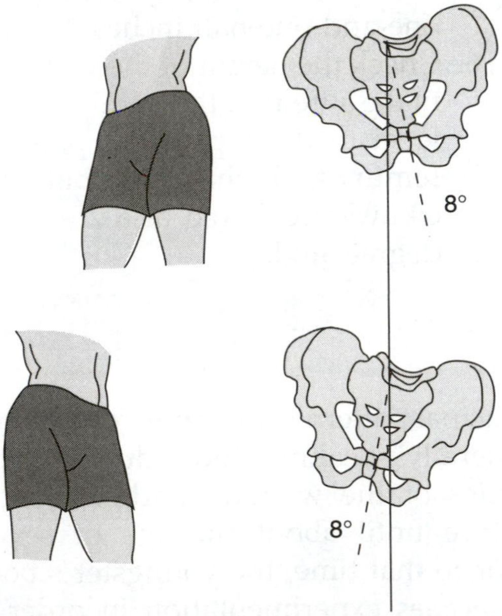

Figure 13-15 Pelvis rotation seen in a normal gait.

The shoulder girdle moves in the horizontal plane with the same degree of excursion as the pelvis, the only difference being that the shoulder moves in reverse order. On the side where the pelvis rotates forward, the shoulder rotates backward.

There is one point in the gait cycle in which there is a period of double support when the two extremities are in contact with the ground at the same time. This occurs between the toe pushoff on one side and the heel strike and midstance phase on the other. The length of time of double support is directly related to the speed of walking; as the walking speed decreases, the length of time spent in double support increases. As speed increases, double support decreases; and as the person changes from walking to running, double support disappears.

As an individual ages, a decreased elasticity of the ligaments and muscles and loss of the smoothness of the joint surfaces bring about some change in the person's gait. Changes in the neurological system also contribute to gait alterations. As aging occurs, the gait loses the appearance of being effortless. The step becomes shorter and wider. The frequent need among the elderly to use a cane oftentimes resembles holding on to a firm object during a child's first attempts at walking. Also, certain diseases of the nervous and musculoskeletal systems may cause gait deviations. One such ailment, frequently found among the elderly, is *osteoarthritis* of the hip joint, which generally results in a painful hip or *coxalgia* gait.

◆ THE COXALGIC GAIT

In osteoarthritis of the hip, the smooth head of the femur becomes uneven. The motion of the hip joint, that is, the motion of the femoral head in the acetabulum, is hampered by increased friction and becomes restricted and painful. In the swing phase, when the hip and knee have to be flexed in order to bring the leg forward and in front of the other foot, flexion of the hip joint may be painful and restricted. The hyperextension of the hip at the end of the stance phase may be diminished; hence, the step becomes shorter.

In order to enable the swing phase leg to clear the ground in a very severe restriction of the hip flexion, the stance phase leg goes up on the toes (Figure 13-16). The width of the step is reduced, depending on the degree of abduction limitation.

When there is pain in the hip joint on only one side, the weight-bearing period on the painful side tends to become shorter than on the normal side (Figure 13-17). The person tries to shorten the burden of weight on the painful hip as much as possible. Therefore, the stance phase becomes shorter and the swing phase longer on the painful side.

The components of the normal gait that may be increased in the painful-hip or coxalgic gait are flexion and extension of the lumbar spine, and, with it, the backward and forward tilting of the pelvis. The lateral shift of the trunk is also oftentimes increased, mainly with one-sided hip pain and restriction. The

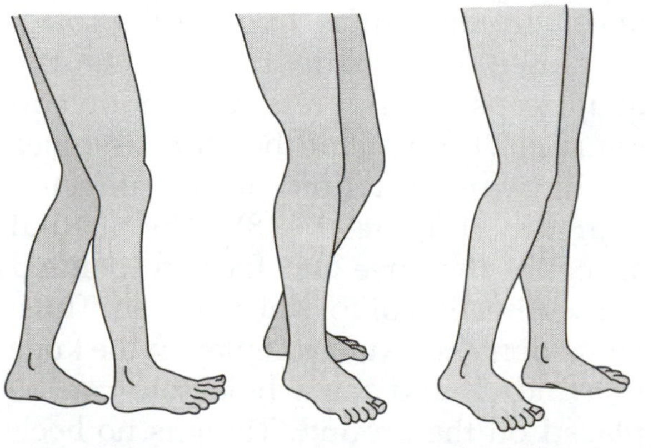

Figure 13-16 The coxalgic gait.

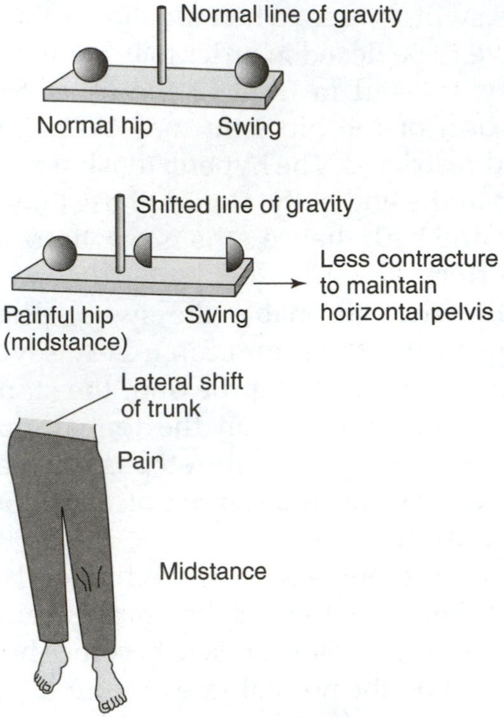

Figure 13-17 Weight shift seen in the painful-hip gait.

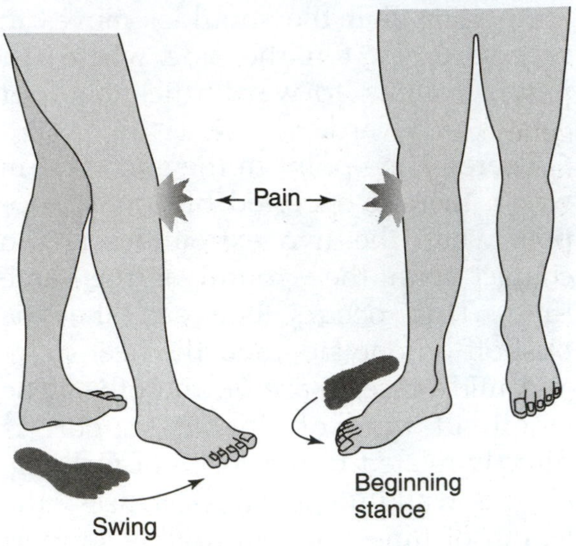

Figure 13-18 The painful-knee gait.

cadence, or measurement of rhythmic motion, may become diminished.

◆ THE PAINFUL-KNEE GAIT

A stiff or painful knee is not infrequent in old age. This may be due to osteoarthritis or other forms of joint affliction. Flexion and extension of the knee become painful. In order to protect the knee, the patient contracts the quadriceps to suppress any motion in the knee. The patient therefore assumes an outward rotation of the affected extremity (Figure 13-18). The medial aspect of the knee and foot are pointed in the direction of forward motion. Thus, all flexion and extension play in the knee is avoided, and the whole sole can be placed on the ground. There is no heel-to-toe motion, and the outward rotation of the affected limb cannot be assumed by external rotation in the hip alone. There is also some increased rotation of the pelvis.

◆ THE SACROILIAC GAIT

During normal gait, there is a motion between the sacrum and the iliac bone. Both of these bones are connected firmly with ligaments. These connections,, however, allow some motion during walking. With increased age, this motion becomes more difficult due to the increased friction and loss of elasticity of the ligaments. Persons who have any affliction or disorder within the sacroiliac joint tend to walk slightly bent forward with a decreased motion of the pelvis. The gait has the appearance of being very cautious and does not have the features of complete relaxation that a normal gait shows. Pain in the sacroiliac region generally leads to a slight shortening of the step because there is no movement between the sacrum and the iliac bone.

THE FLEXED-HIP GAIT

The flexed-hip gait (Figure 13-19) is generally assumed by persons who suffer from flexion contractures of the hip joint capsule. Hip flexion contracture is frequently found in patients who are confined for long periods of sitting because of pain in the lower extremities. The pain does not necessarily have to be caused by an affliction of the hip joint.

THE HEMIPLEGIC GAIT

This gait deviation is most often seen in elderly patients. It is usually caused by the neurological involvement seen in a stroke.

The patient has loss of motion in the arm and leg on one side. Four to six weeks after the onset of the stroke, spasticity often sets in. The loss of partial loss of motion and the onset of the spasticity generally result in a rather severe gait deviation. When the hemiplegia is on the right side, the arm swing on the right is lost. The patient has the arm dangling if it is flaccid, or in a flexed-elbow point if spasticity has set in. In order to clear the ground during the swing phase, the hip has to be abducted and the trunk flexed to the healthy side to gain some elevation of the pelvis on the affected side (Figure 13-20). At the beginning of the stance phase, there is no stride; the patient walks on the outside of her affected foot. The heel may never touch the ground, and when the affected leg is in the swing phase, the patient pushes up on the healthy side by elevating the heel. In essence, the patient actually throws the leg forward.

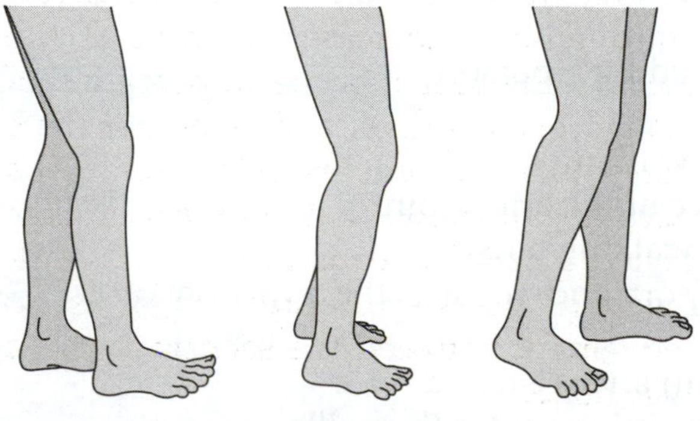

Figure 13-19 The flexed-hip gait.

THE PARKINSONIAN GAIT

One disease of the central nervous system that has a great affect on the patient's gait is Parkinson's disease. It is an ailment that may be controlled

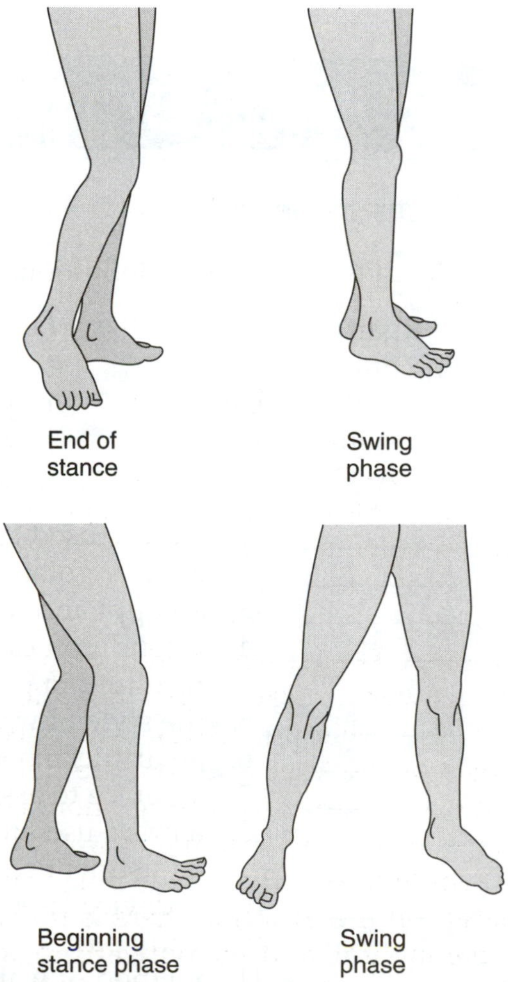

Figure 13-20 The hemiplegic gait.

through drug therapy and that occurs most often in the geriatric, or older, patient.

The patient suffering from Parkinson's disease stands with a slightly forward-flexed trunk and flexed knees and hips. Sometimes there is also a continuous tremor. The base of the step is somewhat widened. When walking, there is generally no arm swing and the trunk oscillates from the right to the left in a block. The legs are advanced rigidly and with hesitation. The swing-phase heel does not pass the toes of the other leg, which is in a stance phase. Generally speaking, the severity of the gait deviation depends upon the severity of the disease.

◆ SUMMARY

In this Chapter we discussed the purpose, preparation, and skills involved in assisting the patient to ambulate. We identified the various devices used in ambulation, as well as the individual gaits patients are generally required to learn. We also discussed the physical therapy aide's role in assisting the patient to walk up and down stairs. We completed our discussion of ambulation and gait training with a brief description and explanation of some of the more common disorders associated with dysfunctional gaits.

◆ ◆ LEARNING ACTIVITY 13-1

Terms to Define

Match the term to its definition.

a. gait
b. brace
c. crutch palsy
d. axillary bar
e. AFO
f. orthosis
g. wing screws
h. prosthesis
i. two-point gait
j. walker

_________ 1. a brace used to stabilize both the knee and the ankle joints
_________ 2. a rectangular frame used as a walking aid
_________ 3. an appliance that supports a specific portion of the body
_________ 4. a condition caused by pressure on the nerves in the axilla resulting in paralysis
_________ 5. the style of walking used by a person
_________ 6. an artificial body part
_________ 7. a device to assist with walking
_________ 8. a brace used to stabilize at the ankle joint
_________ 9. adjustment screws on walking aids
_________ 10. a device used to support and replace the function of a body part
_________ 11. method of walking with an assistive device
_________ 12. upper piece of a crutch fitting under the axilla

◆ ◆ LEARNING ACTIVITY 13-2

Questions to Answer

Answer the following questions:

1. What materials are used to make an orthosis?
2. What may happen if the patient rests on the axillary pads?
3. What is the number one problem encountered when training patients to use equipment?
4. When is the swing-through gait used?
5. What is the primary concern of the therapist when selecting equipment for a patient?
6. List the goals of using the proper physical therapy equipment.
7. How are crutches measured for the patient?
8. On which side should the patient carry the cane?
9. What criteria are considered before the therapist orders equipment for the patient?
10. Which part of the body is critical for the performance of most ADL activities?
11. What key motions of the upper extremities are most important for ADL?
12. What motions of the lower extremities are important for standing and walking?
13. What factors help patients accept and use their therapeutic equipment?
14. Name three types of crutches.
15. A good wheelchair provides two things for a patient. Name these.
16. When is it best to move backwards with a patient in a wheelchair?
17. Describe briefly three pregait-training activities.
18. What must the patient be able to do in order to use a walker?
19. How is a walker adjusted?
20. What is a four-point gait?
21. Describe the procedure for getting into a chair with crutches.
22. What is the rule for going up and down stairs with crutches?

◆ ◆ LEARNING ACTIVITY 13-3

Understanding the Correct Use of Ambulation Equipment

Answer the following questions.

1. When is an ambulatory device used to assist a patient?
2. What is the name of an ambulation device that has metal bars and is attached to a frame that is bolted to the floor?
3. Draw a picture of a walker
4. What is a walker constructed of?
5. Identify three types of crutches.
6. What type of crutch is used by a patient diagnosed with arthritis?
7. Identify at least two types of canes.

REVIEW QUESTIONS

1. The term __________ means to walk.
2. The PTA may use __________ __________ to make walking easier for the patient.
3. The goal of the physical therapy team member is to __________ and __________ proper walking and gait movement to the patient.
4. The type of assistive device used by a patient depends greatly upon her __________.
5. The gait used with crutches that is closest to that of the natural rhythm of walking is called __________ gait.
6. The human gait is a result of __________ alternating movements of the __________, __________, and __________.
7. Generally speaking, walking patterns do not mature until about the age of __________.
8. In the __________-__________ gait, the patient contracts the quadriceps in order to suppress any motion in the knees.
9. The gait deviation most frequently seen in elderly patients, usually caused by neurological involvement as seen in a stroke, is the __________ gait.
10. __________ __________ is almost always accompanied by an abnormal gait and a continuous tremor.

14

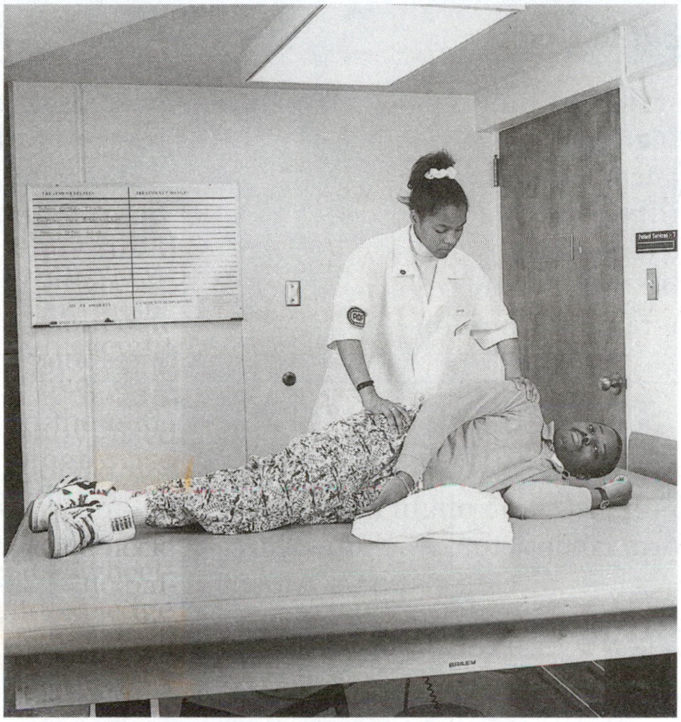

Therapeutic Exercises

OBJECTIVES

Upon completion of this chapter, you should be able to:

1. State the ultimate purpose of any therapeutic exercise program.
2. Discuss the physical therapy aide's role in assisting the patient with therapeutic exercises.
3. Describe the purpose of range-of-motion exercises and explain the difference between passive and active range of motion.
4. Briefly discuss how muscle strength is graded.
5. Compare the difference between skill and coordination exercises.
6. Explain anatomical planes of motion.
7. Briefly discuss diagonal patterns of motion.
8. Identify the seven range-of-motion exercises used on the lower extremities and the thirteen range-of-motion exercises used on the upper extremities.

KEY TERMS

Active range of motion
Coordination
Endurance
Flexibility
Isometric exercise
Mobility
Passive range-of-motion
Progressive resistive
Range-of-motion
Relaxation
Sensory input
Skill
Strength
Therapeutic

As a physical therapy aide, one of the more difficult tasks you might be expected to perform is the actual teaching of an exercise program to your patients. Most of the time, it does not suffice to show the patient just once how to do the exercises. You may have to reemphasize certain very specific details, correct the patient's performance frequently, and adjust to his physical condition at a particular time. Much effort and dedication on the part of the physical therapist and the aide are often necessary in order to improve the patient's performance. In order to assist the patient with his exercise program, you must first have a basic understanding of the importance placed on it.

The ultimate goal of any **therapeutic** exercise program is its ability to assist the patient in achieving symptom-free movement and function. Such a goal can only be met by establishing the positive effects the program has on the patient. These effects include the benefits derived for the patient's development, improvement, and restoration, or maintenance of normal **strength, endurance, mobility** and **flexibility, relaxation, coordination,** and skill.

In order to effectively administer therapeutic exercise to the patient, both the therapist and the aide must know the basic principles and effects of the treatment. While the therapist is the individual responsible for conducting the functional evaluation of a patient prior to beginning the exercise program, it is generally the aide who assists the patient in carrying the exercise program out. While each patient reacts differently to an exercise program and needs individual consideration in the program outline, there are some well-established physiological principles that should always be followed. Let's take a look at some of the most important principles.

First, let's note that the purpose and goal of the exercise program must be very clearly defined for the patient. For example, it has to be decided whether the patient's general physical condition should be improved or whether the range of motion of a specific joint should be increased or a specific muscle be strengthened. The program has to be designed accordingly.

Secondly, the amount of stress that the exercise program places on the patient in general or on a specific joint or muscle must be determined according to the patient's tolerance and the strength of the specific muscle or the condition of the joint.

A third point is that when an exercise program is designed, the type of stress imposed by the exercises should be relevant to the function that is to be enhanced. For example, extending the knee against resistance and gravity will strengthen the quadriceps muscle. There should always be a steady attempt, day by day or week by week, to perform better. In other words, the tolerance of the patient or the strength of the muscle or the range of joint motion should constantly be challenged, but always at a steady pace. If a person only performs the activity he is accustomed to, that person will never increase his strength, tolerance, or skill.

A fourth point to note is that the program should always adhere to well-established physiological principles; that is, intensity and duration of the stress imposed should increase gradually. In order to achieve an increase in strength, tolerance, or endurance, the exercise program has to be performed, if not daily, at least frequently and at regular intervals.

The final physiological principle deals with never allowing your patient to become exhausted. If the patient still feels fatigued the day following the exercise program, it probably means that the program was too strenuous for her or she has to be given additional rest. The same applies to the specific muscle or joint that was exposed to the exercise stress.

Should the muscle become painful or weaker or the joint more swollen and painful the day following the exercises, the program must be eased or decreased temporarily.

Improvement is not entirely a physiological function; psychological factors also play a key role in the patient's exercise program. Many of the problems your patients may be facing are long-lasting and are therefore more apt to be the cause of discouragement. Patients entrusted to your care will need much encouragement. Also remember that a substantial number of patients you will encounter may have ailments that cannot be entirely cured; however, the patient's functioning nearly always can be improved. The patient has to be made aware of this by his or her physician. This potential for improvement only, and not a complete cure, may sometimes hinder the patient's motivation to perform the prescribed program.

◆ FORMS OF EXERCISE

There are various forms of exercises that may be used according to the effect they are designed to achieve. These generally include exercises for range of motion of a joint, exercises to increase strength, and exercises to improve skill or coordination.

Range-of-Motion Exercises

When a joint is not being regularly moved, it may become stiff and the **range-of-motion** is, therefore, decreased. You may have noticed the desire to stretch after you have been lying in one position for a long period of time. With advancing age, tightness and stiffness of the joints sets in more readily, and it becomes more difficult to restore normal range of motion. If a patient is unable to move one arm or leg after a stroke because no impulses are able to travel from the brain to the peripheral motor nerves, the joint's range of motion decreases and the tissue around the joint contracts and shortens. In the case of a temporary or permanent paralysis, the treating person has to move the patient's limb through various ranges of motion. In this instance, one speaks of **passive range-of-motion** exercises. If the patient is able to move the limb by active muscle contraction, we say the exercises are

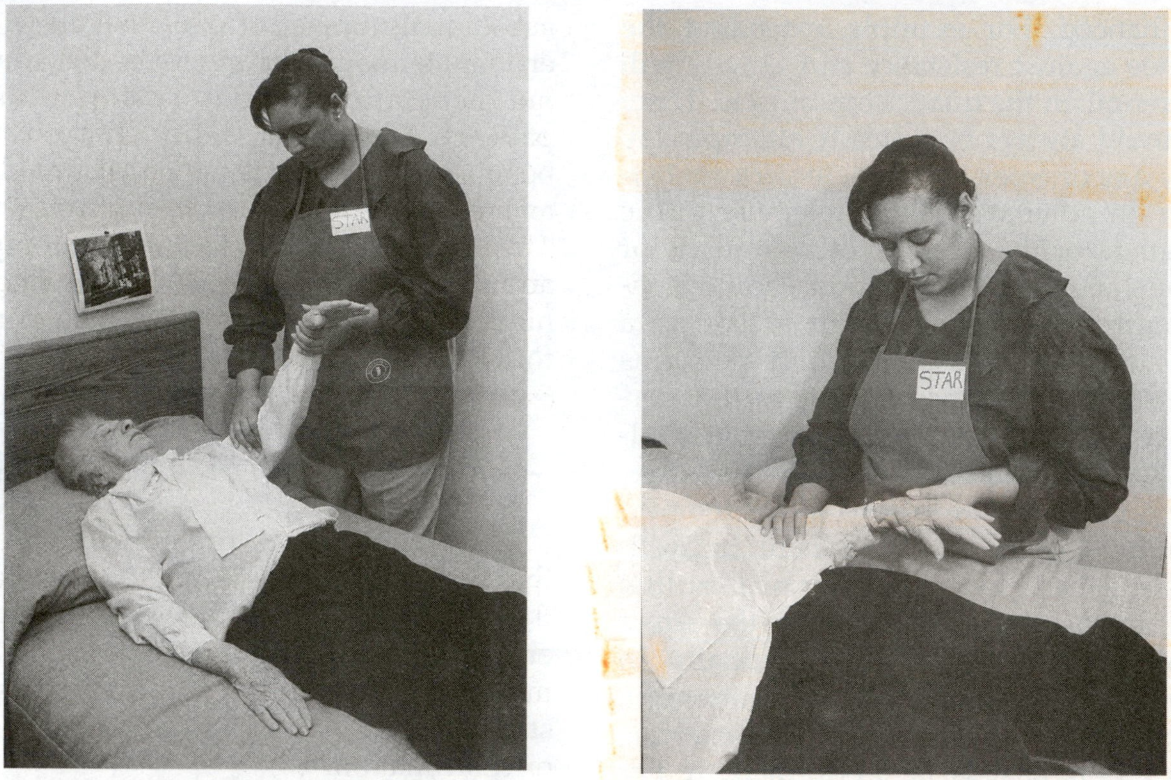

A

B

Figure 14-1 Exercising the shoulder joint.

active range-of-motion.

Range-of-motion exercises can be performed by a physical therapy aide after she has been instructed how to perform them by a physical therapist. Whenever these exercises are to be performed, great care must always be taken not to damage or further contract the involved joints. It is easier to prevent contractures than to restore normal range of motion after the contracture has occurred (Figure 14-1).

Exercises to Increase Strength

Whenever a muscle or a group of muscles are forced into inactivity, the strength of those muscles will gradually fade away. If total inactivity is forced upon a patient, the rate of decrease in muscle strength is approximately 7.5 percent per day.

Muscles that are forced into inactivity become flabby and eventually decrease in size. In case the peripheral nerve or the lower motor neuron is damaged and the muscle cannot contract at all for a long period of time, the muscle fibers which cannot contract are replaced by nonfunctional fibrous tissue. In such instances, the muscle cannot be made stronger.

Progressive resistive exercises are designed to increase the strength of the muscles. The principle is that of repetition of maximal contraction against resistance, with the resistance gradually increasing (Figure 14-2).

Another form of exercise that helps to maintain or, perhaps, even improve the strength of a muscle is called **isometric exercises.** In this type of exercise, the muscle is contracted without bringing about any joint motion. Many claims

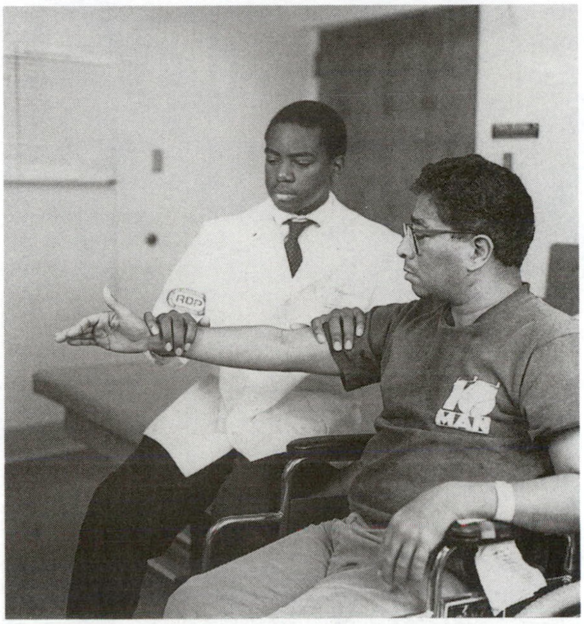

Figure 14-2 Example of resisted exercise for shoulder flexion.

have been made about this form of isometric contraction. It is said that when these exercises are performed several times a day, muscle strength does increase.

The most important value of isometric exercise is that it can be used when active motion in the joint is not possible or desirable. In addition, isometric exercises may also be used to help facilitate active exercises. Out of fear of causing pain in an inflamed joint, the patient often thinks he is unable to contract a muscle. The use of isometric exercises allows you to show the patient that it is still possible to do the exercises without feeling the pain.

◆ MEASURING MUSCLE STRENGTH

There are a great many methods for measuring the strength of a muscle. It can be done manually or with measuring devices. Manual muscle testing is the more widely used method since all it requires is the examiner's knowledge of the tested muscle's origin and insertion and the direction of its maximal force upon the joint. Usually manual muscle testing is performed by an experienced physical therapist, but this skill can also be acquired by the physical therapy aide.

The most widely used grading of muscle strength in manual muscle testing is as follows:

Normal:	complete range of motion against gravity with full resistance
Good:	complete range of motion against gravity with some resistance
Fair:	complete range of motion against gravity
Poor:	complete range of motion with gravity eliminated
Trace:	evidence of slight contractility; no joint motion
Zero:	no evidence of contractility

Grading becomes very difficult if the patient has an upper motor contracture or suffers from any spasticity or rigidity. No adequate testing can be performed when contraction against resistance or even active motion causes pain.

◆ SKILL OR COORDINATION EXERCISES

Each and every skilled motion or movement we use depends upon the intact functioning of various components or parts of our nervous system. The structures that conduct the sensory input, the structures in the brain that integrate the many stimuli to the appropriate organ, and the skeletal muscle fibers all have to be intact. When we speak of improvement of skill, coordination, and balance, what we are really saying is that we are increasing the control that the individual has over various muscle contractions. In order to achieve a high degree of control over the various muscle groups, it takes many years of experience and practice. A young child, for example, has the necessary reflexes, nerve structures, and muscles to perform all the skills adults can perform easily and well; yet the child's movements appear clumsy. The child's gait, or walk, is still broad-based, and therefore, the child tends to fall more frequently than does the adult. When a high degree of precision in muscle control is attained, even strenuous motions appear very easy.

When disease causes movement disorders, there is generally some loss of skill and coordination. Even when a patient loses a limb, such as a leg, there is usually some problem with balance. An artificial limb, regardless of how sophisticated and well-fitting it may be always lacks one component—the **sensory input.**

Various exercise programs and equipment are available in print for specific diseases (Figure 14-3). As with progressive resistive exercise programs, exercises to increase control of muscle action must also be performed. The challenge to improve muscle control has to be steadily increased; otherwise, no improvement can be achieved and the patient stays at the same level of function.

The learning of skills, or, in other words, the acquisition of a better and more precise control of muscle action and muscle coordination, needs constant reinforcement by the person treating the physically limited patient. Control of muscle action can be lost by long-standing disease or after a serious illness. In such instances, skill nearly to the same level as previously achieved can be regained with training. It is always easier to retain for previously acquired skills than to learn new ones.

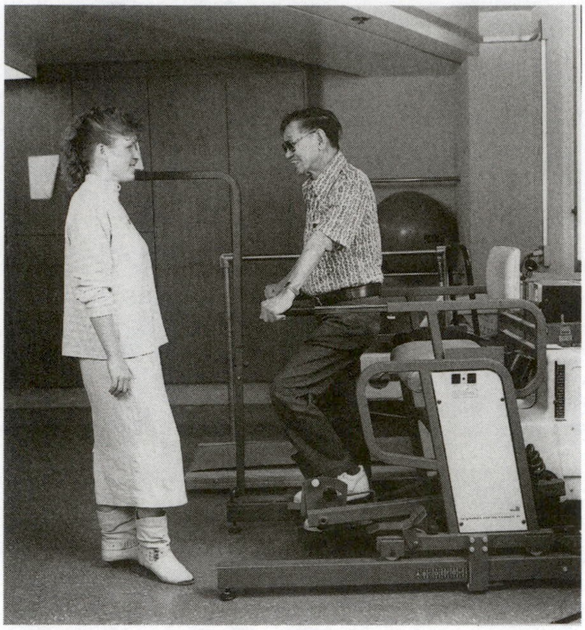

Figure 14-3 Example of using therapeutic exercise equipment.

◆ RANGE-OF-MOTION EXERCISES

Range-of-motion exercises involve performing movements of each joint and muscle through the use of available range of motion. The execution of these exercises prevent the patient from developing contractures, muscle shortening and tightness or adhesions in capsules, ligaments, and tendons that could eventually limit mobility. Range of motion exercises involve two principles. First, the joint is ranged with respect only to its actual movement, and second, it must be ranged so that the length of the muscles actually cross the joint. It should also be noted that range of motion exercises provide the patient with sensory stimulation.

There are two types of range-of-motion exercises. The first, called passive range of motion, is generally used when the patient is unable to move a body part or when movement by the patient produces increased spasticity or other undesirable muscle tone, pain, or excessive cardiopulmonary stress. The second type of range-of-motion exercises are referred to as active range of motion. These exercises may be performed when the patient needs some help due to weakness, pain, cardiopulmonary problems, or decreased muscle tone. Unlike the passive exercises, active range of motion is usually performed independently by the patient, generally with the aide or therapist supervising in order to ensure proper performance of the exercises.

Whenever you are required to perform range of motion, you should always make sure that the body part you are working with is gently but firmly supported. The placement of your hand should allow movement of the body part through the full range with minimal hand repositioning. You should also support all segments distal to the joint at which the motion is to occur. Movements should be slow to moderate through all planes of motion available in the joint.

When performing range-of-motion exercises, remember that each joint should be moved through its full range for both the joint motion and the muscle length. When moving a joint through its full range of motion, multijoint muscles, or muscles that stretch over more than one joint, must not be lengthened across all the joints over which they act.

You should always remember that maximum range is generally achieved when the body part cannot be moved further due to the restriction of tissues or bone or the patient complains of pain. When pain is limiting the range of motion, it is time to stop the exercises.

In some cases, involuntary muscle contractions may occur and interfere with range-of-motion exercises. This generally happens when a patient involuntarily contracts muscles in order to avoid pain. Spasticity may also be felt as gradually increasing resistance to movement occurs. This is followed by a sudden reduction of tone. Movement through the remaining range of motion is then possible. If spasticity does occur, slow maintained movement will usually allow movement through the full range of motion.

◆ ANATOMICAL PLANES OF MOTION

All motions of the body are described in terms of starting from the anatomical position, that is, the position in which a person is standing upright, eyes looking straight ahead, arms at the sides with the palms facing forward, and the feet approximately four inches apart at the heels, with the toes pointing forward (Figure 14-4). In this position, three planes are seen. The first, called the *sagittal* plane, divides the body into two portions through a longitudinal axis of the trunk. The *midsagittal plane* is an imaginary line that divides the body through an anterior-posterior midaxis, thereby dividing it into equal right and left halves. Hence, all motions involving flexion and extension, occur in the sagittal plane.

The second plane is called the *frontal plane.* It divides the body into front and back portions. All motions involving abduction and adduction occur in the frontal plane.

The third and final plane defined in the anatomical position is called the *transverse plane.* It divides the body into

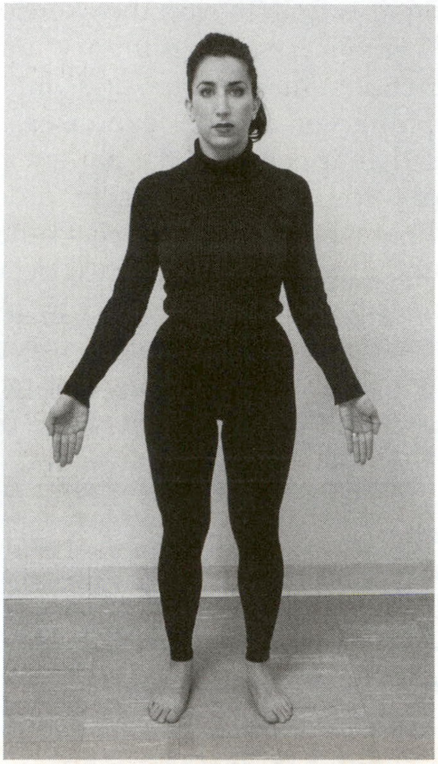

Figure 14-4 The anatomical position.

upper and lower portions and all movements involving rotation occur here.

DIAGONAL PATTERNS OF MOTION

There are two basic diagonal patterns for movements of the extremities, and each of these patterns may be modified by varying the position or movement of the elbow or knee, thereby providing the patient with the ability to perform both joint range of motion and muscular range-of-motion exercises. When combining components of motion are performed, the part may not be taken through as full of a range as when anatomical planes of motion are used. However, the mobility necessary for function is maintained.

RANGE-OF-MOTION EXERCISES: LOWER EXTREMITIES

The following range-of-motion exercises are generally performed on patients who experience diseases or injuries affecting the lower extremities. Refer to Procedure 38.

1. **Body segment:** **Hip and knee** (Figure 14-5)
   Joints being ranged: Hip and knee
   Motion being used: Extension and flexion
   Placement of hands: Heel and behind knee

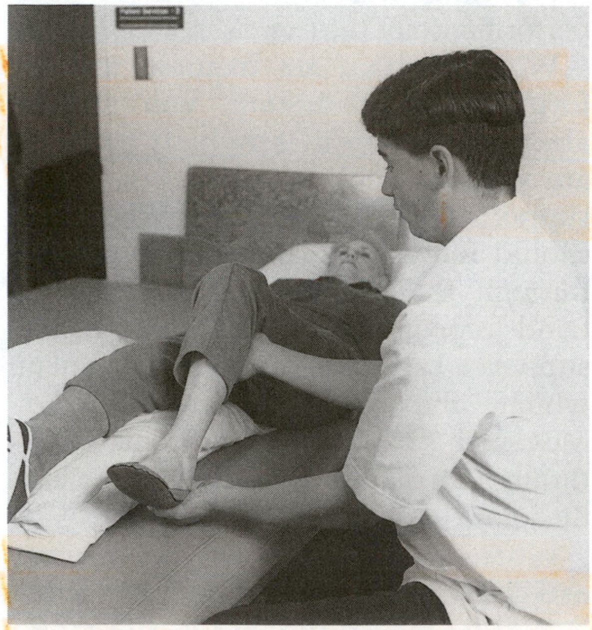

Figure 14-5 Hip and knee flexion and extension.

2. **Body segment:** **Hip** (Figure 14-6)
   Joints being ranged: Hip
   Motion being used: Extension
   Placement of hands: One on the pelvis for stabilization; the other with the forearm, used to support the patient's lower extremity in anatomical position

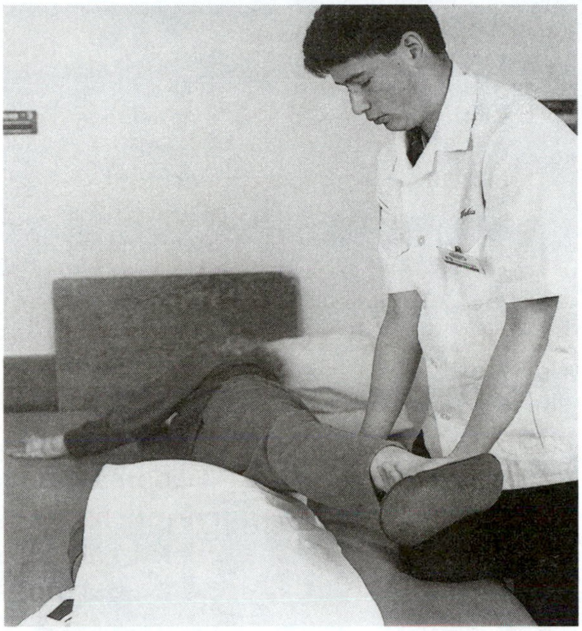

Figure 14-6 Hip extension.

3. **Body segment:** **Hip** (Figure 14-7)
   Joints being ranged: Hip
   Motion being used: Abduction and adduction
   Placement of hands: Heel and behind knee

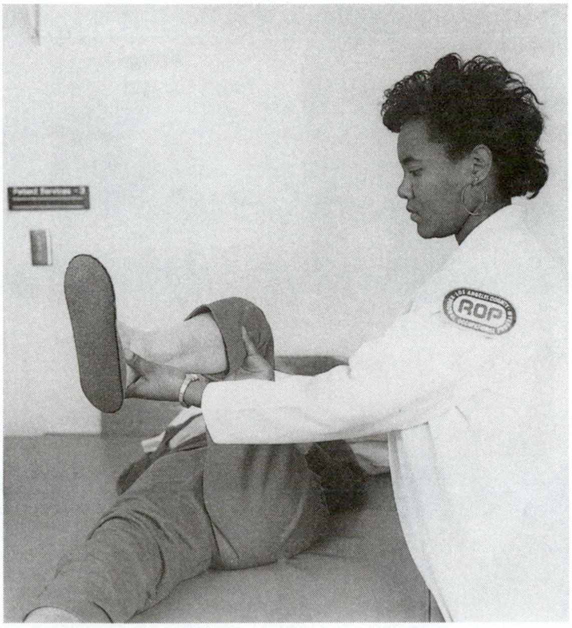

Figure 14-7 Hip abduction and adduction.

4. **Body segment:** **Hip** (Figure 14-8)
   Joints being ranged: Hip
   Motion being used: Internal and external rotation; hip and knee flexed at 90-degree angle
   Placement of hands: Heel and behind knee

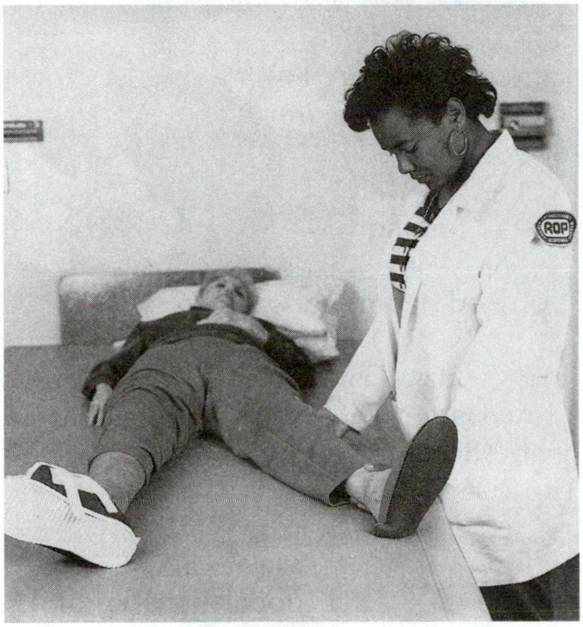

Figure 14-8 Hip rotation.

5. **Body segment:** **Ankle** (Figure 14-9)
   Joint being ranged: Ankle
   Motion being used: Plantar flexion and dorsiflexion
   Placement of hands: Heel and dorsum of foot for plantar flexion; heel and lower leg for dorsiflexion

6. **Body segment:** **Foot** (Figure 14-9)
   Joint being ranged: Foot
   Motion being used: Inversion and eversion
   Placement of hands: One hand stabilizes the lower leg and the other grasps the forefoot

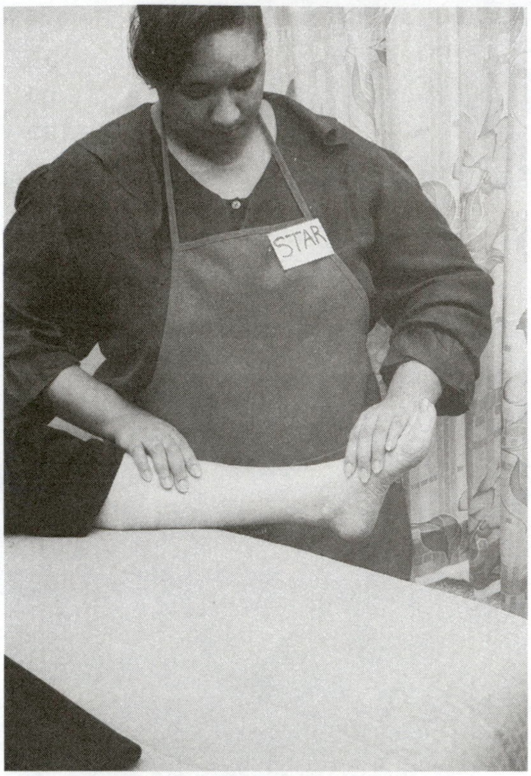

A

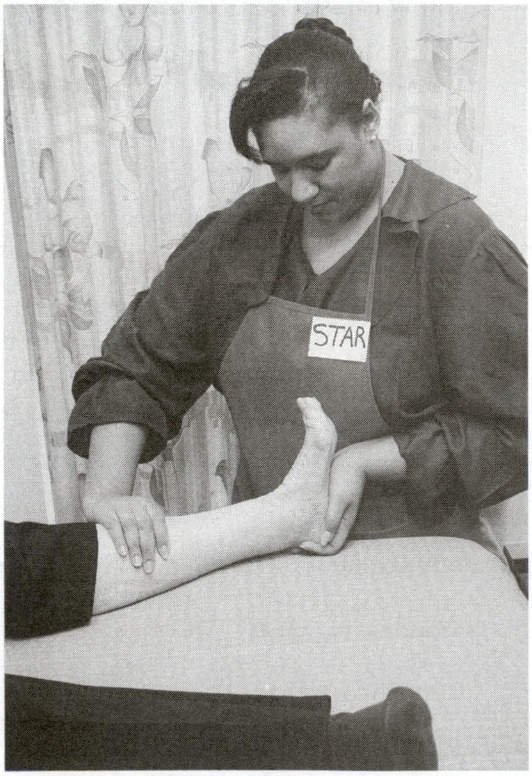

B

Figure 14-9 Exercising the ankle and foot.

7. **Body segment:** **Toes** (Figures 14-10A, B, C, and D)

   Joint being ranged: Toes

   Motion being used: Extension and flexion

   Placement of hands: One hand stabilizes the lower leg and the other grasps the toes

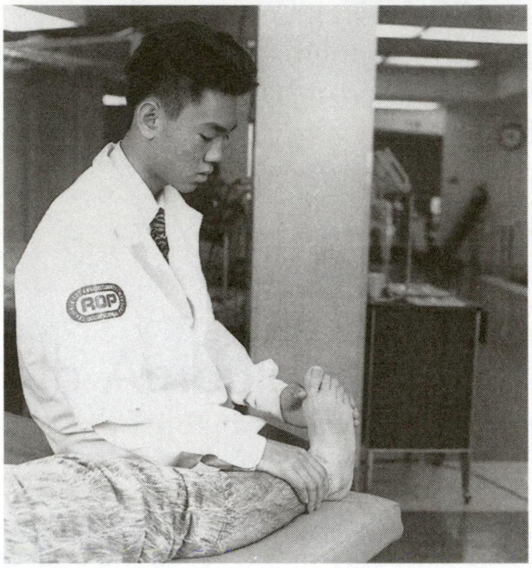

A

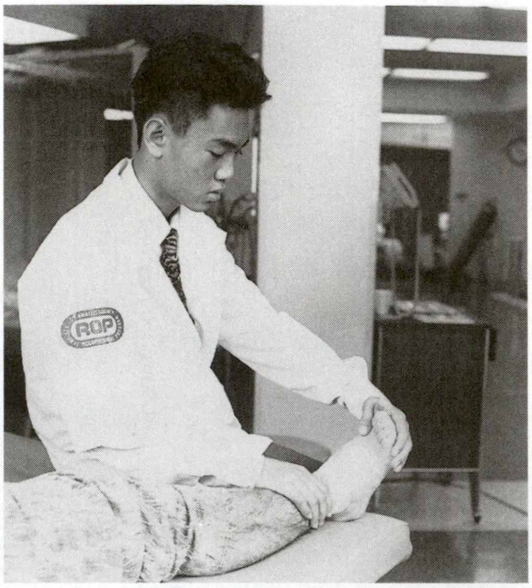

B

Figure 14-10 (A) Foot inversion; and (B) eversion; (C) toe extension; and (D) flexion.

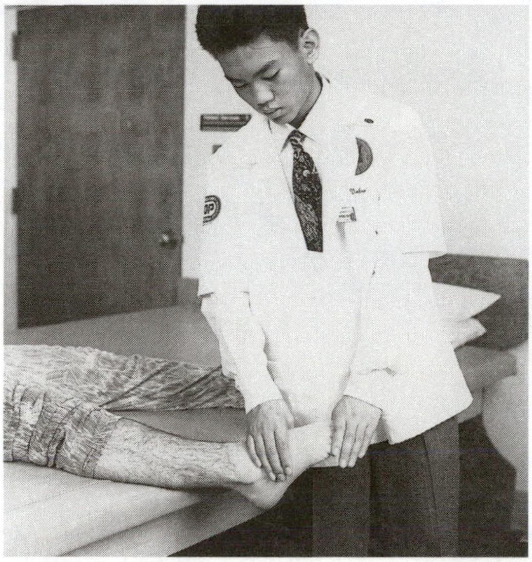

C

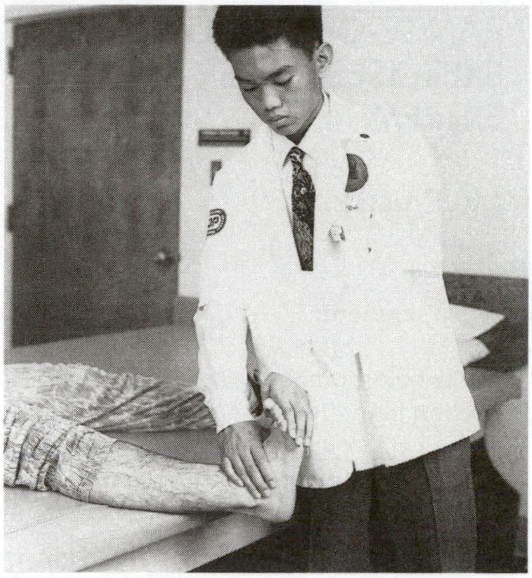

D

Figure 14-10 (A) Foot inversion; and (B) eversion; (C) toe extension; and (D) flexion (continued).

PROCEDURE #38
Performing Passive Range of Motion on the Lower Extremities

1. Wash your hands, identify the patient, and provide for privacy.
2. Explain the procedure to the patient.
3. Adjust the patient's clothing or top covers and only allow for exposure of the affected area.
4. Supporting the knee and ankle, move the entire leg away from the body center (abduction) and toward the body (adduction).
5. Turn to face the bed. Supporting the knee in a bent position (flexion), raise the knee toward the pelvis (hip flexion). Straighten the knee (extension) as you lower the leg to the bed.
6. Supporting the leg at the knee and ankle, roll the leg in a circular fashion away from body (lateral hip rotation). Continuing to support the leg, roll the leg in the same fashion toward the body (medial hip rotation).
7. Grasp the patient's toes and support the ankle. Bring the toes toward the knee (dorsiflexion). Then point the toes toward the foot of the table (plantar flexion).
8. Gently turn the patient's foot inward (inversion) and outward (eversion).
9. Place your fingers over the patient's toes. Bend the toes away from the second toe (abduction) and then toward the second toe (adduction).
10. Cover the leg with clothing or a top cover and move to the opposite side.
11. Move the patient close to you and repeat steps 4 through 9.

◆ RANGE-OF-MOTION EXERCISES: UPPER EXTREMITIES

Refer to Procedure 39.

1. **Body segment:** **Scapulo-thoracic** (Figure 14-11)
   Joints being ranged: Scapulo-thoracic
   Motion being used: Protraction and retraction
   Placement of hands: One hand placed over the acromion and the other placed behind the scapula

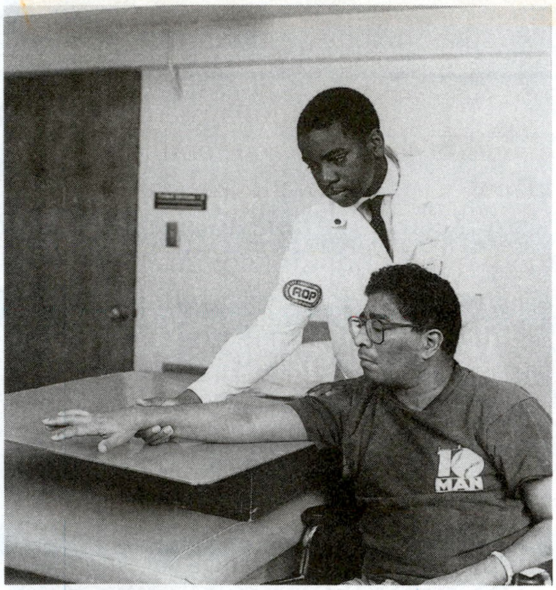

Figure 14-11 Scapulo-thoracic protraction and retraction.

2. **Body segment:** **Shoulder** (Figure 14-12)
   Joints being ranged: Shoulder
   Motion being used: Flexion
   Placement of hands: One hand supports the wrist and hand while the other supports the upper arm

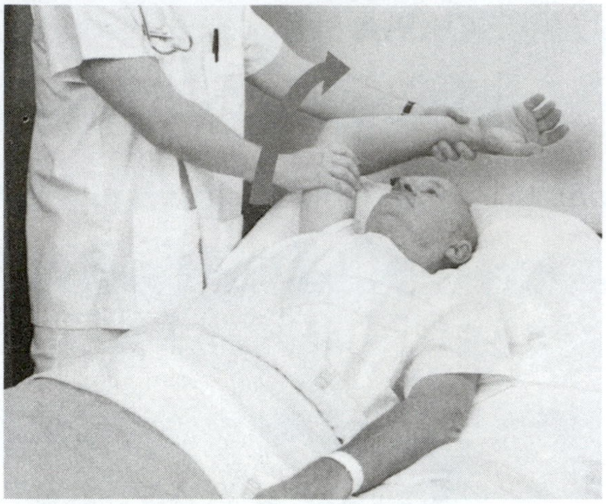

Figure 14-12 Shoulder flexion. With shoulder in abduction, flex elbow and raise entire arm over head.

3. **Body segment:** **Shoulder, elbow and forearm** (see Figure 14-13)
   Joints being ranged: Shoulder and elbow
   Motion being used: Shoulder and elbow extension with pronation; shoulder and elbow flexion with supination

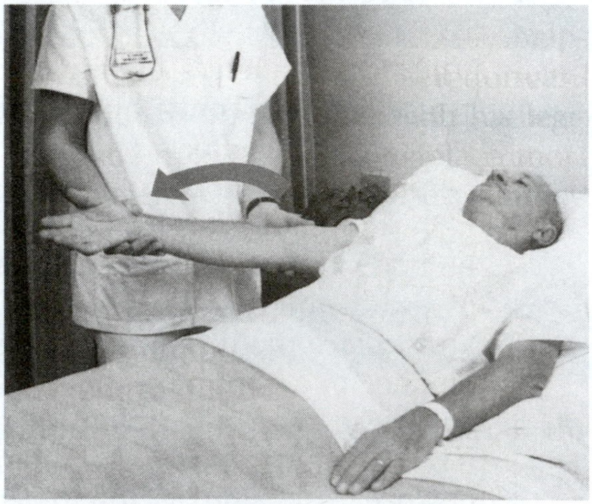

Figure 14-13A Elbow exersion and flexion. Supporting the upper arm and wrist, straighten elbow.

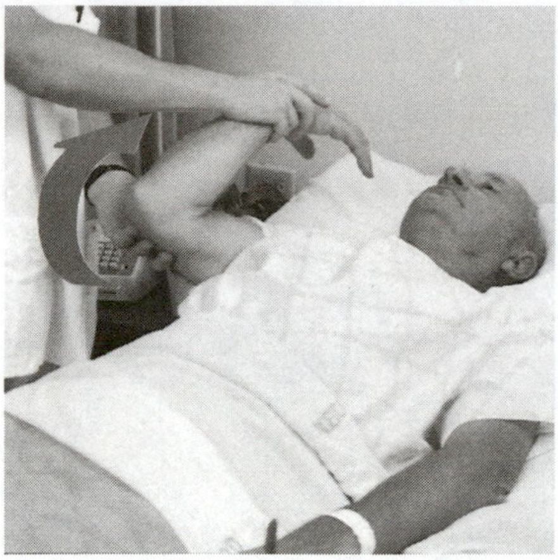

Figure 14-13B Then bring lower arm toward upper arm.

Placement of hands: One hand supports the wrist and hand while the other supports the upper arm; the aide's left hand should support the patient's right wrist and hand

4. **Body segment:** **Shoulder** (Figure 14-14)
   Joints being ranged: Shoulder
   Motion being used: Abduction
   Placement of hands: One hand stabilizes the shoulder girdle while the other hand and forearm

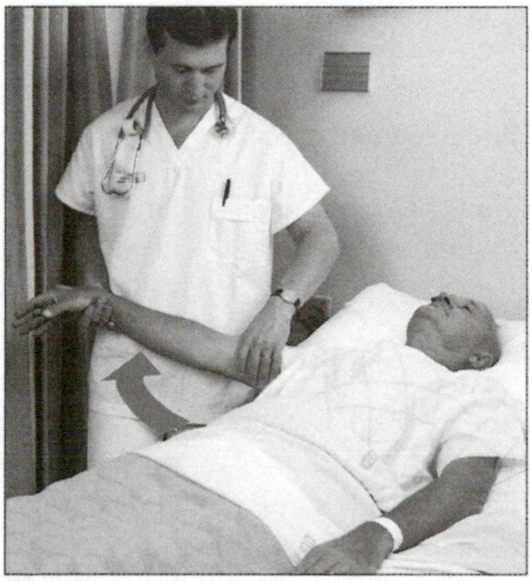

Figure 14-14 Shoulder abduction.

supports the patient's upper extremity

5. **Body segment:** **Shoulder** (Figure 14-15)
   Joints being ranged: Shoulder
   Motion being used: Adduction and flexion; the shoulder is abducted 90-degrees while the elbow is flexed to 90 degrees
   Placement of hands: One hand stabilizes the shoulder girdle while the other grasps the fore-arm

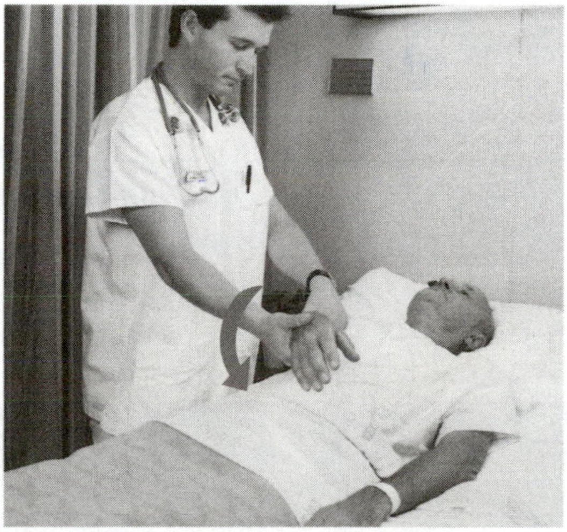

Figure 14-15 Shoulder adduction.

6. **Body segment:** **Shoulder** (Figure 14-16)
   Joints being ranged: Shoulder
   Motion being used: Internal rotation; the shoulder is abducted 90-degrees while the elbow is flexed to 90 degrees
   Placement of hands: One hand stabilizes the shoulder girdle while the other grasps the patient's forearm

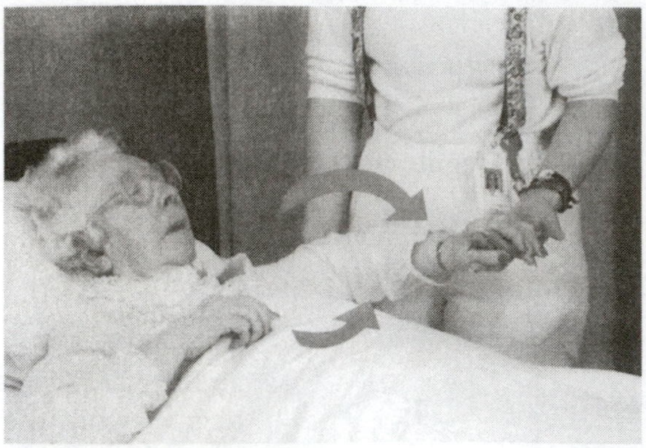

Figure 14-16 Shoulder internal rotation.

7. **Body segment:** **Shoulder** (Figure 14-17)
   Joints being ranged: Shoulder
   Motion being used: External rotation; the shoulder is abducted 90 degrees while the elbow is flexed 90-degrees
   Placement of hands: One hand stabilizes the shoulder girdle while the other grasps the patient's forearm

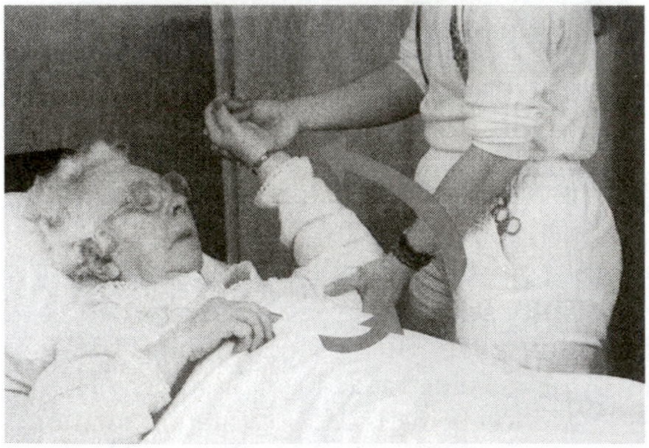

Figure 14-17 Shoulder external rotation.

8. **Body segment:** **Wrist** (Figure 14-18)
   Joints being ranged: Wrist
   Motion being used: Flexion and extension; the elbow is flexed, allowing the fingers to be moved
   Placement of hands: One hand stabilizes the forearm while the other grasps the patient's hand

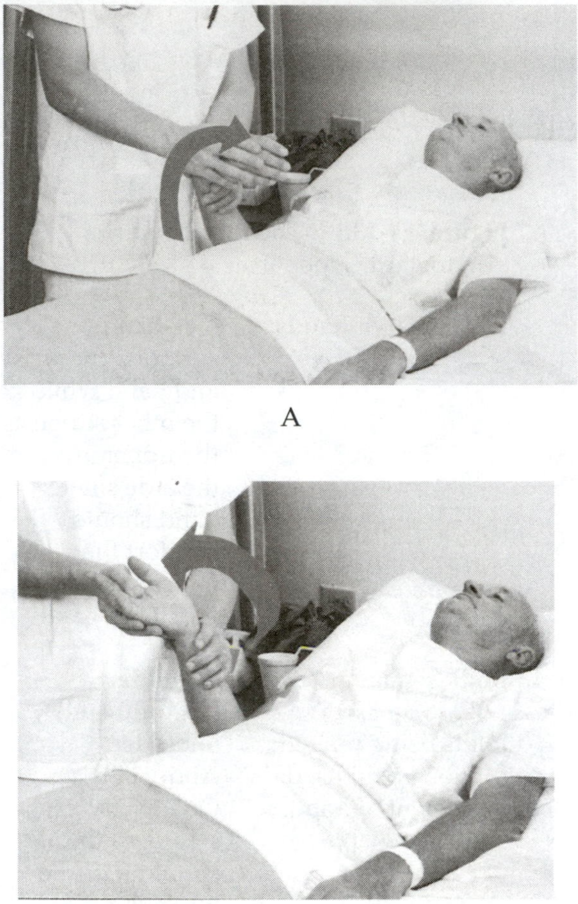

A

B

Figure 14-18 Wrist flexion and extension.

9. **Body segment:** **Fingers** (Figure 14-19)
   Joints being ranged: Fingers
   Motion being used: Flexion and extension; the wrist is in the anatomical position allowing the elbow to be flexed 90 degrees
   Placement of hands: One hand stabilizes the forearm while the other grasps the fingers

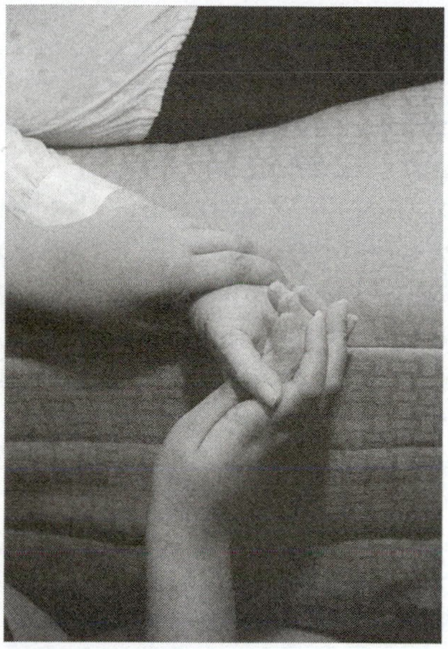

A

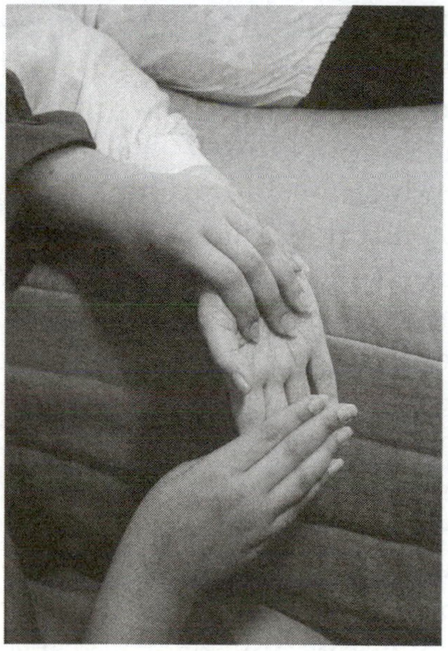

B

Figure 14-19 Fingers flexion and extension.

10. Body segment:	**Wrist and fingers** (Figure 14-20)
Joints being ranged:	Wrist and fingers
Motion being used:	Wrist extension with finger extension; wrist flexion with finger flexion; the elbow is extended
Placement of hands:	One hand grasps the wrist while the other grasps the fingers

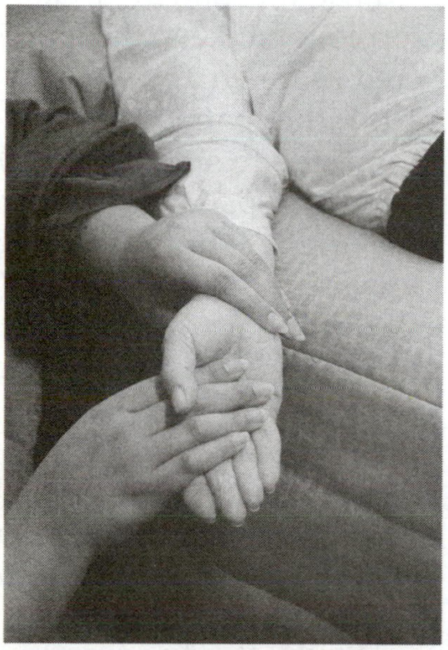

A

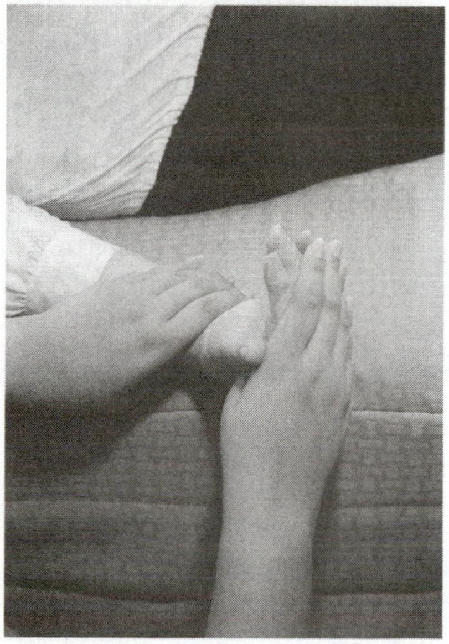

B

Figure 14-20 Wrist and fingers extension and flexion.

PROCEDURE 39: Performing Passive Range of Motion on the Upper Extremities

1. Wash your hands, identify the patient, and provide for privacy.
2. Explain the procedure to the patient.
3. Position the patient on his back close to you.
4. Adjust the patient's clothing or top cover to keep the patient covered as much as possible.
5. Turn the patient's head gently from side to side (rotation).
6. Bend the patient's head toward the right shoulder and then toward the left shoulder (lateral flexion).
7. Bring the chin toward the chest (flexion).
8. Place a pillow under the shoulders and gently support the head in a backward tilt (hyperextension). Return to the straight position (extension). Adjust the pillow under the head and shoulders.
9. Supporting the elbow and wrist, exercise the shoulder joint by bringing the entire arm out at a right angle to the body (horizontal abduction) and returning the arm to a position parallel to the body (horizontal adduction).
10. With the arm parallel to the body, roll the entire arm toward the body (internal rotation of the shoulder). Maintaining the parallel position, roll the entire arm away from the body (external rotation of the shoulder).
11. With the shoulder in abduction, flex the elbow and raise the entire arm over the head (shoulder flexion).
12. With the arm parallel to the body (palm up—supination), flex and extend the elbow.
13. Flex and extend the wrist. Flex and extend each finger joint.
14. Move each finger, in turn, away from the middle finger (abduction), and toward the middle finger (adduction).
15. Abduct the thumb by moving it toward the extended fingers.
16. Touch the thumb to the base of the little finger, then to each fingertip (opposition).
17. Turn the hand palm down (pronation), then turn it palm up (supination).
18. Grasp the patient's wrist with one hand and the patient's hand with the other. Bring the wrist toward the body (inversion) and then away from the body (eversion).
19. Move the patient close to you and repeat steps 5 through 18.

SUMMARY

In this chapter, we discussed the concept of therapeutic exercises as a physical therapy modality and the role of the physical therapy aide in assisting the patient with carrying out these exercises. We also discussed the concept and skills involved in assisting the patient with both passive and active range of motion exercises, including those exercises used on the upper and lower extremities.

◆ ◆ LEARNING ACTIVITY 14-1

Terms to Define

Use your textbook to write the definitions for the following words, which relate to body motion.

1. abduct
2. adduct
3. circumduction
4. extension
5. flexion
6. hyperextension
7. kinesiology
8. pronation
9. rotation
10. supination

◆ ◆ LEARNING ACTIVITY 14-2

Types of Exercise

Describe each category of exercise listed, and state its purpose.

1. Therapeutic exercise:

   Purpose:
2. Passive exercise:

   Purpose:
3. Active exercise:

   Purpose:
4. Range-of-motion exercise:

   Purpose:
5. Active-assistive exercise:

   Purpose:
6. Progressive-resistive exercise:

   Purpose:
7. Isometric exercise:

   Purpose:
8. Stretching exercise:

   Purpose:
9. Functional exercise:

   Purpose:
10. Mat exercise:

    Purpose:
11. Parallel bar exercise:

    Purpose:
12. Crutch exercise:

    Purpose:

◆ ◆ LEARNING ACTIVITY 14-3

Know Your Exercises

Answer the following questions.

1. List at least five exercises that are used in physical therapy.
2. In your own words, describe how a passive exercise is done.
3. What type of exercise is performed by the patient alone?
4. What exercise uses weights and pulleys?
5. In your own words, describe the goal of therapeutic exercise.

REVIEW QUESTIONS

1. Range-of-motion exercises involve performing movements of __________ and __________.
2. __________ range-of-motion is generally used when the patient is unable to move the affected body part.
3. __________ range-of-motion is generally used when the patient is able to assist in moving the affected body part.
4. The physical therapy aide should always remember to __________ all segments farthest away from the origin of the range of motion.
5. In some cases, __________ __________ __________ may interfere with range-of-motion exercises.
6. The __________ position describes the position in which the patient stands upright, eyes looking straight ahead, arms at sides with the palms forward, and feet approximately four inches apart.
7. A __________ plane divides the body into right and left sides.
8. A __________-__________ plane divides the body into exact right and left halves.
9. The __________ plane divides the body into front and back sections.
10. The __________ plane divides the body into upper and lower portions.

11. Match the correct answers in Column A with its appropriate response in Column B:

Column A	Column B
thumb	protraction and retraction
foot	extension and flexion
hand	opposition
ankle	abduction
scapulo-thoracic	abduction and adduction
shoulder	inversion and eversion
hip and knee	internal and external rotation
hip	Plantar flexion and dorsal flexion

15

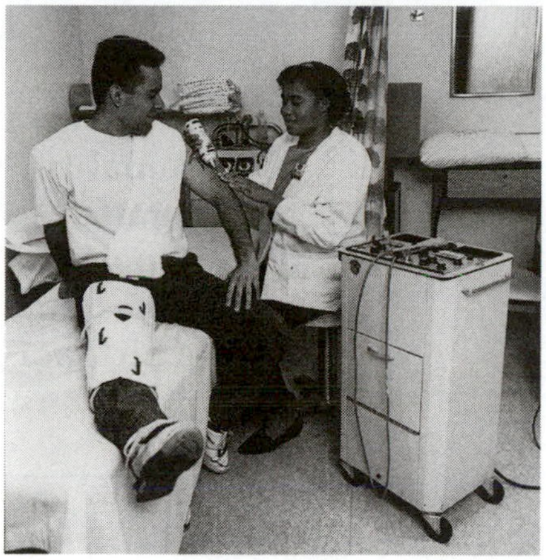

Physical Therapy Agents and Modalities

OBJECTIVES

Upon completion of this chapter, you should be able to:

1. Discuss the purpose of employing different agents and modalities in performing physical therapy.
2. Define hydrotherapy and describe its use in physical therapy.
3. Identify and discuss the three different superficial hearing agents used in physical therapy.
4. Explain the function of diathermy.
5. Differentiate between microwave and shortwave therapy.
6. Define ultrasound and briefly discuss its application in physical therapy.
7. Contrast the difference between cold therapy and heat therapy and briefly discuss when each should be applied.

KEY TERMS

- **Agent**
- **Contraindication**
- **Diathermy**
- **Electromagnetic**
- **Hydrocollator pack**
- **Hydrotherapy**
- **Infrared**
- **Microwave**
- **Modality**
- **Paraffin bath**
- **Superficial**
- **Ultrasound**
- **Whirlpool**

In order to properly prepare the muscles and joints of a body region for exercise or physical therapy, various **modalities,** or **agents,** of heating or cooling these structures may be employed.

Heat helps in the reduction of pain and tightness within the muscles and stiffness in the joints. In the body region in which the temperature is elevated, the blood vessels dilate, making it possible for the flow of blood to that area to increase. All these changes aid in the performance of exercise therapy. Such heat application has basically the same purpose as the warming-up and loosening-up exercises that are used by athletes just before they enter a strenuous event.

Heat can be applied to parts of the body by a number of methods. One such method is by the complete immersion of the body part into heated water. This form of heating is called **hydrotherapy.** In hydrotherapy, the heat delivered to the immersed body part is only one of the therapeutic factors from which the patient can receive benefit.

The goal in the use of heating modalities is to effect a specific temperature elevation and an increased blood flow in the part selected for therapy. Optimal benefit from this type of local application of heat is generally achieved within twenty minutes. After that amount of time, no further local temperature elevation can be achieved. In fact, any more time can cause the increased blood flow to carry the heat away into the entire body.

The various heating agents used in physical therapy can be divided into two types: the one brings heat to the **superficial** structures and the other brings heat to the deeper structures of a body region.

Both temperature elevation and cooling may be used to create a therapeutic environment for the affected body region or structure.. The lowering of tissue temperature is generally achieved through the application of various forms. In essence, the lowering of the temperature of the affected body part helps to decrease the amount of swelling, inflammation, and spasticity to the area involved.

◆ SUPERFICIAL HEATING AGENTS

Modalities found within this group are those that can affect temperature elevation approximately 10 millimeters beneath the skin's surface. They include hydrocollator packs, infrared lamps, and paraffin baths.

Hydrocollator Packs

A **hydrocollator pack** is composed of a silica gel that has been encased in a canvas bag and can be contoured to the various body regions (Figure 15-1A). Silica gel is able to maintain a temperature of 104 degrees Fahrenheit (40 degrees Centigrade) for a period of approximately 30 to 40 minutes. The hydrocollator pack should be placed in a water bath at a temperature of about 170 degrees Fahrenheit. It must then be removed from the water and placed onto the area that afterward will be treated with range-of-motion, active, or resistive exercises. Both the area in which the moist pack will be applied and the packs themselves are generally covered with a thick Turkish towel in order to protect the patient's skin from any possible burns and to reduce any emission of heat from the packs toward the outside. The upper side of the pack can also be covered with a plastic or rubber sheet in order to forestall any heat emission away from the packs, Figure 15-1B.

Generally speaking, it is more advantageous to place the pack on the patient than to make the patient lie on the pack.

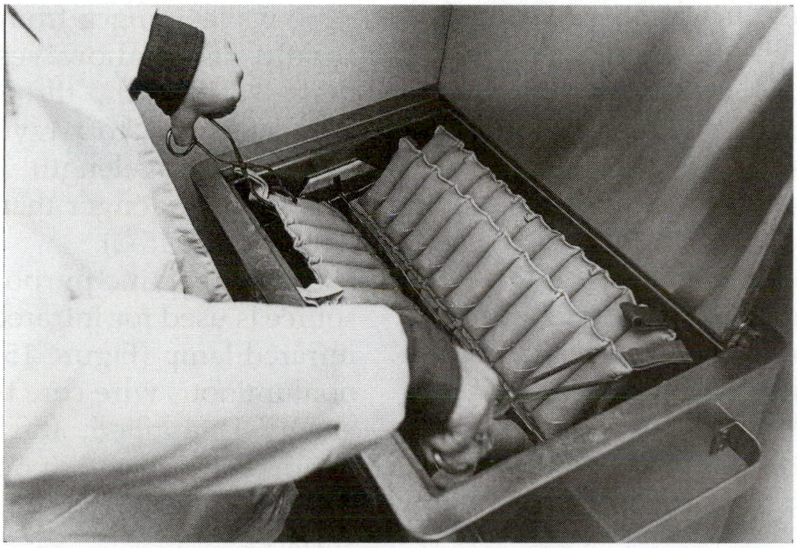

A

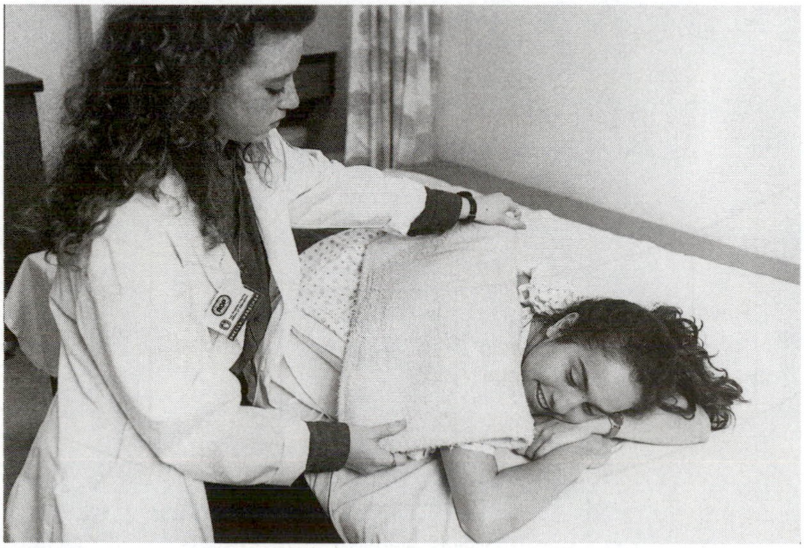

B

Figure 15-1 (A) Hydrocollator packs; (B) in use.

The latter invites greater chance for burns. Sometimes the patient's condition may require the placing of the hydrocollator pack under a part of his or her body. If this is the case, special precautions have to be taken, and you should speak with the physical therapist prior to applying the pack.

Heat delivered from the moist hydrocollator pack to the body is a form of conductive heat. The moisture of the pack serves as the conductor to the skin surface. Water is also a good heat conductor. The counterpart of conductors are the insulators. They are responsible for the hampering of the transfer of heat, and some of the more common types include wood, asbestos, plastics, and rubber.

If a patient suffers from a skin disease, hydrocollator packs should never be used. The same is true for areas of impaired blood supply.

When the hydrocollator pack is used as a therapeutic application, it should be removed after a period of 20 minutes and placed in a reheating bath of 170 degrees Fahrenheit. Thirty minutes later, the packs may again be ready for application.

Infrared Heating

This form of heat is found widely in both nature and in daily life. The most abundant of all infrared sources is the sun. More than half of the sun's total radiation is infrared, and most heated substances emit infrared rays. **Infrared** is a type of radiant heat and can be transmitted to an object or the body from a distance source through a vacuum.

The physical properties of any radiant energy are that of **electromagnetic** waves. The spectrum of the electromagnetic waves ranges from electric power supply and radiowaves, with a very long wavelength, through the visible light spectrum, to x-rays, which have a very short wavelength. The wavelength of infrared is longer than that of visible light (Figure 15-2).

For therapeutic purposes, an artificial source is used for infrared radiation. The infrared lamp (Figure 15-3) consists of a nonluminous wire core to which electric energy is applied. Infrared can affect temperature elevation down to approximately 10 millimeters beneath the skin's surface.

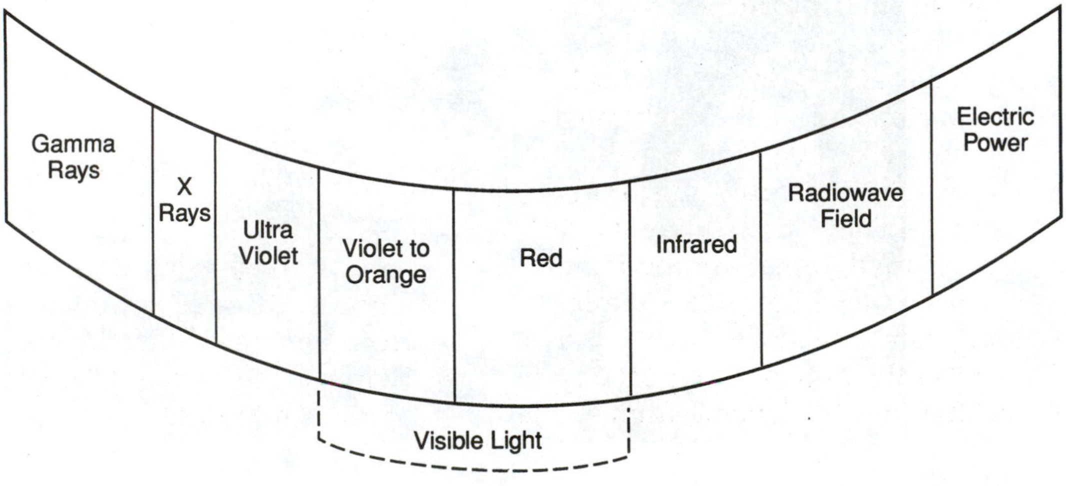

Figure 15-2 The electromagnetic spectrum.

There are several advantages to using infrared heat as a therapeutic modality. There is no pressure on the body, and the aide attending the patient can easily observe the area without interrupting the treatment.

As with other local heating methods, the optimal local temperature is generally achieved within twenty minutes. Any extension of this time frame may lead to sweating and general heating. The effects of infrared are very similar to those of the heat emitted by the hydrocollator packs. It also should not be applied over areas of impaired vascular supply or impaired temperature sensation. Refer to Procedure 40.

THE PARAFFIN BATH

The **paraffin bath** (Figure 15-4), contains a mixture of one part liquid petrolatum to seven parts of paraffin. After these components are placed in the container of the paraffin bath, the mixture has to be heated until the paraffin melts. Before it is ready for use, the temperature of the mixture must drop to approximately 125 to 130 degrees Fahrenheit (51 to 54 degrees Centigrade). A period of two to three hours may be required for this drop to occur.

The paraffin bath is most often used to treat small areas, such as the hands and feet. Arthritic joint pain and stiffness of

PROCEDURE #40: Applying an Infrared Lamp

1. Wash your hands, identify the patient, and provide for privacy.
2. Inspect the lamp for good working condition prior to beginning the procedure.
3. Explain the procedure to the patient.
4. Place the lamp 30 inches (about 45 centimeters) from the body area receiving the rays, Figure 15-3.
5. Drape the surrounding body parts not receiving treatment.
6. Make sure that the infrared lamp has been turned on 20 to 30 minutes prior to its use.
7. Instruct the patient to report any feelings of "hot spots" immediately since they may be warning signals of an imminent burn from the infrared lamp.
8. Remove the infrared lamp after 15 to 20 minutes.

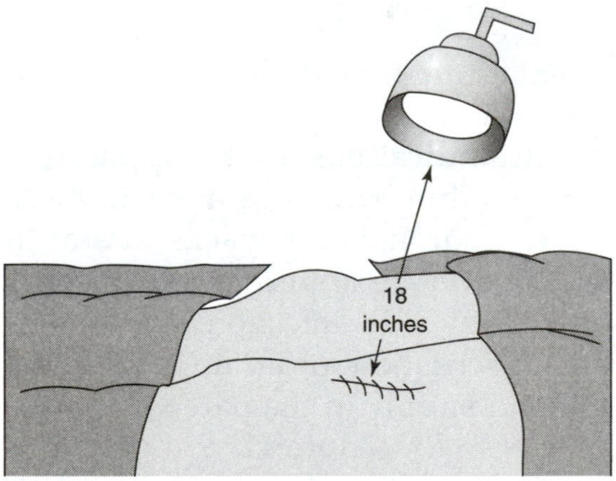

Figure 15-3 Application of the infrared lamp.

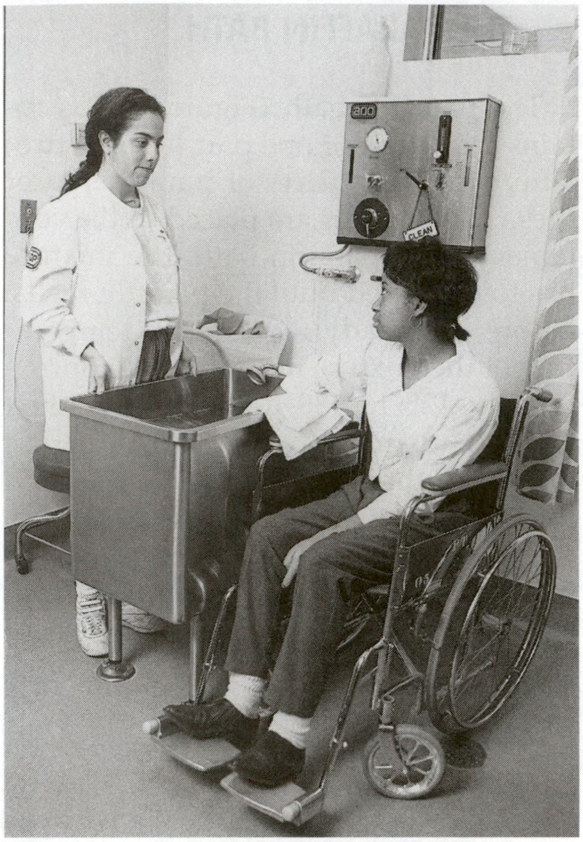

Figure 15-4 Hand immersion into a paraffin bath.

the hands, are frequently indications for paraffin use.

Contraindications for the application of the paraffin bath are similar to those of the hydrocollator packs. Paraffin should never be applied when there is evidence of skin infection, an impairment of sensation, or an impairment of the blood supply in the part to be treated. Refer to Procedure 41.

PROCEDURE #41: Applying a Paraffin Bath

1. Wash your hands, identify the patient, and provide for privacy.
2. Explain the procedure to the patient.
3. Instruct the patient to remove all jewelry from his hands.
4. Cleanse and dry the skin of the hand prior to submission into the bath.
5. Instruct the patient to "dip" the hand (or other affected area) quickly in and out of the paraffin ten to twelve times and to keep the fingers spread in order to allow the paraffin to form a glove.
6. Inform the patient that she may feel a warmth and/or tingling in the fingers and explain that such a sensation is brought on by the dilation of blood vessels from the increased heat.
7. After twenty minutes, the hand is withdrawn from the paraffin, and the glove removed.
8. Remove used paraffin and place it into the paraffin container for future use.

DEEP HEATING AGENTS

These types of heating modalities emit energy in the form of electromagnetic or mechanical waves. These waves have the physical properties necessary to elevate the temperature of the tissue as far down as 30 to 50 millimeters beneath the skin's surface. Electromagnetic waves generate heat by the tissue's resistance to electric current, and mechanical waves cause a form of tissue vibration that is able to generate heat.

Deep heating by electromagnetic or mechanical waves, is called **diathermy.** It is a process of heating the tissue with electromagnetic waves by warming up a wire that conducts electric current. The amount of generated heat depends on several factors and is also governed by a simple law of physics found in the study of electrical current. *Joule's Law* states that "a rise in temperature in a conductor is caused by the passage of an electric current; the degree of temperature rise is therefore dependent on the amount of heat being produced." The law further indicates that the amount of heat produced is dependent upon three proportions: it must be directly proportional to the resistance of the conductor in *ohms;* it must be directly proportional to the square of the strength of the current in *amperes;* and it must be directly proportional to the length of time the current flows.

Deep heating, or diathermy by electromagnetic waves, is accomplished through the means of a microwave or a shortwave generator.

◆ MICROWAVES

One of the most frequently used deep heating or diathermy machines currently in use is the **microwave** diathermy machine (Figure 15-5).

Microwaves are located on the right of infrared in the electromagnetic spectrum since the wavelength is longer than that of infrared rays but shorter than the wavelength of electromagnetic waves, which can supply mechanical power. Microwaves are found within the radiowave field frequency.

A microwave machine consists of a generator, which is operated by electrical power; the director, which emits the microwaves; and a spacing gauge. The generator is a magnetron responsible for generating high-frequency electric energy, or microwaves. No part of the machine comes in contact with the patient.

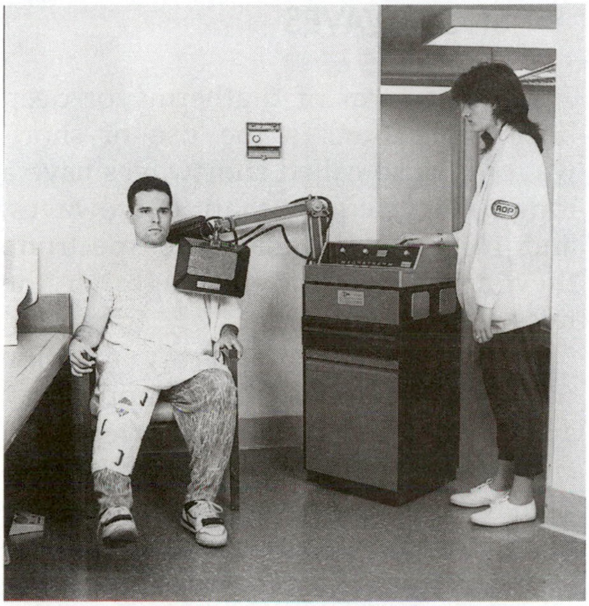

Figure 15-5 Application of microwaves.

The distance of the director from the body part being treated is of importance. It must be calculated accurately by the spacing gauge. The director should be perpendicular to the treated part. The intensity of the microwaves reaching the part to be treated decreases with the square of the distance between the microwave director and the body part.

Prior to microwave application, the skin of the area to be treated should be clean and dry since moisture and grease would increase the skin's resistance, thereby causing a burn. As with other heating agents, the optimal temperature elevation is obtained within twenty minutes.

Microwaves should never be applied to a patient with a cardiac pacemaker. Since the pacemaker rests beneath the patient's skin continuously sending out electrical impulses to the heart in order to maintain a regular heartbeat, microwaves could seriously interfere with the function of the pacemaker and lead to serious complications or even death.

SHORTWAVES

Another form of diathermy or deep heat application, is the use of shortwaves. The so-called shortwaves have a longer wavelength than microwaves, and in the electromagnetic spectrum, they are located to the right of the microwave.

The shortwave diathermy machine consists of an electric power supply unit, an oscillator unit, a shortwave frequency circuit, and a patient output circuit. The widely used household alternating current is transformed by the oscillator unit into electromagnetic waves with the length and frequency of shortwaves. The shortwaves are within the radiowave frequency range.

The application of shortwave diathermy is a bit more difficult than microwave application. The shortwaves are delivered to the patient by contour applicators, inductance cable, or air-spaced electrodes. Therefore, the patient's skin must be protected with a thick Turkish towel since this type of material also absorbs for body's sweat from the surface of the skin.

The body part that is to be treated should be within the electromagnetic field that is generated between the applicator devices (Figure 15-6). A milliampere meter is located on the panel and indicates the amount of energy being "drained" by the body. A specific meter reading will indicate that the patient output circuit has been tuned to the oscillatoir unit. This means that maximal flow in the area to be treated can be achieved.

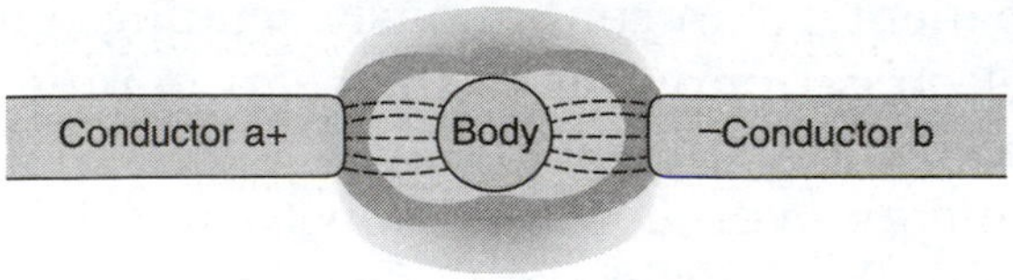

Figure 15–6 The electromagnetic field.

Most recently, the use of shortwave diathermy has decreased, since it is being replaced more and more with microwave therapy. Contraindications for the use of shortwave therapy are generally the same as for microwaves. It must never be used in hemorrhage, acute inflammation or marked circulatory disorders, and never near metallic implants such as cardiac pacemakers.

ULTRASOUND

Another deep heating treatment is the application of ultrasonic waves or **ultrasound.** Ultrasonic waves are not faster than sound but are of a higher frequency than the sound waves that can be heard by the human ear. The principles of the ultrasound wave involve electricity being supplied to a crystal of a certain physical constitution. This crystal, in turn, starts to emit ultrasonic waves that penetrate the superficial tissue and are reflected on the deep tissue. This sets up a very fine vibrating motion within the tissue, which in turn generates heat. A similar effect is the heating up of a wire that is bent back and forth rapidly.

The major difference between electromagnetic waves and ultrasound waves is that the latter are mechanical. The mechanical force of sound and ultrasound waves can be demonstrated by a membrane placed in the course of these waves. A vibrating motion takes place in the membrane. Ultrasound must also be transmitted by a media that is not compressible such as water or mineral oil.

The ultrasound machine contains a power supply and an oscillator circuit (Figure 15-7). The latter transmits the ultrasound waves generated in the crystal to the ultrasound head. The head is moved in a stroking or circular motion over the part to be treated. These motions help to distribute the energy. A commercially available coupling agent or mineral oil must be applied with the ultrasound. Water may also be used. While the therapeutic application of ultrasound is still quite limited, in recent years, it has had great diagnostic use in diseases of the heart and eyes. Refer to Procedure 42.

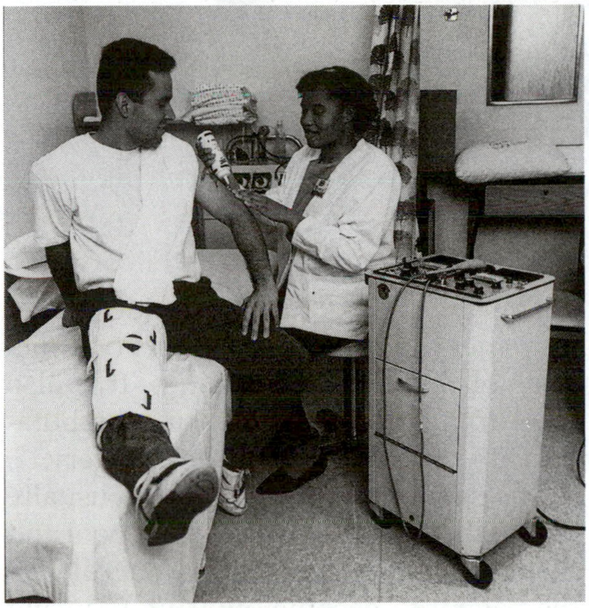

Figure 15-7 Application of ultrasound.

◆ HYDROTHERAPY

Whirlpool Therapy

The **whirlpool** (Figure 15-8) consists of a container filled with water and an agitator. The agitator causes the water to move in a whirling motion that has a massaging effect on the skin and tends to dilate the blood vessels. This massaging effect also soothes pain and is therefore most widely used for disorders related to joints in the wrists, ankles, and knees, as well as in the treatment of bones after a fracture has occurred.

The whirlpool temperature generally ranges from 98 to 104 degrees Fahrenheit (37 to 40 degrees Centigrade). Much care should be exercised in adjusting the temperature of the water since allowing it to become too high may cause the patient to become disoriented or delirious. Also,

PROCEDURE #42: Application of Ultrasound

1. Wash your hands, identify the patient, and provide for privacy.
2. Explain the procedure to the patient.
3. Expose only that area that is to receive the ultrasound and drape the surrounding areas with a towel.
4. Apply a small amount of coupling agent, gel, or mineral oil to the ultrasound head.
5. Turn the machine on and set the timer for 15 to 20 minutes.
6. Apply ultrasound by using a vibrating circular motion of the head against the affected area.
7. Upon completion of the treatment, wipe off any excess oil or gel from the affected area of the body and form the ultrasound head.
8. Turn the machine off.

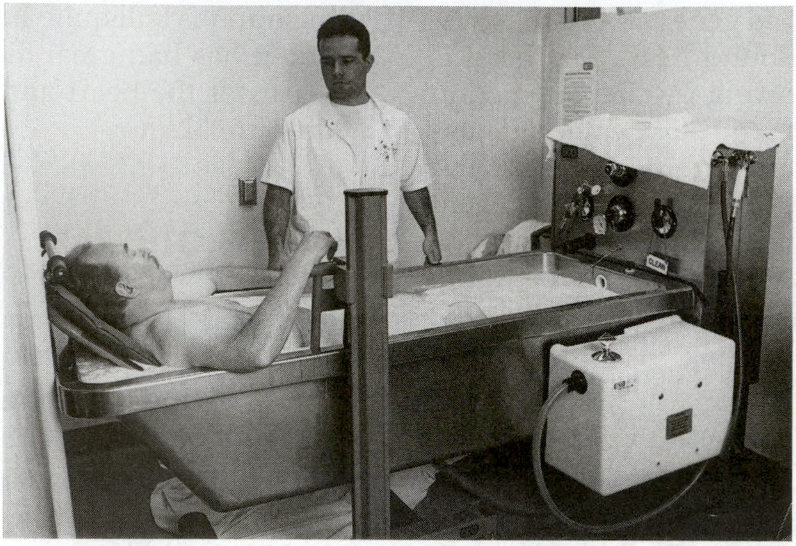

Figure 15-8 Whirlpool application.

submission into the whirlpool bath should never be longer than twenty minutes, and is generally a therapy used most frequently in conjunction with exercise therapy during and after its application. Refer to Procedure 43.

Therapeutic Pool

The therapeutic pool is generally kept at a temperature of 98 degrees Fahrenheit (37 degrees Centigrade). It is usually structured in such a way as to have an inclining bottom so that the patient can be placed either in the deep end or in the shallow water.

This type of pool is most widely used for patients who have disorders or afflictions of the lower extremities. It is also used for gradually increasing ambulation after hip, knee, and back surgery.

The patient receiving treatment usually begins therapy by floating in the pool and then standing in deep water. This allows the patient to become buoyant, reducing the weight of the submerged body parts on the legs. Gradually the patient progresses to the shallow side, and as he goes to the shallow water, the weight on the lower extremities increases.

PROCEDURE #43: Assisting the Patient with a Whirlpool Bath

1. Wash your hands, identify the patient, and provide for privacy.
2. Explain the procedure to the patient.
3. Fill the whirlpool tub with water at a temperature ranging from 98 to 104 degrees Fahrenheit (37 to 40 degrees Centigrade).
4. Assist the patient into the bath.
5. Set the timer for 20 minutes and check on the patient at frequent intervals.
6. Assist the patient out of the whirlpool.

Walking in the therapeutic pool also helps to strengthen the muscles of the lower extremities. To overcome the resistance of the water, increased muscle activity is also required.

The therapeutic pool is a very expedient mode of treating patients, but the same results can be obtained in rehabilitation departments without the use of the pool. If a department does not have one, it does not necessarily mean that the care or treatment is inferior.

◆ COLD THERAPY

Application of cold therapy (Figure 15-9), is generally done with a large ice cube or a plastic pack of ice cubes which have been frozen at 28 to 32 degrees Fahrenheit (0 to 2 degrees Centigrade). The ice is placed or rubbed over the affected area until the patient feels some numbness. This usually takes between ten to fifteen minutes. Shortly afterward, a redness of the skin will appear. This is called *erythema.* Exercise therapy is also generally initiated immediately after the application of the ice packs.

Cold therapy is frequently applied in order to reduce swelling, inflammation and spasticity.

It should always be kept in mind that the use of heating or cooling modalities or agents is considered an axillary measure to therapeutic treatment. Application of head or cold alone usually does not offer the patient any significant benefit. Heat or cold applications are used as precursors of therapeutic programs such as exercises, gait training, or stretching. Refer to Procedure 44.

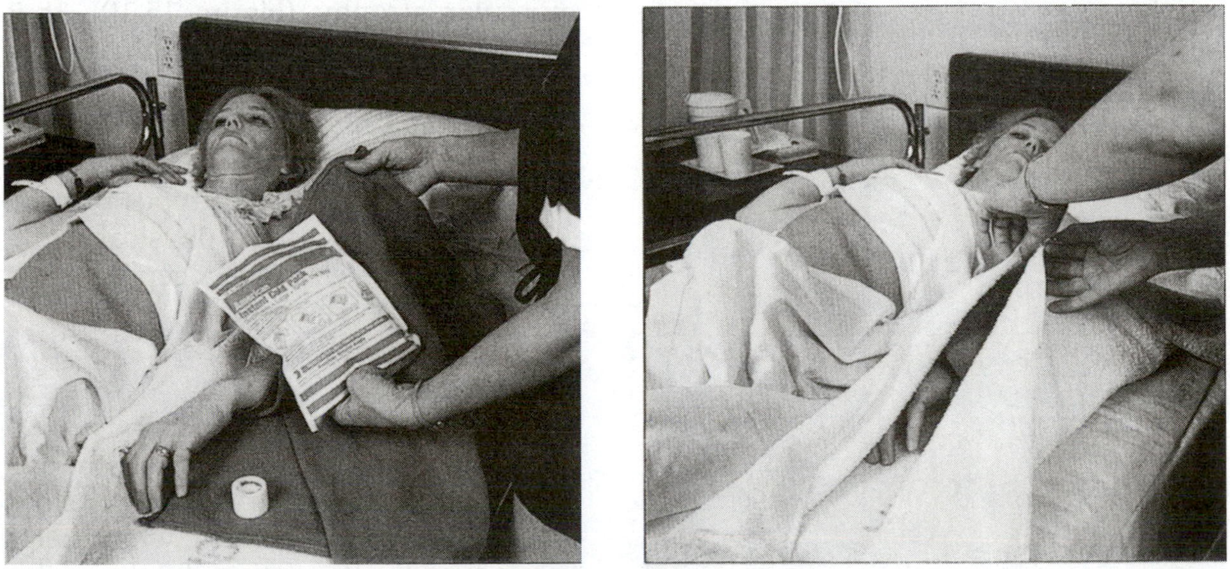

A B

Figure 15-9 Application of cold pack. (A) Cover the disposable cold pack with a towel before applying it to the patient. (B) Cover the cold pack application with another towel.

PROCEDURE #44: Applying a Cold Pack

1. Wash your hands, identify the patient, and provide for privacy.
2. Assemble all necessary equipment.
3. Explain the procedure to the patient.
4. Expose the area to be treated and note its condition.
5. Place the cold pack in a cloth covering.
6. Strike or squeeze the cold pack to activate the chemicals inside it.
7. Place the covered cold pack on the proper area and enclose it with a towel. Note the time of the application.
8. Secure the pack with tape or gauze.
9. Leave the patient in a comfortable position with a call light within reach.
10. Check on the patient at least every ten minutes, and note any changes in the condition of the affected area.
11. If no adverse symptoms occur, remove the pack in thirty minutes.
12. Remove the pack from the cover and dispose of it in the appropriate manner.

MASSAGE

Massage is one of the oldest, most useful, and easily administered forms of treatment for the relief of pain and other symptoms of disease and injury. It is frequently used to increase the supply of blood to an affected part, to help in the drainage from the region of an involved joint that has been diminished by periarticular swelling, to provide muscular relaxation, and to lessen the potential for muscular atrophy (Figure 15-10). It is also helpful in the treatment of arthritis, sprains and contusions, pain caused by sacroiliac strains, and in many orthopedic conditions, including back problems.

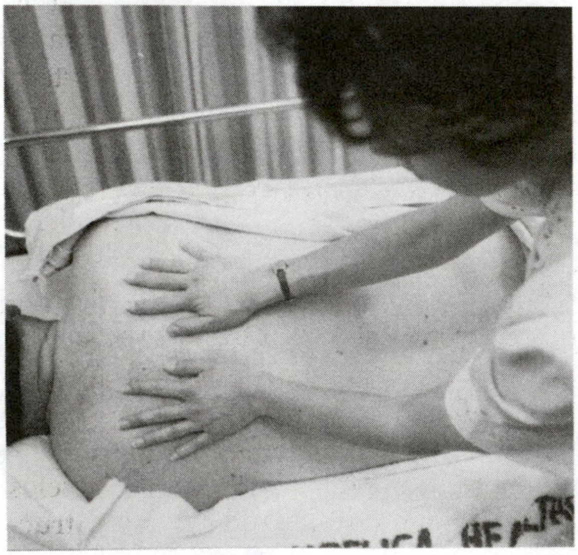

Figure 15-10 Use long, smooth strokes as you apply the lotion.

There are five different types of massage that can be used in physical therapy: effleurage, petrissage, deep stroking, friction, and percussion.

Effleurage

Effleurage involves superficial stroking toward the body or heart, using a slow, gentle, rhythmic movement, which helps to produce a reflex action. To obtain this effect, the pressure must be extremely light and each movement should be repeated in the same direction.

When giving effleurage massage, you can use one of four different types of striking:

- *using one hand*—generally used on the extremities, back of the head, and in single massage of the neck
- *using the thumb*—frequently used between two muscles or between a muscle and a tendon, and often to reach the interossei of the hands and feet
- *using both hands*—frequently used upon the lower extremities on adults, on the chest and back, and when performing double massage of the neck
- *using the tips of the fingers*—principally used around the joints

Deep Stroking Massage

Deep stroking massage, that is, stroking in the same direction of the natural flow of lymph and venous blood, is frequently used to aid in the emptying of veins and lymphatics and in pressing their contents in the direction of their natural flow. When using deep stroking massage, it is essential that you make sure your patient's muscles are relaxed, and that your movements are deep, but not heavy.

Petrissage

Petrissage is a process in which you use kneading, wringing, lifting, or pressing of a part to help assist in the venous and lymphatic circulation. It also helps in stretching retracted muscles and tendons, and in stretching adhesions. The strokes used in petrissage are the same as they are for deep stroking, and one or both hands may be used.

Friction

The goal of friction is to press deeply into a part by way of moving your hand in a circular direction in order to free adherent skin, loosen scars and adhesions located deep, and aid in the absorption of local effusion. Friction is an important type of massage to use around joints for small areas as the hands, feet, and the face. It may also be given with the thumb, the fingertips, or with one hand.

Percussion

Percussion, which is also known as *tapotement,* consists of striking the part to be massaged quickly with the hand. There are four types pf percussion which you can use. They include clapping with the palms of your hands, hacking with the ulnar borders of your hands, tapping with the tips of the fingers, and beating with a clenched fist.

◆ CERVICAL TRACTION

Traction is another modality that is often employed in physical therapy when there is a need to assure a certain amount of immobilization of the spine. It also helps in the relief of muscle spasms. When correctly applied, cervical traction straightens the spine and enlarges the intervertebral foramina to relieve compressive or irritative forces placed upon the nerve roots.

Intermittent traction is the most effective method of traction application. It relieves muscle spasm because of its massage-like effect upon the muscles and the ligamentous and capsular structures. It also reduces swelling, improves circulation in the tissues, and prevents the formation of adhesions between the dural sleeves of the nerve roots and the adjacent capsular structures.

When applying traction, you must always remember to first give the patient hot packs and massage before the traction is started. The patient is then placed in a sitting position with his or her head and neck flexed or bent slightly forward. The traction is then applied, starting with ten pounds, and held for two seconds, followed by a rest period of three seconds. The total treatment time should be no longer than fifteen minutes. As long as the patient can tolerate it, you can gradually increase the weight by two pounds at each treatment until the total weight is between twenty to thirty pounds. The usual protocol for applying cervical traction on the hospitalized patient is once a day, for no longer than fifteen minutes at a time.

◆ THERAPEUTIC EXERCISE

Therapeutic exercise involves movements which are prescribed by a physician or physical therapist to help restore normal function or to maintain a state of well-being. Its application is based upon restoring, improving, or maintaining a muscle's *strength, elasticity,* and *coordination.* All therapeutic exercise programs are developed according to meeting a patient's individual needs, and as such, are based upon a medical evaluation of the person's disability.

Types of Movements Used in Therapeutic Exercises

There are four types of movements which are used in the performance of therapeutic exercises. They include *passive* movements, which are movements performed by someone other than the patient, in which no muscle action occurs and the patient exerts no effort; *active* movements, which are performed by the patient, who voluntarily contract and relax the muscles that control a particular movement; *assistive* movements, in which the patient is helped to perform the movement; and *resistive* movements, in which the patient performs the movement against resistance.

Types of Therapeutic Exercises

There are several different types of therapeutic exercises which you may use to assist your patient to restore, improve, or maintain a specific muscle or group of muscles. The types most frequently employed in the physical therapy department, include the following:

- ❒ *range of motion (ROM)*—movement of the joint through its full range in all the appropriate planes; may employ passive, active, or resistive movements
- ❒ *endurance*—exercises that use low-resistance and high-repetition to help increase one's endurance
- ❒ *relaxation*—exercises that help to promote the release of prolonged muscular contractions
- ❒ *postural*—exercises designed to help maintain a proper relationship between body parts
- ❒ *pressive resistance exercises (PRE)*—exercises to help increase resistance in order to help strengthen a muscle, muscle group, or supportive structures surrounding a joint
- ❒ *muscle reeducation*—exercises that help a muscle or muscle group to relearn its normal function

- ❐ *coordination*—exercises to help improve precision of muscle movement
- ❐ *conditioning*—exercises that help to maintain and/or strengthen some or all of the body's musculature

◆ SUMMARY

In this chapter, we discussed the purpose and function of employing different agents and modalities in performing physical therapy. We defined hydrotherapy and described its use as a modality. We also identified different superficial heating agents that can be used as physical therapy modalities. We discussed the function of diathermy, microwave and shortwave therapy, and ultrasound, and their application as therapeutic modalities. We explained the concept of massage therapy and its effects as a therapeutic agent. And, finally, we discussed the difference between cold therapy and heat therapy and discussed when each should be used.

◆ ◆ LEARNING ACTIVITY 15-1

Cold Therapy and Ultraviolet Therapy

Give brief answers to these questions:

1. Name the conditions that respond well to ultraviolet treatment.
2. For what is cryotherapy used?
3. What methods are used to apply cold therapy?
4. What is the effect of cryotherapy?
5. Name three types of lamps that may be used as sources of ultraviolet rays.
6. What factors affect the absorption of ultraviolet rays?
7. What is the best guide for determining treatment time with ultraviolet therapy?
8. Give two sources of ultraviolet rays.

◆ ◆ LEARNING ACTIVITY 15-2

In Your Own Words

In your own words, briefly answer the questions below.

1. Define hydrotherapy.
2. Discuss two physical therapy modalities that use water.
3. What effect does heat therapy have on body tissue?
4. Discuss three types of heat therapy.
5. Discuss two purposes for traction therapy.
6. Define massage.
7. What does "cryo" mean?
8. Explain two types of cryotherapy.
9. When is paraffin therapy indicated?

◆ ◆ LEARNING ACTIVITY 15-3

Safety Procedures

Answer these questions related to safety precautions used during physical therapy treatments.

1. Why is the patient draped before a treatment?
2. When a patient with crutches masters ambulation and crutch exercises, what other activities should be practiced?
3. On what types of patients should precautions be used with therapeutic heat treatments?
4. What skin sign indicates that more padding is needed for heat treatments?
5. Why are patients cautioned to remain still without moving during treatment with a heat lamp?
6. Why must the temperature of a whirlpool bath be monitored when treating a patient with impaired circulation?
7. How does the physical therapy aide prevent burning a patient when using hydrocollator packs?
8. Why are metal implants, shrapnel, or jewelry prohibited near the treatment area when ultrasound or shortwave diathermy are used?
9. What item is prohibited in the area where microwave diathermy is used?
10. What diseases or conditions prevent the use of massage?

REVIEW QUESTIONS

1. __________ helps to reduce pain and tightness within muscles and stiffness in joints.
2. Complete immersion of a body part into heated water is called __________.
3. A __________ __________ is an example of a superficial heating agent.
4. A __________ __________ is often used to treat small areas, such as the hands and feet, which are afflicted with arthritic joints.
5. __________ __________ __________ emit energy in the form of electromagnetic or mechanical waves, which eventually generate heat beneath the skin's surface.
6. __________ is a process created by the heating of tissues with electromagnetic waves by warming up a wire that conducts electric current.
7. __________ therapy should never be applied to a patient with a cardiac pacemaker.
8. The major difference between electromagnetic and ultrasonic waves is that the latter are __________,
9. A __________ is used to create a massaging effect on the skin and thus tends to dilate the blood vessels, thereby soothing pain in the affected part.
10. A __________ __________ is most widely used for patients suffering from disorders or afflictions of the lower extremities.
11. Cold therapy is frequently applied in order to reduce __________, __________, and __________.

16

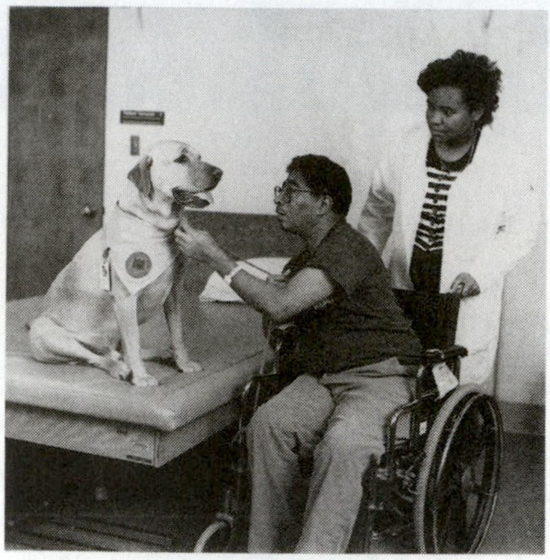

Specialized Clinical Procedures

OBJECTIVES

Upon completion of this chapter, you should be able to:

1. Identify the different types of specialized therapies used for patients with specific physiological needs.
2. Define the term *reduction* and differentiate between open reduction and closed reduction.
3. Describe when a closed reduction may be used.
4. Describe when an open reduction may be used.
5. Discuss the concept of traction and identify various types of traction that can be used to maintain alignment and immobilization of a body part.
6. Discuss the purpose of a cast.
7. Describe instances when the administration of medications might be used as a therapeutic treatment.
8. Discuss how x-rays and tomography are used as therapeutic treatments.
9. Identify specific specialized reflex tests and studies used in diagnosing physical disabilities and in administering therapeutic treatment.
10. Explain the purpose of a lumbar puncture.
11. Explain the purpose of an electroencephalogram.
12. Explain the purpose of magnetic resonance testing.
13. Briefly explain the use of pet therapy as a therapeutic treatment for patients suffering from a physical disability.

KEY TERMS

Achilles reflex
Babinski reflex
Buck's traction
Cast
CAT scan
Closed reduction
EEG
Gout
Immobilization
Lumbar puncture
MRI
Open reduction
Patellar reflex
Reduction
Russell traction
Traction
Vitamin D
X-ray

Depending upon the body part involved and the type of injury or disease sustained, the physical therapy aide may come in contact with any one of several different types of therapies or modalities. These therapies range from the use of immobilization by surgery to immobilization by traction. During this chapter, we will discuss some of the more frequently used of these specialized therapies.

IMMOBILIZATION BY REDUCTION

Whenever a patient fractures a bone, depending upon the type of fracture involved, the physician must determine what type of therapy to use that will promote the healing of the broken bone. It's important to note here that an untreated fracture begins to heal almost immediately. Therefore, the physician has two jobs in treating the break. The first is to place the broken bones so that the restored bone is in the right position to heal in the correct shape. The second is to keep the bone in place as it heals. Placing the bone in position is called **reduction.** It can be done in one of two ways, either by **closed reduction,** in which the physician manipulates the bone into place without opening up the skin, or in **open reduction,** in which an incision or cut into the site of the fracture is necessary to put the broken bone in place.

Holding the bone in place is called **immobilization.** It can usually be done with a cast or a strong bandage. However, in some cases the bone will not heal properly unless it is put in traction, an arrangement of weights and pulleys is set up to put enough tension on the bone and surrounding muscles to hold the bone in place as it begins to heal.

TRACTION

Traction is defined as the pull provided by a series of weights, ropes, and pulleys that are connected to either a frame, wire, or pin or to straps applied over the skin of the patient. *Countertraction* is the force against the traction and is usually supplied by the weight of the patient's body. The application of traction is done by the physician. Maintenance of traction is absolutely necessary. Weights must hang free, ropes and pulleys must be free from interference, and splits and slings must

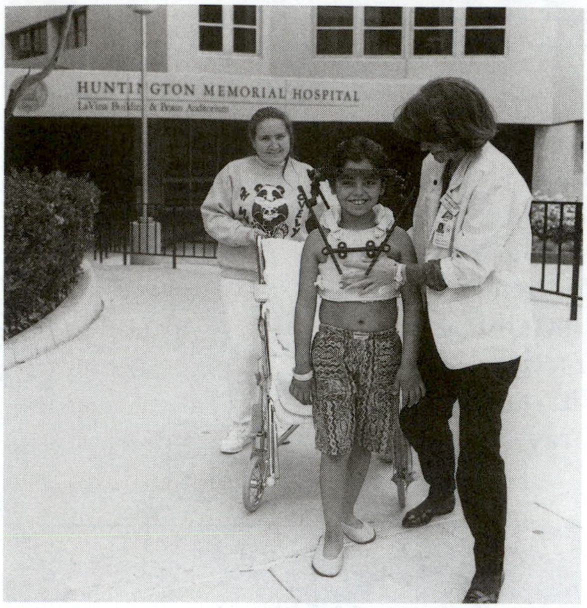

Figure 16-1 Patient with Hare traction.

be suspended without interference.

Several principles are involved in effective traction. First, the traction must be continuous. Second, countertraction must be applied. Third, the traction apparatus must be correctly maintained.

Various types of traction can be used to maintain alignment and immobilization of a fracture or diseased body part. The two most common types are skin traction and skeletal traction. *Skin traction* uses tapes or traction strips attached to the skin, usually by elastic bandages. The tapes or strips are connected to a traction apparatus that consists of ropes, pulleys, and weights. Examples of skin traction are Hare traction (Figure 16-1), **Russell traction,** and **Buck's extension.** *Skeletal traction* uses a wire (Kirschner) or pin (Steinmann) inserted in the bone with pull (traction) applied to the pin or wire. The Thomas splint with the Pearson attachment is often used with the Kirschner wire or Steinmann pin to provide balanced skeletal traction. General anesthesia is required to insert these devices.

Spinal Traction

A rehabilitative modality that is frequently used in physical therapy is spinal traction (Figure 16-2). Correctly performed, spinal traction can produce many positive effects. Among these are distraction of separation of the vertebral bodies and straightening of spinal curves and stretching of the spinal muscles.

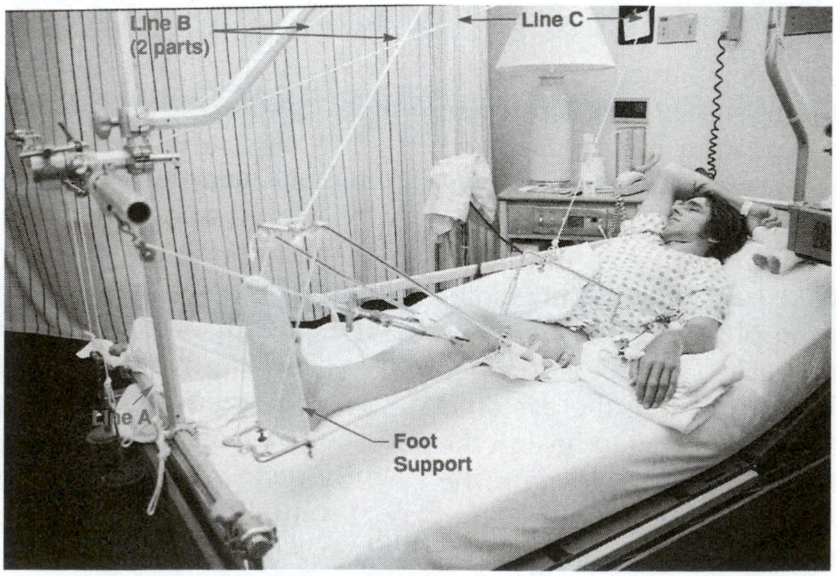

Figure 16-2 A patient in traction *(Photo courtesy of Leona Mourad).*

Indications for Spinal Traction

Spinal traction is generally indicated for patients suffering from herniated disks, degenerative disk joint disease, and joint stiffness associated with hypomobility. However, it should never be used on patients diagnosed with structural disease secondary to tumor or infection, in patients with vascular compromise, and in any condition for which movement is contraindicated.

When applying spinal traction, precautions include conditions such as acute strains, sprains, and inflammation that would be aggravated by traction. Traction applied to patients with joint instability of the spine may cause further strain. Other situations in which spinal traction may be contraindicated include pregnancy, osteoporosis, hiatal hernia, and claustrophobia.

Types of Spinal Traction

When assisting the therapist, depending on the patient's diagnosis or disability, you may encounter any number of spinal traction techniques. The following list will help to provide you with an understanding of which types of these traction techniques are used for various clinical situations:

- *continuous traction*—Continuous spinal traction can be applied for as long as several hours at a time. This extensive duration requires that only small amounts of weight be used, since the patient's skin cannot tolerate prolonged traction at high poundages. Therefore, it is generally accepted that when properly applied to the lumbar spine, this form of traction is ineffective in achieving separation of the vertebrae.
- *sustained (static) mechanical traction*—Sustained traction involves application of a constant amount of traction for periods varying from a few minutes to one-half hour. The shorter duration is usually coupled with heavier weights. Sustained lumbar traction is most effective if a split table is used to reduce friction, and the traction source can be either hanging weights or a mechanical device specially made to produce the traction force. Mechanical devices must maintain constant tension. In other words, as the patient relaxes during treatment, the desired amount of traction must be maintained automatically.
- *intermittent mechanical traction*—This type of traction utilizes a mechanical device that alternately applies and releases traction every few seconds. When applied to the lumbar area, a split table is generally used in order to reduce friction. This is considered by most physical therapists to be the most popular form of traction currently used in the United States.
- *positional traction*—When this technique is used, the patient is placed in various positions, using pillows, blocks, or sandbags to effect a longitudinal pull on the spinal structures. Positional traction usually incorporates lateral bending and only one side of the spinal segment is affected.
- *manual traction*—When this technique is used, the therapist grasps the patient and manually applies a traction force. Manual traction is often applied for a few seconds, but it can be applied as a sudden, quick thrust. This hands-on traction allows the therapist literally to feel the patient's reaction. Sometimes it is more difficult for the patient to relax during manual traction than during

mechanical traction because the exact amount of force that will be applied cannot be anticipated.

- *autotraction (lumbar)*—When this type of traction is applied, a special traction bench composed of two sections that can be individually angled and rotated, must be used. Patients apply the traction by pulling with their own arms, and they can alter the direction of the traction as treatment progresses. Treatment sessions can last one hour or longer, however, they must be supervised by the therapist.
- *gravity lumbar traction*—With gravity lumbar traction, the lower border and the circumference of the rib cage are anchored by a specially made vest which is secured to the top of the bed. The patient is placed on a circular bed or specially made table that is tilted into a vertical or nearly vertical position. In this position, the free weight of the legs and hips exerts a traction force of the lumbar spine by gravity. Two other types of gravity traction have recently become very popular. One technique uses special boots that attach to the patient's ankles. The patient is then able to suspend himself or herself from a frame into a fully inverted position. The other technique involves a device in which the patient is supported on the anterior thighs and is able to hang inverted in a hip and knee flexed position. Both techniques will achieve a traction force of approximately half of the patient's total body weight on the lumbar spine.

◆ ELECTRONEURAL STIMULATION

Electroneural stimulation, or ES, has been used for more than 100 years in the laboratory and in the clinical setting. The control of treatment parameters, however, has been expanded in an effort to produce better results with less discomfort. Today, clinicians and therapists who may select and adapt frequencies, pulse durations, intensities, and other parameters for individualized regimens. The equipment currently available to practitioners offers documentation of progress and monitoring of patient conformity to the prescribed procedures at home.

Purpose of Electroneural Stimulation

Electroneural stimulation is designed to offer the patient a type of therapy that can increase circulation by means of the pumping action of muscles upon the vessels, while at the same time, produce mild heating with all of the benefits accrued from increased temperatures within the tissues. It is usually indicated for muscles requiring assistance for relaxation, as in the case of spasms; for exercise, when the patient is suffering from atrophy, weakness, and paralysis; for pain, when it is secondary to any of the afflictions previously noted; and as an adjunct to the healing process of the body, such as with fractures or open wounds. However, electroneural stimulation should never be used in the presence of active hemorrhage, because the pumping motion of stimulated muscles would tend to increase the blood flow and thus exacerbate the hemorrhage. Nor should it be used at spontaneous fracture sites where undesired movements may increase stress on weakened bone; in patients with severe cardiac arrhythmias; in patients with phlebitis where the danger of embolism may be present; and in certain instances when the patient has a pacemaker in place.

◆ TRANSCULTANEOUS ELECTRICAL STIMULATION

Transcultaneous electrical stimulation, or TENS, is a special type of electrical stimulation that has been designed to modify pain (Figure 16-3). It is specifically oriented to the stimulation of nerve fibers known to be involved with transmitting signals to the brain that are interpreted by the thalamus as pain. Although electrodes are placed on the surface of the patient's skin and electrical impulses are transmitted transcultaneously, the particular waveforms used with TENS equipment are targeted to be received by large-diameter, myelinated-A fibers, which are reserved for proprioceptive transmission.

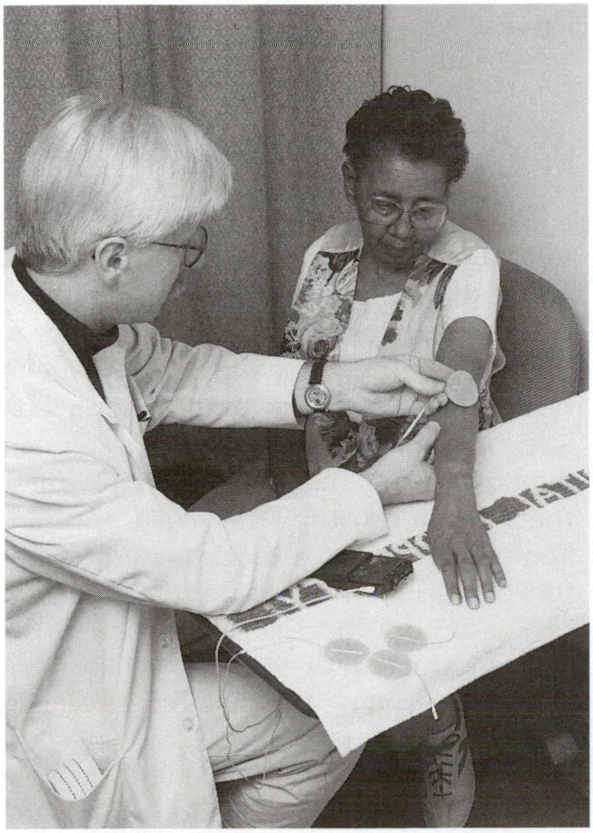

Figure 16-3 A TENS unit is used to relieve pain.

◆ ULTRASOUND

While ultrasound is generally categorized as being an *electrotherapy*, it is not. Sound waves are not electrical, however, their behavior suggests many electrical qualities and traditionally ultrasonic procedures have been identified with other electrotherapies. Ultrasound differs in that sound waves require a medium for transmission. Air itself is a very poor conduction medium for sound wave transmission; thus, physical therapists use water, mineral oil, and specially designed coupling gels to assure sufficient transmission of the therapeutic sound waves.

Recommended treatment times for ultrasound application are frequently offered by most manufacturers of the ultrasound equipment. However, the ideal length of treatment is generally between two to four minutes of ultrasound administered twice or three times weekly. When administered under water, the timing is increased to six to eight minutes, because the dispersion and resistance of the water reduces the driving force of the wave front.

Ultrasound Technique and Effects

The techniques of administration of ultrasound consist of slowly moving the soundhead in a circular pattern over the area to be treated while simultaneously advancing along a lineal track so as to cover a large area (Figure 16-4). When the treatment is administered under water, it is highly recommended by all manufacturers and qualified sources that the whirlpool tank or other metallic receptacles *not* be used for this purpose. Rather, fiberglass or plastic receptacles should be used. Placement of the transducer under water may be either adjacent to and directed at the target site, or

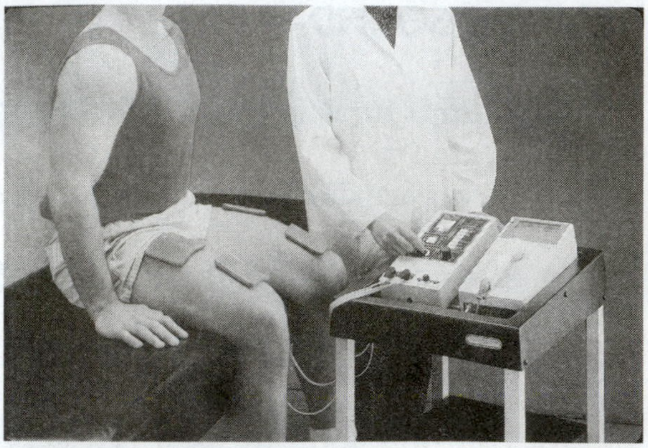

A

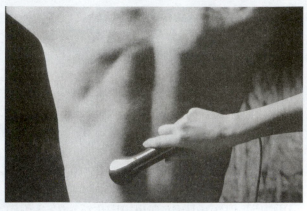

B

Figure 16-4 (A) Ultrasound treatment being applied to a patient. *(Courtesy of Mettler Electronics Corp.)* (B) Ultrasound is an effective form of treatment for chronic pain or acute injuries. *(Courtesy of Mettler Electronics Corp.).*

at a slight distance from and parallel to the target site, therefore allowing the sound wave front to be dispersed and reflected, reverberating from the walls of the receptacle.

The physiological effects of ultrasound have traditionally been divided into four phases: mechanical, chemical, biological, and thermal. Some clinicians consider it to also have a deep heating mechanism. However, the majority of physical therapists who use this form of treatment, consider ultrasound primarily as a mechanical modality rather than a heating modality. Heat is produced with absorption of ultrasound energy, however, this heat is confined to circumscribed areas under the transducer head at the time of application.

Indications for Ultrasound Application

Ultrasound is indicated primarily for right or spasmodic musculature, tendons, and the like. It has also been found to be useful as an analgesic when the discomfort is based upon spasm, adhesions, and scar tissue. Underwater techniques are also being used in the treatment and management of disorders at bony prominences and anatomically inaccessible locations, such as the elbow, wrists, fingers, ankles, and toes.

Ultrasound should never be used on the eye, on a pregnant uterus, and on areas prone to hemorrhage or hypersensitivity.

◆ APPLICATION OF A CAST

Some disorders, such as those of the musculoskeletal system, may require the application of a **cast** as part of the therapeutic treatment and healing process. Casts hold the bone in place while it heals and permit early ambulation when a leg is broken. In some cases, a patient may be given a narcotic or general anesthetic before the cast is applied. Sometimes, a nerve block is performed, for example, infiltrating the brachial plexus with a local anesthetic agent for closed reduction of a fracture of the arm.

When applying the cast, the physician positions the patient in a way that ensures the proper alignment of the part to be immobilized. An aide holds the arm or leg exactly in place. A cast applied to an area that includes a joint usually is applied with the joint flexed to lessen stiffness.

ADMINISTRATION OF MEDICATIONS

Many disorders of the musculoskeletal and nervous systems may require the administration of medications or drugs as part of therapeutic treatment. Some joint diseases, for example, may require the use of aspirin or other anti-inflammatory and pain-relieving drugs. **Gout,** another disease of the joints, can be virtually eliminated with medication. And osteoporosis, a common disorder of the bone, is always treated by providing the patient with supplements of **vitamin D** and calcium, pain-relieving drugs, and hormones to promote ossification and protection of the back.

A great many of the diseases affecting the muscles can also be treated through the administration of certain muscle relaxant medications, while other disorders of the nervous system generally use a number of drugs to relieve pain, treat bacterial infections, and reduce inflammation and swelling.

SPECIALIZED THERAPIES USED IN DIAGNOSING

X-rays

Many specialized therapies and tests may be used in the diagnosing and treatment of disorders of the musculoskeletal and nervous systems. One of the most frequently used is **x-ray** (Figure 16-5).

X-rays are often used to diagnose bone diseases and injuries. In general, they are only done when necessary to diagnose or treat a particular problem.

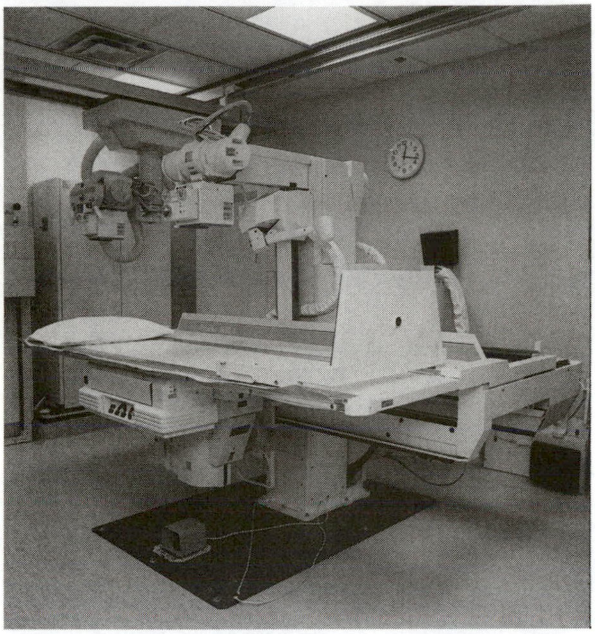

Figure 16-5 The x-ray machine.

The x-ray machine bombards a photographic film with radiation through the part of the body that is injured. The rays can penetrate through the skin and connective tissue but not through bone, so wherever the bone intervenes between the rays and the film, which becomes dark when the rays penetrate it, stays white.

Computerized Axial Tomography (CAT) Scan

Computerized axial tomography, or the **CAT scan,** has largely replaced previous forms of x-rays that were used to visualize specific structures and provides better information than ordinary x-rays in many cases. The CAT scan gives a clear picture of the structure or organ being viewed. It does so by using a series of pictures of the crosssections of the structure that were put together with a computer. The procedure is low-risk and gives information otherwise unobtainable except by surgery (Figure 16-6).

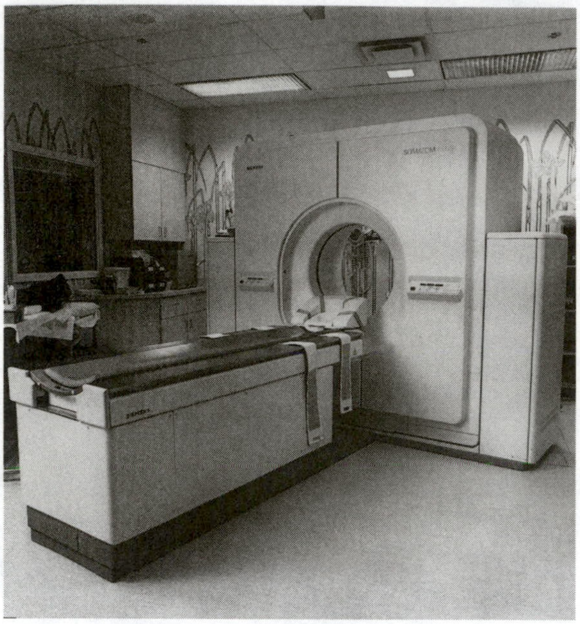

Figure 16-6 The CAT scan machine.

◆ SPECIALIZED REFLEX TESTS AND STUDIES

As a physical therapy aide, you may encounter certain specialized reflex tests and diagnostic studies that may be used in the treatment of disorders of the musculoskeletal and nervous systems. Several reflexes can be tested quickly and easily to get general information about motor neuron function. In some facilities, the physical therapist or the physician may be responsible for conducting these tests. The role of the physical therapy aide is to assist the therapist or the physician in carrying out the tests.

The **patellar reflex,** or knee-jerk reflex, is tested by striking the patient's knee just below the kneecap, or patella. Normally the lower leg will automatically extend. This indicates a complete two-neuron reflex arc at the second, third, and fourth lumbar nerves and proper function of the related muscles.

The **Babinski reflex** is generally conducted by the physician and is performed by using a blunt object to stroke the outside of the sole of the patient's foot. Normally this causes the toes to flex immediately. An abnormal response is for the big toe to extend and the other toes to fan out. This is known as the positive *Babinski sign* and it usually indicates impairment of the spino cortical nerve pathways.

The **Achilles reflex,** or ankle jerk, is similar to the patellar reflex. On tapping the Achilles tendon in the ankle, the foot should flex. The centers for this reflex are in the first and second sacral nerves.

◆ OTHER TESTS

If it has been established that the patient is likely to have a neurological problem, other tests may be used to pinpoint the problem more exactly. The most common of these include the previously discussed CAT scan, lumbar puncture and examination of cerebrospinal fluid, electroencephalography (EEG), and nuclear magnetic resonance imaging (MRI).

Lumbar Puncture

A **lumbar puncture** is performed to measure pressure in the central nervous system and to obtain fluid for examination and laboratory testing. The fluid can be tested for blood, other foreign cells, infection, and chemical imbalances. The same technique is used to inject medications, anesthetics, or contrast media for x-ray studies into the spinal canal.

Electroencephalograph (EEG)

The **EEG** is a painless procedure used for measuring the electrical activity of the brain. Electrodes are attached to both the patient's skull and a recording device that makes a tracing of electrical impulses from many areas of the brain. The patient should be awake, alert, and calm and should have eaten recently.

The EEG can also be used on patients in a coma to determine brain activity. A patient who has a "flat" EEG, that is one that shows no activity, and who has no reflexes, breathing, or muscle activity for six hours or more is considered dead, even if circulation can be mechanically maintained. This is because the brain tissue is almost all dead and cannot be regenerated.

Magnetic Resonance Imaging (MRI)

Magnetic resonance imaging, **MRI,** is a relatively new technique and its usefulness in neurology and orthopedics has not been fully established. Using this procedure, it is possible to look at soft tissue rather than at bones or blood vessels; therefore, growths in the white or gray matter are easier to detect than they are with other tests.

◆ PET THERAPY

Another type of therapy being used more frequently than ever before because of its great physiological as well as psychological benefits is pet therapy (Figure 16-7). Physicians and physical therapists are discovering that pairing patients with disabilities with highly trained and emotionally socialized pets, results in a soothing, therapeutic effect on the patient's well-being. By doing so, such therapy has the ability to increase the patient's rehabilitative capacity, thereby making his recovery and ultimate healing process much more efficient.

◆ SUMMARY

In this chapter, we discussed some of the more specialized therapies currently available to patients undergoing rehabilitative and therapeutic treatment. First we discussed treatment by immobilization and reduction. This was followed by a discussion on traction, electroneur-

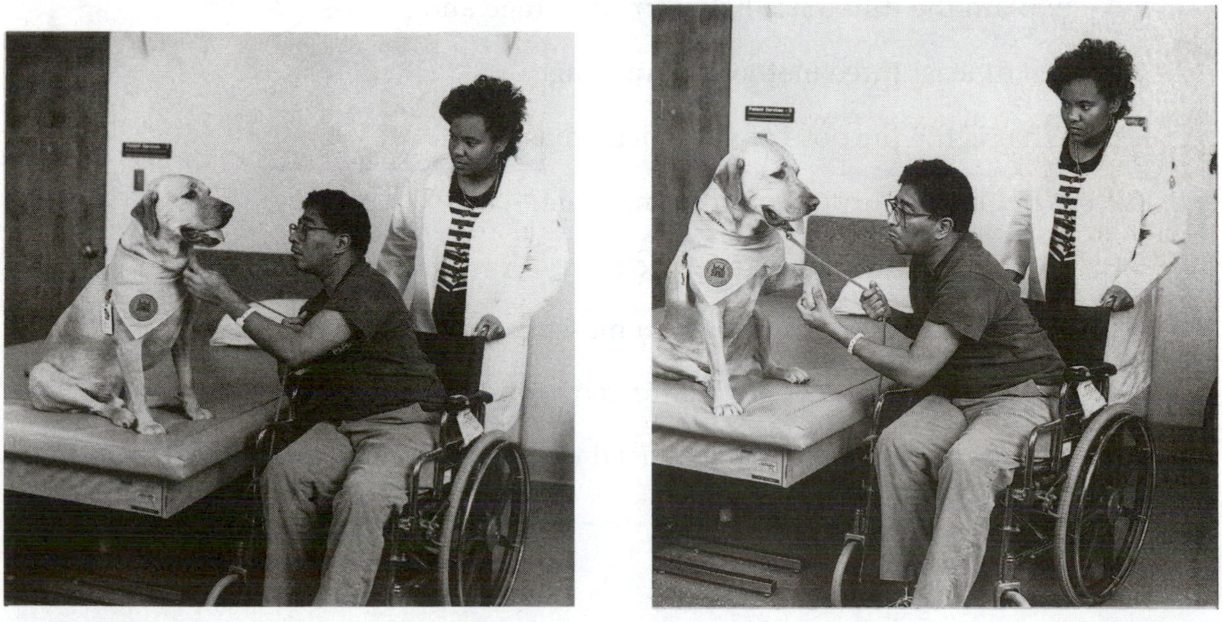

A B

Figure 16-7 Patient with a dog during a pet therapy session.

al stimulation, transcultaneous electrical stimulation (TENS), and the application of ultrasound. We also discussed the purpose of casting as a therapeutic treatment, and the role radiology and tomography play as a means of diagnosing physical disabilities. We explained the purpose of lumbar punctures, electroencephalography, and magnetic resonance imaging as additional means of identifying physical trauma and disabilities that might require therapeutic treatment. We also talked about the role medications play as a therapeutic treatment. Finally, we explained the use of pet therapy as a therapeutic treatment for patients suffering from a physical disability.

◆ ◆ LEARNING ACTIVITY 16-1

Electrotherapy and Massage

Use your textbook and medical dictionary to give brief answers to these questions.

1. Define electrotherapy.
2. What two types of body tissue does electrotherapy treat?
3. Electrotherapy is used primarily for three purposes. Name these.
4. Define massage.
5. State the rules to apply for the best results from massage.
6. Explain the difference between effleurage and petrissage.
7. List at least three methods of massage.
8. What is the purpose of superficial massage?
9. What is the purpose of deep massage?
10. How is friction massage applied?
11. Give one purpose of friction in massage therapy.
12. What types of disorders are treated with vibration and percussion?
13. In general, what are the beneficial uses of massage?

◆ ◆ LEARNING ACTIVITY 16-2

Questions to Answer

Match each term to its definition.

a. alternating current
b. cryotherapy
c. radiation
d. direct current
e. superficial
f. vasodilation
g. vasoconstriction
h. ultraviolet rays

__________ 1. Shallow, surface, or external

__________ 2. Narrowing of a blood vessel

__________ 3. An electrical current in which the flow of electrons moves in one direction only

__________ 4. Invisible source of energy in the violet end of the light spectrum; emitted by the sun and special lamps

__________ 5. Widening of a blood vessel

__________ 6. An electrical current in which the flow of electrons changes from one direction to another

__________ 7. To issue in waves around a source

__________ 8. Cold therapy

Answer the following questions as briefly as possible.

9. Identify at least three reasons for using heat treatments.
10. Give at least five methods/devices for delivering heat therapy.
11. What is the usual treatment time for a superficial heat treatment?
12. What is the depth of penetration for superficial heat?
13. What is the advantage of hydrotherapy over radiant heat therapy?
14. Contrast the portions of the body treated by a whirlpool bath and by a Hubbard tank.
15. What is a contrast bath?
16. List three types of deep heating available in physical therapy.
17. Name at least two physiological effects produced by ultrasound.
18. What is the coupling medium used in ultrasound therapy?

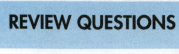

REVIEW QUESTIONS

1. Placing a bone in position is called __________.
2. __________ __________ involves manipulating a bone without opening the skin, and __________ __________ involves making an incision into the site and putting the broken bone in place.
3. Holding a bone in place is called __________.
4. Briefly define the term *traction.*
5. Briefly define the term *countertraction.*
6. List two types of traction frequently used in the hospital setting:

   a. __________

   b. __________
7. Briefly explain the purpose of applying a cast.
8. What disorder of the musculoskeletal system frequently calls for the administration of vitamin D as part of the treatment?
9. What diagnostic tool is often used to diagnose bone diseases and injuries?
10. Briefly define the difference between a CAT scan and an MRI.
11. What is the patellar reflex test used for?
12. The __________ is a painless procedure used for measuring the electrical activity of the brain.

APPENDICES

APPENDIX

A

The Human Skeleton

I. Divisions of the Skeleton

A. **Axial skeleton:** section of the skeleton that includes the bony framework of the head and the trunk

B. **Appendicular skeleton:** section of the skeleton that forms the framework for the arms and legs, commonly referred to as the extremities

II. The Framework of the Head: The Skull

A. **Cranium:** a rounded box enclosing the brain and composed of eight cranial bones, including:

1. **Frontal bone:** forms the forehead
2. **Parietal bones:** form most of the top and side walls of the cranium
3. **Temporal bones:** form part of the sides and some of the base of the skull
4. **Ethmoid bone:** located between the eyes in the orbital cavities
5. **Sphenoid bone:** located at the base of the skull in front of the temporal bones
6. **Occipital bone:** forms the back and a part of the base of the skull

B. **Facial portion**

1. **Mandible:** lower jaw; the only movable bone in the skull
2. **Maxillae:** forms the upper jaw
3. **Zygomatic bones:** form the prominence of the cheek
4. **Nasal bones:** form the bridge of the nose
5. **Lacrimal bones:** lie near the inside corner of the eye
6. **Vomer:** forms the lower part of the nasal septum
7. **Palatine bones:** paired, forming the back part of the hard palate
8. **Interior nasal conchae:** paired, lying alongside the lateral wall of the nasal cavities

III. Framework of the Trunk

A. **Vertebral column:** made up of a series of irregularly shaped bones, numbering twenty-six in the adult; names according to their location

1. **Cervical:** seven in number, located in the neck
2. **Thoracic:** 12 in number, located in the thorax

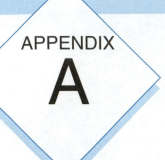

3. **Lumbar:** five in number, located in the small of the back
4. **Sacral:** five separate bones in the child, but eventually they fuse together in the adult, and is referred to as the sacrum
5. **Coccyx:** the tailbone, consisting of four or five tiny bones in the child, which fuse together in the adult to become one

B. **The thorax**
1. **True ribs:** the first seven pairs, attached directly to the sternum by costal cartilage
2. **False ribs:** include the remaining five pairs; eighth, ninth, and tenth pairs attach to the cartilage of rib above; last two pairs have no attachment and are known as "floating ribs"

IV. The Bones of the Extremities

A. **Upper extremities**
1. **Shoulder girdle:** consists of two bones, the clavicle, or collarbone, and the scapula, or shoulder blade
2. **Humerus:** the arm bone
3. **Ulna and radius:** make up the forearm
4. **Carpals:** eight small bones making up the wrist
5. **Metacarpal bones:** make up the bones of the hand
6. **Phalanges:** fourteen bones, making up the bones of the fingers

B. **Lower extremities**
1. **Pelvic girdle:** strong bony ring forming the walls of the pelvis
2. **Femur:** the thighbone; longest and strongest bone in the body
3. **Patella:** the kneecap
4. **Tibia and fibula:** two bones making up the lower portion of the leg
5. **Tarsal bones:** seven bones making up the ankle
6. **Metatarsal bones:** form the framework of the instep
7. **Phalanges:** bones of the toes

V. Joints

A. **Articulation (joint):** area or junction or union between two or more bones

B. **Kinds of joints**
1. **Synarthroses:** referring to an immovable joint
2. **Amphiarthroses:** referring to a slightly movable joint
3. **Diarthroses:** referring to a freely movable joint

C. **Joint function**
1. **Flexion:** bending motion that decreases the angle between bones
2. **Extension:** straightening motion that increases the angle between bones
3. **Abduction:** movement away from the midline of the body
4. **Adduction:** movement toward the midline of the body
5. **Rotation:** a twisting or turning of a bone on its own axis
6. **Supination:** turning the palm up or forward
7. **Pronation:** turning the palm down or backward
8. **Inversion:** turning the sole inward
9. **Eversion:** turning the sole outward

APPENDIX B

Major Muscles of the Body

I. Muscles of the Head and Neck

A. **Orbicularis oculi:** encircles the eyelids; function is to close the eye

B. **Levator palpebrae superioris:** located behind the orbit to the upper eyelid; function is to open the mouth

C. **Orbicularis oris:** encircles the mouth; functions to close the lips

D. **Buccinator:** the fleshy part of the cheek; function is to flatten the cheek and help in eating

E. **Temporal:** located above and near the rear of the cheek; function is to close the jaw

F. **Masseter:** located at the ankle of the jaw; function is to close the jaw

G. **Sternocleidomastoid:** located along the side of the neck next to the mastoid process; function is to flex and rotate the head toward the opposite side

II. Muscles of the Upper Extremities

A. **Trapezius:** located at the back of the neck and upper back to the scapula; function is to raise shoulders and pull them back; also extends the head

B. **Latissimus dorsi:** middle and lower back to the humerus; function is to extend and adduct the arm behind the back

C. **Pectoralis major:** upper, anterior chest to the humerus; function is to flex and adduct arm across the chest and to pull the shoulders forward and downward

D. **Deltoid:** covers the shoulder joint to the lateral humerus; function is to abduct the arm

E. **Biceps brachii:** anterior arm to the radius; function is to flex the forearm and supinate hand

F. **Triceps brachii:** posterior arm to the ulna; function is to extend the forearm

G. **Flexor and extensor carpi groups:** located at anterior and posterior forearm to the hand; function is to flex and extend the hand

H. **Flexor and extensor digitorum groups:** located at anterior and posterior forearm to the finger; function is to flex and extend the fingers

III. Muscles of the Trunk

A. **Diaphragm:** dome-shaped partition located between the thoracic and abdominal cavities;

dome descends to enlarge thoracic cavity from top to bottom

B. **External intercostals:** located between the ribs; function is to elevate the ribs and enlarge the thoracic cavity

C. **Rectus abdominis, obliquus, transversus:** located anteriolateral to the abdominal wall; function is to compress the abdominal cavity and expel substances from the body; also flexes the spinal column

D. **Levator ani:** the pelvic floor; function is to aid in defecation

E. **Sacrospinalis:** located deep in the back; function is to extend vertebral column and to assist in erect posture

IV. **Muscles of the Lower Extremities**

A. **Gluteus maximus:** the superficial buttock closest to the femur; function is to extend the thigh

B. **Gluteus medius:** the deep buttock closest to the femur; function is to abduct the thigh

C. **Iliopsoas:** crosses in front of the hip joint to the femur; function is to flex the thigh

D. **Adductor group:** the medial thigh to the femur; function is to adduct the thigh

E. **Sartorius:** winds down the thigh, ilium, and tibia; function is to flex the thigh and leg

F. **Quadriceps femoris:** the anteri or thigh to the tibia and fibula; function is to flex the leg

G. **Hamstrings group:** the posterior thigh to the tibia and fibula; function is to flex the leg

H. **Gastrocnemius:** the calf of the leg closest to the calcaneus; function is to extend the foot

I. **Tibialis anterior:** the anterior and lateral shin closest to the foot; function is to allow for dorsiflexion and inversion of the foot

J. **Peroneus longus:** the lateral leg, closest to the foot; function is to evert the foot

K. **Flexor and extensor digitorum groups:** the posterior leg, closest to the foot; function is to flex and extend the toes

APPENDIX

C

Procedure Evaluations

PROCEDURE EVALUATION

Student ______________________________

PROCEDURE*	Satisfactory	Marginal	Unsatisfactory
Answering the Telephone			
Screening Telephone Calls			
Taking Callback Messages			
Scheduling an Appointment			
Completing a Medical Record			
Completing a 2-Minute Handwash			
Measuring Blood Pressure			
Measuring a Radial Pulse			
Obtaining a Respiratory Rate			
Descending and Ascending a Wheelchair from a Curb			
Turning Patient from Supine to Prone			
Turning Patient from Prone to Supine			
Turning Patient on a Floor Mat			
Turning patient from a Supine to a Side-lying Position			

*Procedures required for HOSA Evaluation are indicated by a >.

PROCEDURE EVALUATION Student ____________________

PROCEDURE*	Satisfactory	Marginal	Unsatisfactory
Returning Patient from a Sitting to a Supine Position			
Assisting Patient from Bed to a Wheelchair			
Assisting Patient from Wheelchair to Parallel Bars			
Assisting Patient from Bed to a Wheelchair			
>Applying a Hot (hydrocollator) Pack			
>Applying a Cold Pack			
Performing Range-of-Motion on a Patient's Lower Extremities			
Performing Range-of-Motion on a Patient's Upper Extremities			
Assist a Patient to Ambulate Using a Walker			
>Assist a Patient with a 3-point Gait Using Crutches			
>Assist a Patient with a 2-point Gait Using Crutches			

*Procedures required for HOSA Evaluation are indicated by a >.

PROCEDURE EVALUATION

Student ______________________________

PROCEDURE*	Satisfactory	Marginal	Unsatisfactory
>Assist a Patient with a 4-point Gait Using Crutches			
>Assist a Patient with a Swing-to Gait Using Crutches			
>Assist a Patient with a Swing-through Gait Using Crutches			
Assist Patient to Walk Upstairs and Downstairs with Crutches			
>Assist a Patient to Walk Using a Standard Cane			

*Procedures required for HOSA Evaluation are indicated by a >.

APPENDIX

D

Practice Evaluation Test

Directions: For the questions given below, provide the answers you believe are most correct.

1. Define physical therapy.

2. Identify at least two goals of a physical therapy department.
   a.
   b.

3. Identify at least two goals of a rehabilitation department.
   a.
   b.

4. Of the agents listed below, circle at least four that would be used in a physical therapy department.

heat	radiology	antibiotics	asepsis
running	exercise	noise	anger
suntan oil	balance	energy	gas
electricity	light	water	enemas

5. Generally speaking, most physical therapy aides are employed in __________ and __________.

6. Identify at least six diseases or disabilities that are treated by the physical therapy department.
   a. __________ d. __________
   b. __________ e. __________
   c. __________ f. __________

7. Duties that could be performed by the physical therapy aide include all of the following, *except:* (circle the letters that are not included below)
   a. acts as a receptionist
   b. tests patients for evaluation
   c. maintains equipment
   d. determines amounts of weights to be used for traction
   e. helps prepare patients for treatment
   f. transports patients to and from the physical therapy department in a hospital

8. Circle those professionals listed below who are members of the rehabilitation team:
   a. hygienist
   b. social worker
   c. psychologist
   d. orthotist
   e. occupational therapist
   f. cardiologist
   g. pediatrician
   h. speech therapist
   i. audiologist
   j. gynecologist

9. Read the following statements. If the statement is more true than false, write true beside the statement; if the statement is more false than true, write false beside the statement
   _____ a. To be a physical therapy aide, the applicant must be a graduate of an accredited training program.
   _____ b. The physical therapy aide should be in good health since the job requires a high level of energy.
   _____ c. The physical therapy aide must be licensed to work in a physical therapy department.
   _____ d. The physical therapy aide must work under the direction of a licensed physical therapist.

10. Circle the desired qualities for a physical therapy aide:
    a. be in good health
    b. be good in math
    c. type at least 50 words per minute
    d. have common sense
    e. be sincere with others
    f. be tactful
    g. be attractive
    h. be strong
    i. be tall

11. List at least two ways the physical therapy aide can prevent falls in the physical therapy department.
    a.
    b.

12. Guarding techniques and safety belts are used to ________________.

13. List two safety observations the physical therapy aide can make while working with physical therapy equipment.
    a.
    b.

14. In case a fire breaks out, the physical therapy aide should know where the __________ is located, the __________ plan of the facility, and the __________ routes.

15. Briefly define the following terms:
    a. supination: ______________________________
    b. erect: ______________________________
    c. eversion: ______________________________
    d. inversion: ______________________________
    e. flexion: ______________________________
    f. extension: ______________________________
    g. proximal: ______________________________
    h. inferior: ______________________________
    I. distal: ______________________________
    j. pronation: ______________________________

16. What is another term for the back-lying position?

17. What is another term for the face-lying position?

18. What is another term for the side-lying position?

19. Turning the palm of the hand downward is called __________.
    a. supination
    b. rotation
    c. pronation
    d. adduction

20. Identify at least five modalities that the physical therapy aide might use in the treatment of patients. For each modality listed, briefly explain what the treatment is trying to accomplish:

	Modality	**Result of Modality**
a.	____________________	____________________
b.	____________________	____________________
c.	____________________	____________________
d.	____________________	____________________
e.	____________________	____________________

21. Explain the difference between passive and active range-of-motion exercises.

22. List three methods of applying heat for physical therapy treatments.
    a.
    b.
    c.

23. Briefly explain hydrotherapy.

24. Briefly explain the procedure for applying a paraffin bath.

25. Matching: Place the correct letter in the space beside the correct answer:
    _____ 1. heat therapy
    _____ 2. cryotherapy
    _____ 3. massage
    _____ 4. traction
    _____ 5. active-assistive exercise

    A. patient performs the exercise with an aide's assistance
    B. examples are ice packs and cold water immersion
    C. reduces pain and increases circulation
    D. involves squeezing and pressing the muscles
    E. reduces pain and restores range-of-motion using weights and pulleys

26. List two goals of the guarding techniques.
    a.
    b.

27. Briefly describe the purpose of a gait belt.

28. In your own words, briefly discuss why it is important to use good body mechanics when guarding a patient.

29. Identify three safety factors to be considered while guarding a patient.
    a.
    b.
    c.

30. **Matching:** Place the letter of the correct standing position in front of the correct number.

_____ 1. guarding on level ground
_____ 2. guarding a patient with a weak side and balance problems
_____ 3. guarding a patient going up a staircase
_____ 4. guarding a patient going down a staircase
_____ 5. guarding while transferring a patient

A. Standing in front of the patient
B. Standing behind the patient

31. If a patient begins to fall, the physical therapy aide should try to control certain parts of the body. The __________, hips, and __________ are the best body points to control.

32. In your own words, briefly describe the gait or walking belt.

33. If a patient does fall, it is important to protect her __________ from hard or sharp objects.

Glossary

abduction. Movement away from the midline of the body, as in moving the arms straight out to the sides.

acromegaly. A disease of adults that results from hyperactivity of the anterior pituitary in which the bones of the face, hands, and feet, widen.

active range of motion. Occurs when the patient is able to move his limb by active muscle contraction, on his own.

adduction. Movement toward the midline of the body, as in bringing the arms back to their original position.

alignment. The positioning and supporting of the body in such a way that all body parts are in correct anatomical position.

amphiarthroses. A slightly movable joint.

anterior. Referring to the front.

aponeurosis. A tendonlike expansion that connects a muscle with the parts that it moves.

appendicitis. Inflammation of the appendix.

appendicular skeleton. Section of the skeleton that forms the framework for those parts usually referred to as the arms and legs, but commonly called the extremities.

arthritis. Inflammation of a joint.

articular cartilage. Covers the epiphyses in areas where the ends of separate bones meet in order to form a joint.

articulation. The place of a union, as in the union of a joint.

atrophy. A wasting or decrease in the size of a muscle when it cannot be used.

axial skeleton: Section of the skeleton that includes the bony framework of the head and the trunk.

axilla. The armpit or the area under the arms.

body mechanics. A term used to refer to the way in which the body moves and maintains its balance by the most efficient use of all of its parts.

bursitis. Inflammation of the bursa.

cancellous bone tissue. A type of bone tissue that has many open spaces, thus giving a spongy appearance.

caudal. Something being inferior or away from the head.

cerebralvascular accident (CVA). Often referred to as a *stroke,* in which there is a destruction of brain tissue as a result of hemorrhage from blood vessels of the brain.

compact bone tissue. A type of bone tissue that is more dense then cancellous bone tissue, and on microscopic examination, appears to have many circles.

contractility. The capacity of a muscle fiber to become shorter as its response to a stimuli.

contracture. A tightening or shortening of a muscle.

cranial. Nearest the head.

deep stroking massage. A type of massage that involves stroking in the same direction of the natural flow of lymph and venous blood, and which is frequently used to aid in the emptying of veins and lymphatics and in pressing their contents in the direction of their natural flow.

defamation. Any verbal statement which is considered as an attack on a person's reputation.

diabetes mellitus. A disease associated with the endocrine system, which results from a lack of insulin being produced in the *islet of Langerhans.*

diaphysis. The long, main portion or shaft of a bone.

diarthroses. A freely movable joint.

dislocation. A derangement of the parts of a joint.

distal. Farthest from a point of reference.

dorsal. Near the back of the body.

duty of care. A process that entitles a patient to safe care by making it mandatory that he be treated by meeting the common or average standards of practice expected in the community under similar circumstances.

dysmenorrhea. Painful menstruation.

effleurage. A type of massage that involves superficial stroking toward the body, using a slow, gentle, rhythmic movement, which helps to produce a reflex action.

electroneural stimulation (ES). Used to increase circulation by means of the pumping action of muscles upon the vessels, while at the same time, produce mild heating with all the benefits accrued from increased temperature.

empathy. The ability to understand another's feelings and the sensitivity to be able to respond to those feelings.

endosteum. A thin membrane that lines the marrow cavities of bone and is a source of cells which aid in the growth and repair of bone tissue.

endomysium. Membrane that covers individual muscle cells.

epimysium. A fibrous sheath surrounding a muscle.

epiphyses. The ends of a long bone.

erythrocyte. Red blood cell.

ethical behavior. Behavior that represents the ideal conduct for a certain group.

eversion. Turning the sole outward, away from the body.

excitability. The capacity of a muscle to respond to a stimuli.

exercise physiologist. Health care technician responsible for designing a physical activity program that is tailored to the specific needs of the individual participant.

extension: A straightening motion that increases the angle between bones, as in straightening the fingers in order to open the hand.

fertilization. The union of the female's ovum with the male's sperm.

flexion. A bending motion that decreases the angle between bones, as in bending the fingers in order to close the hand.

foramen. A natural opening or passageway; used as a general term for describing a passage into or through a bone.

fracture. A break, usually referring to a break in a bone.

Good Samaritan Law. A law which states that if a physician or any health care worker comes upon the scene of an accident, he or she may render care without fearing the possibility of a malpractice suit.

gout. A form of arthritis that generally affects only one joint, usually the big toe, and is characterized by crystal deposits in and around the affected point.

Guillain-Barre Syndrome. A disorder of the nervous system characterized by the absence of fever, pain or tenderness in the muscles, motor weakness, and the interruption or lack of motor reflexes.

Haversian canals. Tiny channels, or canals, of which compact bone wraps itself around.

health maintenance organization (HMO). A medical group that generally consists of several primary physicians and medical specialists. Usually the patient must be referred to a specialist from a primary physician.

holding. A telephone's capability of keeping a call waiting on one line while a second call is on another line.

immobilization. Holding a bone in place, either with a cast or a strong bandage.

informed consent. The process by which a patient fully understands what care and/or treatment he or she will receive.

insertion. The place of attachment of a muscle to the bone that it moves.

inversion. The act of turning the sole inward, so that it faces the opposite foot.

irritability. The capacity of a muscle to respond to a stimulus.

isometric contraction. Contractions in which there is no change in muscle length, but there is a great increase in muscle tension.

isotonic contraction. Contractions in which the bone or tension within the muscle remains the same, but the muscle as a whole shortens, producing movement.

joint. An articulation or area of junction or union between two or more bones.

kyphosis. An exaggeration of the natural posterior curve, thus causing the patient to walk with a hunchbacked appearance.

leukocyte. White blood cell.

libel. A defamatory statement that is written.

ligament. A band of fibrous tissue connecting bones.

lordosis. An exaggerated inward curvature of the lumbar region of the spinal column.

malpractice. Any misconduct or lack of skill resulting in the patient's injury.

medial. Near the midline of the body.

medical ethics. Concerned with whether the health care worker's actions are right or wrong.

medical law. Concerned with focusing on whether one acted legally or illegally.

Medical Practice Acts. Statutes dealing with individual licensing and certification of individual health care professionals.

medical specialist. A physician who devotes himself to a single branch of medical knowledge.

medullary cavity. The hollow shaft of a long bone.

multiple sclerosis. A highly complex, chronic, progressive neurological disease that is caused by changes in the white matter of the brain and spinal cord.

muscular dystrophy. A degenerative disorder of the muscular system which is caused by a degeneration of the muscle cells, eventually causing the muscles to waste away and atrophy.

muscle tone. A partially contracted state of the muscles, which is normal even though the muscles may not be in use at the time.

myasthenia gravis. A poorly understood disease of the muscular system that causes great muscle weakness and fatigue. In myasthenia gravis, the nerve impulses fail to initiate normal muscle contractions, eventually causing the patient to have the appearance of drooping eyelids and an inattentive appearance.

negligence. The failure to give reasonable care or the giving of unreasonable care.

nonverbal communication. Messages sent without words or in addition to words.

origin. The less movable attachment of a muscle.

oral (verbal) communication. Oral messages, including face-to-face encounters, announcements, questions, offhand remarks, telephone conversations, gossip, and other forms of communication.

orchitis. An inflammatory condition of the male's testes.

orthopedics. The study or branch of medicine/surgery that deals with the treatment of diseases and deformities of the bones, muscles, and joints.

osteoarthritis. A form of arthritis, also known as *degenerative joint disease,* thought to be caused by gonococcus.

osteoblast. A cell involved in the production of bone.

osteoclast. A large cell involved in the absorption and removal of bone.

osteocyte. Bone cells.

passive range of motion. Occurs when the health care worker assists the patient through various ranges of motion.

Patient's Bill of Rights. The intent of this document is to make both members of the health care system and patients aware of what the patient has a right to expect in terms of his care and treatment.

percussion. Also known as *tapotement,* when used in the application of physical therapy, involves a striking of the part to be massaged quickly with the hand. There are four types of percussion: clapping with the palms of the hands; hacking with the ulnar borders of the hands; tapping with the tips of the fingers, and beating with the clenched fist.

perimysium. Once the epimysium surrounds each individual muscle bundle, it becomes the perimysium.

periosteum. The outer cover of bone.

petrissage. A type of massage that involves a process of kneading, wringing, lifting or pressing of the part in order to help assist in the venous and lymphatic circulation.

physical therapist (PT). A licensed technician who is a graduate of a four-year college program with a bachelor's degree, and in some cases, a master's degree in health sciences. Responsible for performing treatments that require special training in therapeutic exercises, hydrotherapy, and electrotherapy, and for carrying out procedures dealing with individual muscles and muscular movement.

physical therapy aide (PTA). Health care worker generally responsible for carrying out nontechnical duties of physical therapy, such as preparing treatment areas, ordering devices and supplies, and transporting patients. Works under the direction of the physical therapist.

physical therapy assistant. Health care worker who is a graduate of a two-year associate of arts or applied sciences community college program, and who is certified according to the American Physical Therapy Association. Works under the direction of the physical therapist and is responsible for assisting with patient care and performing selected treatments such as ultrasound.

physical therapy. Treatment by physical means, such as heat, cold, water, massage, and electricity.

physician. Licensed medical doctor who has overall responsibility for outlining the rehabilitation program for the patient and for ordering any special physical therapy treatments.

posterior. Referring to the back.

prefix. A word fragment placed in front of the basic or root word.

process. A prominence or part extending from an organ.

pronation. The act of turning the palm down or backward.

prone. Position in which a person is lying with the face down or on the abdomen.

prosthesis. Replacement of a natural part with an artificial part, such as a limb.

proximal. Nearest to a point of reference.

occupation therapist (OT). A licensed technician who is a graduate of a school for occupational therapy and has acquired expertise in making special equipment in order to facilitate the performance of a patient's daily activities.

radiology. Branch of medicine dealing with x-rays and radioactive substances.

range of motion. Movement of a joint through its full range of all the appropriate planes. May employ passive, active, or resistive movements.

reasonable care. Protection of the health care professional by law if it can be proven that he acted reasonably as compared to fellow workers of the same or similar training in a situation of the same nature.

reduction. Holding a broken bone in place so that the restored bone is in the right position to heal in the correct shape. Can be either a *closed reduction,* in which the bone is manipulated by the physician without breaking the skin, or an *open reduction,* in which an incision into the site of the fracture is made in order to put the broken bone in place.

rheumatoid arthritis. A type of arthritis that affects the bones and joints plus other body systems such as the lungs, muscles, skin, blood vessels, and the heart.

Rule of Personal Liability. In health care, under this rule, all individuals are held responsible for their own personal conduct.

root word. The main body of a word.

sciatica. A common neurological disorder that is associated with rheumatism and arthritis and with prolapse of an intervertebral disk. Treatment involves relief of pain through physical therapy.

scoliosis. A side to side curvature of the spine.

slander. A defamatory statement that is spoken.

SOAP notes. A four-point system for keeping medical or nursing notes in a patient's medical record.

sprain. An injury of a joint with a stretching or tearing of the ligaments.

strain. An injury caused by excessive stretching, overuse, or misuse of a muscle.

suffix. A word fragment added at the end of the basic or root word.

superior. Above, or being in a higher position.

supination. The act of turning the palm up or forward

supine. Lying flat on the back, with the face upward.

synarthroses. An immovable joint.

tact. Saving or doing the proper thing at the proper time.

tendon. A fibrous cord that attaches a muscle to a bone.

therapeutic exercise. Movement prescribed by a physician or physical therapist to help restore normal function or to maintain a state of well-being.

therapy. Treatment of a disease or disorder, as in physical therapy.

traction. The pull provided by a series of weights, ropes, and pulleys that are connected to either a frame, wire, or pin or to straps applied over the skin of the patient.

transcultaneous electrical stimulation. A special type of electrical stimulation designed to help modify pain.

ultrasonic unit. A piece of equipment that uses sound waves as treatment.

ultrasound. The process by which sound waves are used to produce deep muscle relaxation.

urinary calculi. Stone found in the urinary bladder.

ventral. The same as anterior; pertaining to something being located near the belly surface or front of the body.

vital signs. Includes blood pressure, temperature, pulse, and respiration.

Volkmann's canals. Microscopic channels extending from the periosteum to the Haversian canals and to the inner or medullary cavity of bones.

xiphoid process. The small bony projection at the lower end of the sternum or breastbone.

Index

References in bold are illustrations

C

D

P

R